Influence of Nutrients, Bioactive Compounds, and Plant Extracts in Liver Diseases

Influence of Nutrients, Bioactive Compounds, and Plant Extracts in Liver Diseases

Edited by

Seyed Moayed Alavian
Middle East Liver Disease Center (MELD), Tehran, Iran

Seyed Mohammad Nabavi
Applied Biotechnology Research Center,
Baqiyatallah University of Medical Sciences, Tehran, Iran

Seyed Fazel Nabavi
Applied Biotechnology Research Center,
Baqiyatallah University of Medical Sciences, Tehran, Iran

Ana Sanches Silva
National Institute of Agrarian and Veterinary Research, Vila do Conde, Portugal
Center for Study in Animal Science (CECA), University of Oporto, Oporto, Portugal

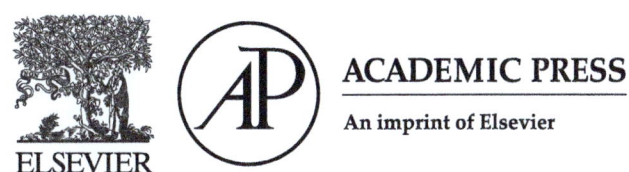

ELSEVIER

ACADEMIC PRESS
An imprint of Elsevier

Academic Press is an imprint of Elsevier
125 London Wall, London EC2Y 5AS, United Kingdom
525 B Street, Suite 1650, San Diego, CA 92101, United States
50 Hampshire Street, 5th Floor, Cambridge, MA 02139, United States
The Boulevard, Langford Lane, Kidlington, Oxford OX5 1GB, United Kingdom

Notices
Knowledge and best practice in this field are constantly changing. As new research and experience broaden
our understanding, changes in research methods, professional practices, or medical treatment may become
necessary.

Practitioners and researchers must always rely on their own experience and knowledge in evaluating and
using any information, methods, compounds, or experiments described herein. In using such information or
methods they should be mindful of their own safety and the safety of others, including parties for whom they
have a professional responsibility.

To the fullest extent of the law, neither the Publisher nor the authors, contributors, or editors, assume any
liability for any injury and/or damage to persons or property as a matter of products liability, negligence or
otherwise, or from any use or operation of any methods, products, instructions, or ideas contained in the
material herein.

Library of Congress Cataloging-in-Publication Data
A catalog record for this book is available from the Library of Congress

British Library Cataloguing-in-Publication Data
A catalogue record for this book is available from the British Library

ISBN 978-0-12-816488-4

For information on all Academic Press publications
visit our website at https://www.elsevier.com/books-and-journals

Publisher: Charlotte Cockle
Acquisitions Editor: Megan R. Ball
Editorial Project Manager: Ruby Smith
Production Project Manager: Joy Christel Neumarin Honest Thangiah
Cover Designer: Victoria Pearson

Typeset by SPi Global, India

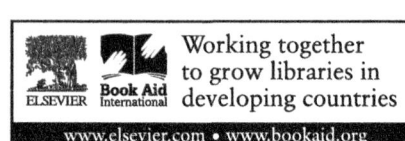

Dedication

With the memory of Seyed Ali Asghar Nabavi, I dedicate this book to my family
Seyed Mohammad Nabavi
Seyed Fazel Nabavi

To my wife Shahnaz and my son Amir Ali
Seyed Moayed Alavian

To my sweet and loving children, Maria Inês and João, and to my husband,
Ricardo Pessoa
Ana Sanches Silva

Contents

Contributors .... *xiii*

Preface .... *xv*

Chapter 1: Introduction *1*
Fatma Tugce Guragac Dereli, Ali Guragac, and Tarun Belwal

PART 1 HEPATOPROTECTIVE ACTIVITY OF NATURAL COMPOUNDS AND PLANT EXTRACTS IN LIVER DISEASES

Chapter 2: Hepatitis B *19*
Umair Younas, Sana Tehseen, Fazlullah Khan, and Kamal Niaz

2.1	Introduction	19
2.2	*Rheum palmatum* L.	20
2.3	*Ganoderma lucidum* (Curtis) P. Karst.	22
2.4	*Oenanthe javanica* (Blume) DC.	23
2.5	*Curcuma longa* L.	23
2.6	Phyllanthus amarus Schum. and Thonn.	24
2.7	Phyllanthus niruri L.	24
2.8	Swertia patens Burkill	26
2.9	Boehmeria nivea (L.) Gaudich.	26
2.10	Role of natural compounds in ameliorating hepatitis B ..	27
	2.10.1 Terpenoids	27
	2.10.2 Lignans	28
	2.10.3 Phenolic acids	29
	2.10.4 Polyphenols	30
	2.10.5 Alkaloids	32
2.11	Conclusion	33
	Acknowledgments	33
	Conflict of interest	33
	References	33
	Further reading	39

Chapter 3: Hepatitis C **41**

Abdullah, Kamal Niaz, and Fazlullah Khan

    3.1   Introduction 41

    3.2   Etiology 42

    3.3   Signs and symptoms 42

    3.4   Genotypes and serotypes of HCV....................................43

    3.5   Diagnosis (serology, biopsy, and screening)........................43

    3.6   Serology 43

    3.7   Screening tests 44

          3.7.1   Enzyme immunosorbent assay (EIA) 44

          3.7.2   The rapid test (point of care test) 44

    3.8   Biopsy..45

    3.9   Screening 46

    3.10 Prevention 46

    3.11 Treatment 46

    3.12 Hepatoprotective activity of natural compounds and plant

          extracts in Hepatitis C...47

          3.12.1   Silymarin..47

          3.12.2   Naringenin..48

          3.12.3   Quercetin...48

          3.12.4   (−)-Epigallocatechin-3-gallate (EGCG)................48

          3.12.5   Luteolin and apigenin 49

          3.12.6   Honokiol..49

          3.12.7   3-Hydroxy caruilignan C (3-HCL-C) 49

          3.12.8   Ladanein..49

          3.12.9   Plumbagin 50

          3.12.10 Corilagin 50

    3.13 Conclusion...51

    Conflict of interest 51

    References..51

Chapter 4: Alcoholic liver disease **57**

Anna Blázovics

    4.1   Introduction...57

    4.2   The cause and consequences of alcohol toxicity 58

          4.2.1 Alcohol metabolism and oxidative stress.....................58

          4.2.2 Genetic alterations in developing of alcoholic liver diseases 61

          4.2.3 The role of cytokines, chemokines, and adipocytokines in alcoholic

               liver disease...62

          4.2.4 Sex differences in alcohol sensitivity.........................64

    4.3   Alcohol as a depressant 66

    4.4   Complex treatment of alcohol disease 66

          4.4.1 Treatment of alcoholic liver diseases with vitamin supplements, nutrition,

               and medicaments with natural ingredients: Favorable and adverse effects 67

4.4.2 Some traditional herbal medicines in complex treatment of alcoholists:
Favorable and adverse effects 71

4.5 Conclusions...74

References...75

Chapter 5: Hepatoprotective activity of natural compounds and plant extracts
in nonalcoholic fatty liver disease **83**

Antoni Sureda, Xavier Capó, and Silvia Tejada

5.1 Introduction...83

5.2 Nonalcoholic fatty liver disease pathogenesis and
progression..84

5.3 Oxidative stress and lipotoxicity...86

5.4 Mediterranean diet and nonalcoholic fatty liver disease....................88

5.5 Natural compound effects on nonalcoholic fatty liver
disease..90

5.6 Conclusions..97

Acknowledgments 98

References...98

Chapter 6: Liver cancer **105**

Ismail Shah, Sajjad Ali Khan, Sadiq Hussain, Fazlullah Khan, and Kamal Niaz

6.1 Introduction..105

6.2 Classification of hepatic cancers...106

6.2.1 Benign tumors...106

6.2.2 Malignant tumors...106

6.3 Causes of liver cancer...107

6.4 Diagnosis 111

6.4.1 Nuclear medical imaging 112

6.4.2 Single photon emission computed tomography (SPECT)......112

6.4.3 Liver puncture biopsy...113

6.4.4 Serological molecular markers for liver cancer.......................113

6.4.5 Pathological diagnosis of liver cancer......................................113

6.4.6 Prevention...114

6.4.7 Treatment...114

6.5 Conclusion 122

Conflict of interest 123

References...123

Chapter 7: Chronic liver diseases **129**

Renald Blundell and Joseph Ignatius Azzopardi

7.1 Introduction..129

7.2 Primary sclerosing cholangitis..129

7.3 Hepatic steatosis 130

7.4 Primary biliary cirrhosis 131

7.5 Liver fibrosis..132

7.6 The use of bioactive compounds and plant extracts in chronic liver diseases..........132
7.7 Nutritional support in CLD...134
References...135

Chapter 8: Drug-induced hepatotoxicity..141
Amandeep Singh, Sneha Joshi, Ashima Joshi, Pooja Patni, and Devesh Tewari

8.1 Background...141
8.2 Hepatotoxicity: An overview 142
8.3 Drug metabolic pathways of the liver and hepatotoxicity 144
8.4 Drug-induced hepatotoxicity: Mechanisms and risk factors 145
8.5 Epidemiological aspects 147
8.6 Hepatoprotective activity of natural compounds and plant extracts
    in drug-induced hepatotoxicity 148
8.7 Conclusion 154
References...154

PART 2 INFLUENCE OF NUTRIENTS, PLANT EXTRACTS AND NATURAL COMPOUNDS IN LIVER DISEASES

Chapter 9: Influence of omega-3 fatty acids and monounsaturated fats in liver diseases..161
Abdullah, Maqsood Ur Rehman, Fazlullah Khan, and Kamal Niaz

9.1 Introduction..161
9.2 Chemistry and classification of omega fatty acids 162
9.3 Conversion of ALA to EPA and DHA 165
9.4 Chemistry and classification of MUFA 166
9.5 Sources of omega-3 fatty acids and MUFAs 166
9.6 Metabolism of omega-3 fatty acids and monounsaturated fats 166
9.7 Role of omega-3 fatty acids and monounsaturated fats in various liver diseases......167
    9.7.1 Nonalcoholic fatty liver disease (NAFLD) 167
    9.7.2 Nonalcoholic steatohepatitis (NASH)..169
    9.7.3 Fibrosis...170
    9.7.4 Hepatocellular carcinoma (HCC) 170
9.8 Conclusion 170
Conflict of interest 170
References...171

Chapter 10: Influence of vitamins (C, B_3, D, and E) in liver health........................175
H.G. Ağalar

10.1 Introduction 175
10.2 Vitamin C...175
10.3 Vitamin B_3 (niacin)...177
10.4 Vitamin D...178
10.5 Vitamin E...182

10.6 Vitamin combinations and liver health 185
10.7 Conclusion 186
References..186

Chapter 11: Influence of other nutrients (e.g., L-arginine, taurine, and choline) on liver diseases.. 193

Jaime López-Cervantes, Dalia I. Sánchez-Machado, Olga N. Campas-Baypoli, Ernesto U. Cantú-Soto, and Gabriela Servín de la Mora-López

11.1 Introduction 193
11.2 Liver diseases..194
11.3 Arginine 195
        11.3.1 Structural characteristics and metabolism................................195
        11.3.2 Functional links with the liver...196
        11.3.3 Evidence of hepatoprotective functions 196
11.4 Taurine 197
        11.4.1 Chemical structure and biological functions............................197
        11.4.2 Potential effects as a therapeutic agent 198
        11.4.3 Clinical studies linked to liver diseases 199
11.5 Choline..200
        11.5.1 Its metabolites and dietary sources 200
        11.5.2 Aspects of its metabolism 202
        11.5.3 Clinical evidence of the effect on liver health........................203
11.6 Conclusions 204
References..205

Chapter 12: Antioxidants with hepatoprotective activity 209

Gökçe Şeker Karatoprak

12.1 Introduction 209
12.2 Natural hepatoprotective agents..210
        12.2.1   Ursodeoxycholic acid 210
        12.2.2   Choline...210
        12.2.3   Betaine 211
        12.2.4   *S*-Adenosyl-L-methionine 211
        12.2.5   Melatonin 212
        12.2.6   Glutathione...212
        12.2.7   *N*-Acetylcysteine 213
        12.2.8   Minerals in antioxidant enzymes 214
        12.2.9   Vitamins E and C 215
        12.2.10 Lycopene 216
        12.2.11 Beta-carotene 217
        12.2.12 Silymarin...217
        12.2.13 Alpha-lipoic acid...218
        12.2.14 Coenzyme Q10..219
        12.2.15 Curcumin..219
        12.2.16 Other natural antioxidants with hepatoprotective effects..............220

12.3 Synthetic hepatoprotectors with antioxidant activity 221
    12.3.1 Pentoxiyfylline..221
    12.3.2 Angiotensin-converting enzyme inhibitors 221
12.4 Conclusion 222
References...222

Chapter 13: Plant extracts with putative hepatoprotective activity 227

Esra Köngül Şafak

13.1 Introduction 227
13.2 Conclusion 242
References...246

Chapter 14: Plant extracts with putative hepatotoxicity activity 259

Palaniappan Saravanapriya and Kasi Pandima Devi

14.1 Introduction 259
14.2 General concepts of hepatotoxicity 261
    14.2.1 Types of hepatotoxicity 262
    14.2.2 Causes of hepatotoxicity 264
    14.2.3 Mechanisms of hepatotoxicity 265
14.3 Hepatotoxicity induced by plant extracts and mushrooms 267
    14.3.1 *Atractylis gummifera* L. 269
    14.3.2 *Morinda citrifolia* L. 269
    14.3.3 *Camellia sinensis* L. 270
    14.3.4 *Aloe vera* L. 270
    14.3.5 *Teucrium chamaedrys* L. 271
    14.3.6 *Chelidonium majus* L. 272
    14.3.7 *Piper methysticum* G. Forst...272
    14.3.8 *Larrea tridentata* (Sess. & Moc. ex DC.) Cov. 273
    14.3.9 *Mentha pulegium* L. 274
    14.3.10 *Amanita phalloides* (Vaill. ex Fr.: Fr.)................................274
    14.3.11 *Viscum album* L..275
    14.3.12 *Xanthium strumarium* L...275
    14.3.13 *Scutellaria biacalensis* Georgi 276
    14.3.14 *Callilepis laureola* DC. 277
    14.3.15 *Valeriana officinalis* L...277
    14.3.16 *Hypericum perforatum* L. 277
    14.3.17 *Cascara sagrada* DC. 278
    14.3.18 *Cassia acutifolia* Delile...278
    14.3.19 *Actaea racemosa* L. 279
    14.3.20 *Echinaceae purpurea* L..279
14.4 Conclusion 280
Acknowledgments 280
References...281

Index 289

Contributors

Abdullah   Department of Pharmacy, University of Malakand, Chakdara, Pakistan

H.G. Ağalar   Pharmacognosy Department, Faculty of Pharmacy, Anadolu University, Eskişehir, Turkey

Joseph Ignatius Azzopardi   Department of Physiology and Biochemistry, Faculty of Medicine, University of Malta, Msida, Malta

Tarun Belwal   College of Biosystems Engineering and Food Science, Zhejiang University, Hangzhou, China

Anna Blázovics   Department of Pharmacognosy, Semmelweis University, Budapest, Hungary

Renald Blundell   Department of Physiology and Biochemistry, Faculty of Medicine, University of Malta, Msida; American University of Malta, Bormla, Malta

Olga N. Campas-Baypoli   Sonora Institute of Technology, Ciudad Obregon, Sonora, Mexico

Ernesto U. Cantú-Soto   Sonora Institute of Technology, Ciudad Obregon, Sonora, Mexico

Xavier Capó   Research Group on Community Nutrition and Oxidative Stress (NUCOX), Department of Fundamental Biology and Health Sciences, Health Research Institute of the Balearic Islands (IdISBa), and CIBEROBN (Physiopathology of Obesity and Nutrition CB12/03/30038), University of the Balearic Islands, Palma, Spain

Ali Guragac   Urology Department, Private Denizli Tekden Hospital, Denizli, Turkey

Fatma Tugce Guragac Dereli   Department of Pharmacognosy, Faculty of Pharmacy, Süleyman Demirel University, Isparta, Turkey

Sadiq Hussain   Department of Pharmacy, Abdul Wali Khan University, Garden Campus, Mardan, Pakistan

Ashima Joshi   MojoLab Foundation, New Delhi, India

Sneha Joshi   Department of Pharmaceutical Chemistry, PCTE Group of Institutions, Ludhiana, Punjab, India

Fazlullah Khan   Department of Toxicology and Pharmacology, The Institute of Pharmaceutical Sciences, School of Pharmacy, Tehran University of Medical Sciences, Tehran, Iran; Department of Allied Health Sciences, Bashir Institute of Health Sciences, Bhara Kahu, Islamabad, Pakistan

Sajjad Ali Khan   Department of Pharmacy, Abdul Wali Khan University, Garden Campus, Mardan, Pakistan

Esra Köngül Şafak   Department of Pharmacognosy, Faculty of Pharmacy, Erciyes University, Kayseri, Turkey

Gabriela Servín de la Mora-López   Sonora Institute of Technology, Ciudad Obregon, Sonora, Mexico

Jaime López-Cervantes   Sonora Institute of Technology, Ciudad Obregon, Sonora, Mexico

Kamal Niaz   Department of Pharmacology and Toxicology, Faculty of Bio-Sciences, Cholistan University of Veterinary and Animal Sciences (CUVAS), Bahawalpur, Pakistan

Kasi Pandima Devi   Department of Biotechnology, Alagappa University [Science Campus], Karaikudi, Tamil Nadu, India

Pooja Patni   Department of Pharmaceutics, School of Pharmaceutical Sciences, Lovely Professional University, Phagwara, Punjab, India

Maqsood Ur Rehman   Department of Pharmacy, University of Malakand, Chakdara, Pakistan

Dalia I. Sánchez-Machado   Sonora Institute of Technology, Ciudad Obregon, Sonora, Mexico

Palaniappan Saravanapriya   Department of Biotechnology, Alagappa University [Science Campus], Karaikudi, Tamil Nadu, India

Gökçe Şeker Karatoprak   Department of Pharmacognosy, Faculty of Pharmacy, Erciyes University, Kayseri, Turkey

Ismail Shah   Department of Pharmacy, Abdul Wali Khan University, Garden Campus, Mardan, Pakistan

Amandeep Singh   Department of Pharmacognosy, Khalsa College of Pharmacy, Amritsar, Punjab, India

Antoni Sureda   Research Group on Community Nutrition and Oxidative Stress (NUCOX), Department of Fundamental Biology and Health Sciences, Health Research Institute of the Balearic Islands (IdISBa), and CIBEROBN (Physiopathology of Obesity and Nutrition CB12/03/30038), University of the Balearic Islands, Palma, Spain

Sana Tehseen   Department of Botany, Government College Women University Faisalabad, Faisalabad, Pakistan

Silvia Tejada   Laboratory of Neurophysiology, Department of Biology, Health Research Institute of the Balearic Islands (IdISBa), and CIBEROBN (Physiopathology of Obesity and Nutrition CB12/03/30038), University of the Balearic Islands, Palma, Spain

Devesh Tewari   Department of Pharmacognosy, School of Pharmaceutical Sciences, Lovely Professional University, Phagwara, Punjab, India

Umair Younas   Department of Livestock Management, Faculty of Animal Production and Technology, Cholistan University of Veterinary and Animal Sciences, Bahawalpur, Pakistan

Preface

Impressive advances have emerged in therapeutics related to liver diseases, including new chirurgic and pharmacology approaches. Hepatitis, cancer, and cirrhosis are among the most prevalent liver diseases. These diseases can often remain undiagnosed and untreated for years. Nowadays, interest in the use of natural compounds in the prevention and treatment of diseases is increasing, mainly due to their wide spectrum of biological activities including antioxidant, antimicrobial, anticancer, and antiinflammatory activities as well as modulation of the intracellular signal cascade and immunological response and a good safety profile. However, there is still a lack of scientific-based knowledge to assure the biological effects claimed by these substances, namely regarding liver diseases.

The aim of this book is to provide reliable, up-to-date information on nutrients, bioactive compounds, and plant extracts that have protective or toxic effects in liver diseases. Extensive coverage is given to the mechanism of action of these compounds and on the structure-function relationship of nutrients, bioactive compounds, and plant extracts in hepatitis B, hepatitis C, alcoholic fatty liver disease, nonalcoholic fatty liver disease, liver cancer, biliary cirrhosis, and primary sclerosing cholangitis. Moreover, their effect in the hepatotoxicity of drugs is also addressed.

The book *Influence of Nutrients, Bioactive Compounds, and Plant Extracts in Liver Diseases* is divided into two parts. The first part is dedicated to the hepatoprotective activity of natural compounds and plant extracts in liver diseases and each of the chapters addresses different liver diseases, including hepatitis B and C, alcoholic and nonalcoholic fatty liver disease, liver cancer, and chronic liver diseases (e.g., steatosis, fibrosis, primary sclerosing cholangitis, biliary cirrhosis). The final chapter of the first part of the book is dedicated to drug-induced hepatotoxicity. The second part of the book is dedicated to the influence of nutrients, plant extracts, and natural compounds in liver diseases. In this part of the book, special emphasis is given to the influence of omega-3 fatty acids and monounsaturated fats, vitamins (C, B3, D, and E), and other nutrients (e.g., L-arginine, taurine, and choline) in the liver. Finally, this part of the book also focuses on the antioxidants with hepatoprotective activity and on the plant extracts with hepatoprotective and hepatotoxic effects.

Health professionals have to face new challenges daily in a field that is in rapid growth, with a continuous increase in the number of compounds discovered and in the update of the health-promoting properties of a wide range of compounds, namely natural compounds.

This book will provide the most valuable and consistent information currently available on nutrients, bioactive compounds, and plant extracts that have protective or toxic effects in liver diseases. Therefore, we hope it will be a welcome resource for medical doctors, pharmacists, nutritionists, food chemists, natural product researchers, and pharmacognosists, helping health professionals to offer better therapeutic and nutritional advice.

Seyed Mohammad Nabavi[a], Seyed Fazel Nabavi[a], Seyed Moayed Alavian[b], and Ana Sanches Silva[c,d]

[a]*Applied Biotechnology Research Center, Baqiyatallah University of Medical Sciences, Tehran, Iran*
[b]*Middle East Liver Disease Center (MELD), Tehran, Iran*
[c]*National Institute of Agrarian and Veterinary Research, Vila do Conde, Portugal*
[d]*Center for Study in Animal Science (CECA), University of Oporto, Oporto, Portugal*

CHAPTER 1

Introduction

Fatma Tugce Guragac Dereli[a], Ali Guragac[b], and Tarun Belwal[c]

[a]Department of Pharmacognosy, Faculty of Pharmacy, Suleyman Demirel University, Isparta, Turkey
[b]Urology Department, Private Denizli Tekden Hospital, Denizli, Turkey [c]College of Biosystems Engineering and Food Science, Zhejiang University, Hangzhou, China

The liver, the largest organ as well as the largest parenchymatous gland in the human body, is critically important for several vital physiological processes (Fig. 1.1), especially the regulation of immunity and the metabolism (Carotti et al., 2020; Nemeth et al., 2009).

The anatomy of the liver seems to be specifically designed to maximize its functional properties. It comprises nonparenchymal and parenchymal cells (hepatocytes, HCs). The nonparenchymal cells include sinusoidal endothelial cells (SECs), hepatic stellate cells (myofibroblast-like cells, HSCs), Kupffer cells (hepatic macrophages, KCs), smooth muscle cells (SMCs), dendritic cells (DCs), pit cells (PCs), and oval cells (OCs). All these cells have different structural characteristics and cytokines are responsible for their communication among each other. The activation of signaling cascades, the metabolism of nutrients, and the clearance of toxins and infectious agents are modulated in this way (Carotti et al., 2020; Jenne and Kubes, 2013; Juza and Pauli, 2014).

HCs are predominant cell types in the liver (80% by volume) that provide the main contribution to liver functions, including synthesis, distribution, detoxification and, storage (Si-Tayeb et al., 2010). HSCs are known for their characteristic star-like morphology and they serve as a storehouse for vitamin A. The activation of HSCs results in myofibroblastic differentiation to produce collagens and extracellular matrix proteins (ECM) This production process triggers the formation of liver fibrosis (Friedman, 2008; Geerts, 2001; Gressner and Weiskirchen, 2006). KCs are mononuclear phagocytes involved in the pathogenesis of injury. Activated KCs are responsible for the release of chemokines and proinflammatory cytokines. This event promotes inflammatory cascades. The major role of KCs is the clearance of foreign materials from portal circulation (Bilzer et al., 2006; Naito et al., 2004). PCs are liver-specific natural killer cells (NKs) that contribute to immunity in the liver with potent cytolytic activity. Upon activation, PCs produce interferon-gamma (IFN-γ) and promote changes in the liver. The modulation of T cell responses and cell lysis or hepatocyte death is induced by PCs (Dong et al., 2007; Luo et al., 2000).

Influence of Nutrients, Bioactive Compounds, and Plant Extracts in Liver Diseases. https://doi.org/10.1016/B978-0-12-816488-4.00011-5

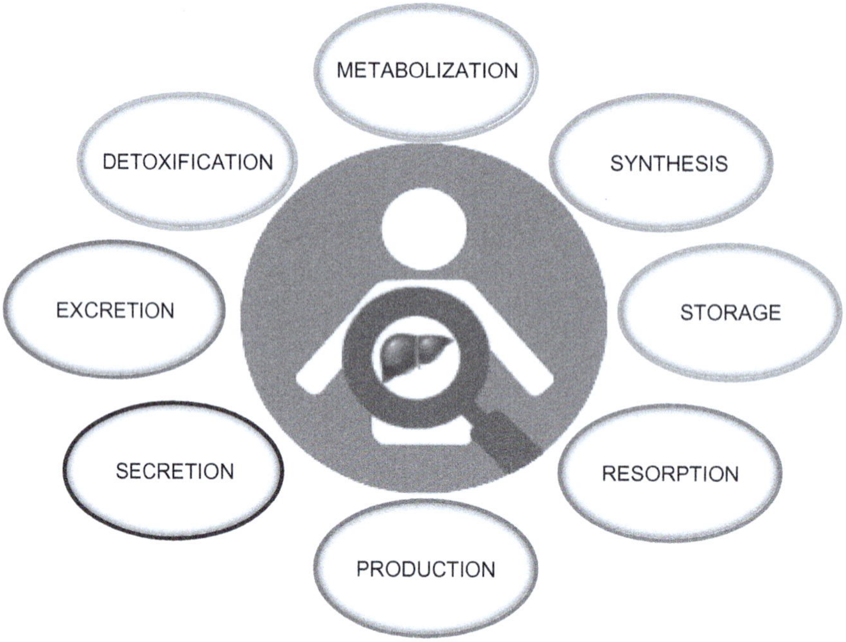

Fig. 1.1
Main functions of the liver.

The liver, a well-vascularized organ, has a dual blood supply that comes from systemic circulation via the hepatic arterial flow and the gastrointestinal tract via the hepatic portal venous flow (Carotti et al., 2020). Due to its anatomic location, the liver is the first organ to be faced with nutrients, pathogens, drugs, and toxins absorbed from the intestine (Guicciardi et al., 2013). It takes the front line in host defence, and this situation makes the liver susceptible to a whole range of pathological conditions. It is able to clear blood flowing from the pancreas and intestine to the rest of the body. Therefore, one of the most important functions of the liver is detoxification (Duncan, 2000). As a multifunctional organ, the liver takes important roles in the regulation of blood clotting, immune responses, and blood glucose-lipid-ammonia levels (Juza and Pauli, 2014). It is responsible for the production and secretion of enzymes, cholesterol, hormones, cofactors, cytokines, bile, plasma proteins, and apolipoproteins (Si-Tayeb et al., 2010). The other multifold function of the liver is storing iron and vitamins such as A, B12, and D (Ramadori et al., 2008). This crucial organ is also important for the maintenance of the metabolic homeostasis of urea, lipids, triglycerides, vitamins, carbohydrates, and several ingested nutrients (Si-Tayeb et al., 2010). All these life-saving functions of the liver may be compromised by various diseases and by overexposure to viruses, toxins, and drugs. Liver dysfunction can impair the quality of life by causing several pathological symptoms in the digestive, cardiovascular, respiratory, hematopoietic, endocrine, and central nervous systems (De Wolf, 2006; Soleimanpour et al., 2015).

Liver diseases may be classified as focal liver diseases (FLDs) and diffuse liver diseases (DLDs) (Bansal et al., 2019). In the case of FLDs, the anomaly is concentrated in a little part of the liver tissue. Some of the most prevalent FLDs are hemangioma, liver cysts, and hepatocellular cancer (HCC). Hemangioma is known as the most frequently seen tumor in infancy. Liver cysts are benign malformations in the liver. The underlying pathogenic event of this disease is isolated aberrant intrahepatic bile ducts (Diez et al., 1998). Among cancers of the liver, HCC is one of the most frequently occurring in individuals. The most common cause of HCC is chronic infections caused by hepatitis B (HBV) and C viruses (HCV) (Kew, 2002). DLDs are characterized by an abnormality distributed throughout the liver tissue. Steatosis (fatty liver disease), hemochromatosis, hepatitis, cirrhosis, and fibrosis are among the most common DLDs (Luersen et al., 2015). Steatosis, namely fatty liver disease, is an abnormal condition of lipid accumulation within the hepatocyte. It is a common histopathological finding of the infection caused by HCV (Adinolfi et al., 2001). Hepatitis is a liver infection that causes inflammation and cell damage. Several viruses such as HBV and HCV are considered the main reasons for this occurrence (Tahir et al., 2015). Hemochromatosis is an iron-overload disease characterized by the overabsorption of iron from the gastrointestinal tract that reaches toxic levels in some endocrine organs, including the liver (Wallace et al., 2002). The formation of liver fibrosis begins in response to damage (infections, toxic chemicals, etc.) and causes the accumulation of ECM, particularly interstitial collagens. The scarring process leads to alterations in liver morphology and functions (Hernandez-Gea and Friedman, 2011). Cirrhosis, a late-stage version of fibrosis, involves irreversible liver degeneration. It is a consequence of long-term injury by viruses or the use of alcohol (Zhou et al., 2014).

The aforementioned liver diseases are among the most frequently encountered in clinical practices. According to epidemiological surveys, the progression of chronic liver diseases (Fig. 1.2) leads to high rates of morbidity and mortality (Asrani et al., 2019). Unfortunately, currently available allopathic therapeutics are far from ideal due to their low therapeutic efficacy, high cost, and common adverse effects. Consequently, the investigation of alternative therapeutic options with more efficacy and lower or no toxicity is vital. In this context,

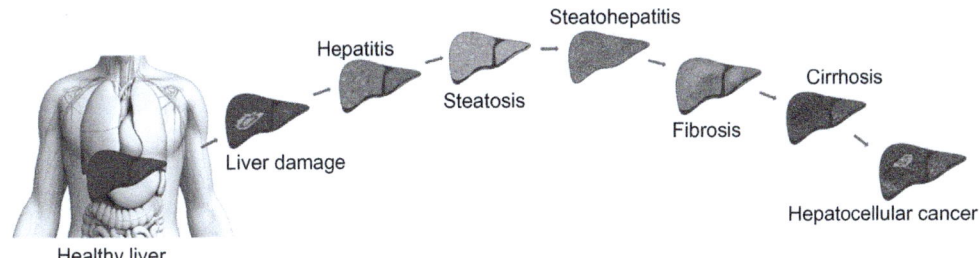

Fig. 1.2
Stages of chronic liver diseases related to damage.

nutrients, bioactive compounds, and plant extracts, mainly from medicinal plants, seem like an option worth exploring (De Smet, 2002; Stickel and Schuppan, 2007). In recent decades, medicinal plants have received increasing interest among researchers for their safety profile and therapeutic value in the management of diverse diseases related to the liver. Increasing evidence from experimental investigations has indicated that various medicinal plants could be useful in this regard by virtue of their antioxidant, antilipid peroxidative, antiinflammatory, antiviral, anticancer, antifibrotic, phagocytic, free radical scavenging, and immunomodulatory properties (Ezhilarasan, 2020; Li et al., 2020; Yao et al., 2016). Several nutrients, bioactive components, and plant extracts have been reported as being healthy for the liver and mitigate the liver and associated disease conditions (Table 1.1) with a wide range of mechanisms. This book addresses in the following chapters both the hepatoprotective and hepatotoxic effects of natural compounds (nutrients, bioactives, and plant extracts).

Table 1.1: List of nutrients, bioactive compounds, and plant extracts for maintaining liver health and mitigating disease conditions with their sources and underlying mechanism of action.

Bioactive compounds	Plant species	Treated liver disease, beneficial for the liver	Main mechanism of action	Reference
Anastatin A Anastatin B	*Anastatica hierochuntica* L.	· Hepatoprotective	· Decreasing CYP2E1 expression · Exhibiting antioxidant property · Showing cytotoxic activity	Xiang et al. (2020) and Yoshikawa et al. (2003)
Apigenin	*Apium graveolens* L.	· Steatosis · Hepatoprotective	· Decreasing the activity of hepatic enzymes · Regulating the esterification of cholesterol and synthesis of triglyceride · Increasing the expression of several hepatic genes related to fatty acid oxidation and cholesterol homeostasis · Decreasing the expression of several hepatic genes related to lipogenesis and lipolysis · Lowering plasma proinflammatory cytokine levels	Jung et al. (2016) and Wang et al. (2017)
Berberine	*Berberis aristata* DC *Berberis vulgaris* L.	· Fibrosis · Nonalcoholic steatosis	· Regulating CYP2E1-dependent oxidant stress · Inhibiting HSC proliferation · Inducing apoptosis · Regulating the hepatic lipid metabolism · Decreasing the expression of fibrosis markers · Controlling cholesterol homeostasis · Inhibiting COX2-prostaglandin production · Exhibiting antioxidant property · Promoting antiinflammatory activity	Eissa et al. (2018), Sun et al. (2018), Sun et al. (2009), and Yan et al. (2015)
Caffeine	*Coffea arabica* L. *Coffea canephora* P.	· Fibrosis · Nonalcoholic steatosis	· Inducing HSC apoptosis · Inhibiting HSC adhesion and activation · Dampening the cAMP/PKA/CREB cascade	Birerdinc et al. (2012), Molloy et al. (2012), Shim et al. (2013), and Wang et al. (2015a)
Colchicine	*Colchicum autumnale* L.	· Cirrhosis · Hepatitis · Fibrosis	· Exhibiting antifibrotic and antiinflammatory activity · Inhibiting transcellular movement of collagen and lipoperoxidation	Cedillo et al. (1996), Kershenobich et al. (1988), Malawista (1968), Mourelle and Meza (1989), and Muriel et al. (2005)

Continued

Table 1.1: List of nutrients, bioactive compounds, and plant extracts for maintaining liver health and mitigating disease conditions with their sources and underlying mechanism of action—cont'd

Bioactive compounds	Plant species	Treated liver disease, beneficial for the liver	Main mechanism of action	Reference
Curcumin	Curcuma longa L.	· Fibrosis · Nonalcoholic steatosis · Metabolic syndrome	· Inhibiting the activation and migration of HSCs · Protecting the hepatocytes from mitochondrial dysfunction and lipoapoptosis · Decreasing oxidative stress-induced hepatic fibrosis · Reducing harmful cytokines · Exhibiting antifibrotic activity	Panahi et al. (2017), Qin et al. (2018), Selmanovic et al. (2017), and She et al. (2018)
Ellagic acid	Phyllanthus urinaria L.	· Fibrosis	· Reducing the levels of hepatic hydroxyproline and lipid peroxide	Buniatian (2003) and Thresiamma and Kuttan (1996)
Epigallocatechin-3-gallate (EGCG)	Camellia sinensis L.	· Fibrosis · Nonalcoholic steatosis	· Inhibiting the cell entry of HCV · Suppressing the TGF-β1, collagen, TNF-α, α-SMA, IL-1β, and MMP-9 expressions as well as the NF-κB pathway · Improving fat infiltration	Ciesek et al. (2011), Sakata et al. (2013), Ying et al. (2017), and Yu et al. (2015)
Esculetin	Cichorium intybus L. Bougainvillea spectabillis Willd.	· Hepatitis · Hepatoprotective	· Preserving the structural integrity of the hepatocellular membrane · Inhibiting xanthine oxidase and 5-lipoxygenase · Exhibiting antiinflammatory activity	Gilani et al. (1998)
Forsythiaside A	Forsythia suspensa Vahl	· Hepatoprotective	· Enhancing Nrf2 signaling · Suppressing NF-κB activity	Pan et al. (2015)
Gallic acid	Acacia confusa Merr.	· Hepatoprotective	· Modulating antioxidant enzyme activities · Inhibiting lipid peroxidation and CYP2E1 activation	Tung et al. (2009)
Geniposide	Gardenia jasminoides Ellis	· Steatosis · Hepatoprotective	· Regulating adipocytokine release and expression of PPARα · Exhibiting antioxidant activity	Ma et al. (2011)

Compound	Source	Application	Activities	References
Gingerol	*Zingiber officinale* Roscoe	· Nonalcoholic steatosis · Hepatocellular carcinoma · Hepatoprotective	· Increasing insulin sensitization · Activating PPAR-γ · Downregulating proinflammatory cytokines · Showing antioxidant and antidyslipidemic activity · Reducing hepatic triglyceride load · Regulating lipid homeostasis and inflammation · Lengthening of the doubling time of hepatoma cells	Sahebkar (2011), Tzeng et al. (2015), and Yagihashi et al. (2008)
Glycyrrhizic acid 18α-Glycyrrhizin	*Glycyrrhiza glabra* L.	· HCV-related cirrhosis · Hepatitis · Fibrosis · Hepatocellular carcinoma	· Increasing the apoptosis rate · Inducing HSC apoptosis and suppressing its activation · Reducing the biochemical markers of fibrosis · Reducing portal hypertension · Preventing HCV progression · Exhibiting antiinflammatory and antioxidant activity	Ikeda et al. (2014), Kumada (2002), Liang et al. (2015), Qu et al. (2012), Qu et al. (2015), and Tu et al. (2012)
Hydroxysafflor yellow A	*Carthamus tinctorius* L.	· Fibrosis · Hepatocellular carcinoma · Cirrhosis	· Attenuating macrophage activation · Inducing heme oxygenase-1 expression · Inhibiting NF-κB activity · Altering membrane fatty acid composition	Hu and Wang (2015), Jiang et al. (2014), Jun et al. (2011), Okuno et al. (1998), and Zhang et al. (2011b)
Kaempferol 3-O-glucoside Kaempferol 3-O-rutinoside	*Carthamus tinctorius* L.	· Hepatoprotective	· Preventing the increase of MDA, ALP, and AST in serum · Restoring GSH, CAT, and SOD activities · Attenuating the histopathological damage	Wang et al. (2015b)
Matrine	*Sophora flavescens* Ait. (Kushen)	· Acute liver injury · Hepatocellular carcinoma	· Exhibiting antiinflammatory and antioxidative properties · Inhibiting cell apoptosis · Inhibiting the expression of matrix metalloproteinase-9	Yu et al. (2011) and Zhang et al. (2011a)
Phyllanthin	*Phyllanthus amarus* Shum and Thonn	· Fibrosis · HBV infection	· Downregulating of TNF-α/NF-κB and TGF-β1 signaling pathways · Inhibiting HBV replication	Krithika et al. (2015), Krithika et al. (2016), and Xin-Hua et al. (2001)

Continued

Table 1.1: List of nutrients, bioactive compounds, and plant extracts for maintaining liver health and mitigating disease conditions with their sources and underlying mechanism of action—cont'd

Bioactive compounds	Plant species	Treated liver disease, beneficial for the liver	Main mechanism of action	Reference
Resveratrol	*Polygonum cuspidatum* Sieb. et Zucc. *Veratrum album* L.	· Intrahepatic endothelial dysfunction · Nonalcoholic steatosis · Fibrosis · Cirrhosis	· Blocking HSC activation · Inducing antiproliferative activity · Decreasing oxidant stress · Suppressing the production of fibrosis markers · Normalizing of protein kinase C responses · Reducing portal hypertension · Exhibiting antiinflammatory and immunomodulatory activity · Regulating glucose and lipid metabolism · Modulating of α-fetoprotein levels	Ahmad and Ahmad (2014), Di Pascoli et al. (2013), Faghihzadeh et al. (2014), Hessin et al. (2017), Lee et al. (2010), Rotman (2015), Souza et al. (2008), and Zhang et al. (2016)
Salvianolic acid B	*Salvia miltiorrhiza* Bunge	· Fibrosis · HBV infection	· Blocking HSC activation · Modulating profibrogenic TGF-β1/SMAD signaling · Reducing cirrhosis-associated portal hypertension · Resolving fibrosis	Liu et al. (2002), Tao et al. (2013), and Xu et al. (2012)
Sarmentosin	*Sedum sarmentosum* Bunge	· Hepatic failure	· Regulating the levels of TNF-α, aspartate aminotransferase, and alanine aminotransferase · Inhibiting of caspase-3 activation · Suppressing the expression of TLR4 · Inhibiting NF-κB activity	Lian et al. (2010)
Schisandrin B	*Schisandra chinensis* (Turcz.) Baill	· Alcohol-related liver diseases · Fibrosis · Hepatoprotective	· Regulating glutathione redox state · Regulating TGF-β/Smad and Nrf2-ARE signaling cascades	Chen et al. (2017), Ip et al. (1996), and Park et al. (2014)
Silymarin Silybin	*Silybum marianum* L.	· HCV infection · Cirrhosis	· Blocking HSC activation, proliferation, and migration · Decreasing the oxidative stress · Reducing the activation of KCs, HSCs, TGF-β1, and α-SMA · Inhibiting cell entry of HCV · Exhibiting antiinflammatory and antifibrogenic properties	Blaising et al. (2013), Ezhilarasan et al. (2017), Fathalah et al. (2017), and Trappoliere et al. (2009)

Compound	Source	Disease/Use	Mechanism	References
Thymoquinone	*Nigella sativa* L.	· Nonalcoholic steatosis · Fibrosis	· Blocking TLR4 expression and PI3K phosphorylation on the activated HSCs · Suppressing oxidant stress and inflammation while reducing the apoptosis rate	Bai et al. (2013) and Awad et al. (2016)
Ursolic acid	*Clerodendrum serratum* L.	· Hepatoprotective	· Reducing the serum bilirubin · Exhibiting antioxidant activity · Inhibiting the activation of toxins · Enhancing body defense system	Vidya et al. (2007)
Wogonin	*Scutellaria baicalensis* Georgi	· Alcohol-related liver diseases · HBV infection · Hepatocellular carcinoma	· Modulating PPAR-γ · Suppressing secretion of the HBV surface antigen · Decreasing the HBV DNA polymerase reaction products · Activating caspase-3 cascade	Chen et al. (2002), Guo et al. (2007), and Li et al. (2017)

References

Adinolfi, L.E., Gambardella, M., Andreana, A., Tripodi, M.F., Utili, R., Ruggiero, G., 2001. Steatosis accelerates the progression of liver damage of chronic hepatitis C patients and correlates with specific HCV genotype and visceral obesity. Hepatology 33 (6), 1358–1364.

Ahmad, A., Ahmad, R., 2014. Resveratrol mitigate structural changes and hepatic stellate cell activation in N′-nitrosodimethylamine-induced liver fibrosis via restraining oxidative damage. Chem. Biol. Interact. 221, 1–12.

Asrani, S.K., Devarbhavi, H., Eaton, J., Kamath, P.S., 2019. Burden of liver diseases in the world. J. Hepatol. 70 (1), 151–171.

Awad, A.S., Abd Al Haleem, E.N., El-Bakly, W.M., Sherief, M.A., 2016. Thymoquinone alleviates nonalcoholic fatty liver disease in rats via suppression of oxidative stress, inflammation, apoptosis. Naunyn Schmiedebergs Arch. Pharmacol. 389 (4), 381–391.

Bai, T., Lian, L.H., Wu, Y.L., Wan, Y., Nan, J.X., 2013. Thymoquinone attenuates liver fibrosis via PI3K and TLR4 signaling pathways in activated hepatic stellate cells. Int. Immunopharmacol. 15 (2), 275–281.

Bansal, S., Chhabra, G., Chandra, B.S., Virmani, J., 2019. A hybrid CAD system design for liver diseases using clinical and radiological data. In: Dey, N., Ashour, A.S., Fong, S.J., Borra, S. (Eds.), U-Healthcare Monitoring Systems. Elsevier Science, San Diego, United States, pp. 289–314.

Bilzer, M., Roggel, F., Gerbes, A.L., 2006. Role of Kupffer cells in host defense and liver disease. Liver Int. 26 (10), 1175–1186.

Birerdinc, A., Stepanova, M., Pawloski, L., Younossi, Z.M., 2012. Caffeine is protective in patients with non-alcoholic fatty liver disease. Aliment. Pharmacol. Ther. 35 (1), 76–82.

Blaising, J., Levy, P.L., Gondeau, C., Phelip, C., Varbanov, M., Teissier, E., Ruggiero, F., Polyak, S.J., Oberlies, N.H., Ivanovic, T., Boulant, S., Pecheur, E.I., 2013. Silibinin inhibits hepatitis C virus entry into hepatocytes by hindering clathrin-dependent trafficking. Cell. Microbiol. 15 (11), 1866–1882.

Buniatian, G.H., 2003. Stages of activation of hepatic stellate cells: effects of ellagic acid, an inhibiter of liver fibrosis, on their differentiation in culture. Cell Prolif. 36 (6), 307–319.

Carotti, S., Morini, S., Carpino, G., Gaudio, E., 2020. Liver histology. In: Radu-Ionita, F., Pyrsopoulos, N., Jinga, M., Tintoiu, I., Sun, Z., Bontas, E. (Eds.), Liver Diseases. Springer, Cham, pp. 17–28.

Cedillo, A., Mourelle, M., Muriel, P., 1996. Effect of colchicine and trimethylcolchicinic acid on CCl_4-induced cirrhosis in the rat. Pharmacol. Toxicol. 79 (5), 241–246.

Chen, Y.C., Shen, S.C., Lee, W.R., Lin, H.Y., Ko, C.H., Shih, C.M., Yang, L.L., 2002. Wogonin and fisetin induction of apoptosis through activation of caspase 3 cascade and alternative expression of p21 protein in hepatocellular carcinoma cells SK-HEP-1. Arch. Toxicol. 76 (5–6), 351–359.

Chen, Q., Zhang, H., Cao, Y., Li, Y., Sun, S., Zhang, J., Zhang, G., 2017. Schisandrin B attenuates CCl_4-induced liver fibrosis in rats by regulation of Nrf2-ARE and TGF-β/Smad signaling pathways. Drug Des. Devel. Ther. 11, 2179–2191.

Ciesek, S., von Hahn, T., Colpitts, C.C., Schang, L.M., Friesland, M., Steinmann, J., Manns, M.P., Ott, M., Wedemeyer, H., Meuleman, P., Pietschmann, T., Steinmann, E., 2011. The green tea polyphenol, epigallocatechin-3-gallate, inhibits hepatitis C virus entry. Hepatology 54 (6), 1947–1955.

De Smet, P.A., 2002. Herbal remedies. N. Engl. J. Med. 347 (25), 2046–2056.

De Wolf, A.M., 2006. 6/2/06 Perioperative assessment of the cardiovascular system in ESLD and transplantation. Int. Anesthesiol. Clin. 44 (4), 59–78.

Di Pascoli, M., Divi, M., Rodriguez-Vilarrupla, A., Rosado, E., Gracia-Sancho, J., Vilaseca, M., Bosch, J., Garcia-Pagan, J.C., 2013. Resveratrol improves intrahepatic endothelial dysfunction and reduces hepatic fibrosis and portal pressure in cirrhotic rats. J. Hepatol. 58 (5), 904–910.

Diez, J., Decoud, J., Gutierrez, L., Suhl, A., Merello, J., 1998. Laparoscopic treatment of symptomatic cysts of the liver. Br. J. Surg. 85 (1), 25–27.

Dong, Z., Wei, H., Sun, R., Tian, Z., 2007. The roles of innate immune cells in liver injury and regeneration. Cell. Mol. Immunol. 4 (4), 241–252.

Duncan, S.A., 2000. Transcriptional regulation of liver development. Dev. Dyn. 219 (2), 131–142.

Eissa, L.A., Kenawy, H.I., El-Karef, A., Elsherbiny, N.M., El-Mihi, K.A., 2018. Antioxidant and anti-inflammatory activities of berberine attenuate hepatic fibrosis induced by thioacetamide injection in rats. Chem. Biol. Interact. 294, 91–100.

Ezhilarasan, D., 2020. Lead compounds with the potentials for the treatment of chronic liver diseases. In: Egbuna, C., Kumar, S., Ifemeje, J., Ezzat, S., Kaliyaperumal, S. (Eds.), Phytochemicals as Lead Compounds for New Drug Discovery. Elsevier Science, Amsterdam, pp. 195–210.

Ezhilarasan, D., Evraerts, J., Sid, B., Calderon, P.B., Karthikeyan, S., Sokal, E., Najimi, M., 2017. Silibinin induces hepatic stellate cell cycle arrest via enhancing p53/p27 and inhibiting Akt downstream signaling protein expression. Hepatobiliary Pancreat. Dis. Int. 16 (1), 80–87.

Faghihzadeh, F., Adibi, P., Rafiei, R., Hekmatdoost, A., 2014. Resveratrol supplementation improves inflammatory biomarkers in patients with nonalcoholic fatty liver disease. Nutr. Res. 34 (10), 837–843.

Fathalah, W.F., Abdel Aziz, M.A., Abou El Soud, N.H., El Raziky, M.E.S., 2017. High dose of silymarin in patients with decompensated liver disease: a randomized controlled trial. J. Interferon Cytokine Res. 37 (11), 480–487.

Friedman, S.L., 2008. Hepatic stellate cells: protean, multifunctional, and enigmatic cells of the liver. Physiol. Rev. 88 (1), 125–172.

Geerts, A., 2001. History, heterogeneity, developmental biology, and functions of quiescent hepatic stellate cells. Semin. Liver Dis. 21 (3), 311–335.

Gilani, A.H., Janbaz, K.H., Shah, B.H., 1998. Esculetin prevents liver damage induced by paracetamol and CCl_4. Pharmacol. Res. 37 (1), 31–35.

Gressner, A.M., Weiskirchen, R., 2006. Modern pathogenetic concepts of liver fibrosis suggest stellate cells and TGF-β as major players and therapeutic targets. J. Cell. Mol. Med. 10 (1), 76–99.

Guicciardi, M.E., Malhi, H., Mott, J.L., Gores, G.J., 2013. Apoptosis and necrosis in the liver. Compr. Physiol. 3 (2), 977–1010.

Guo, Q.L., Zhao, L., You, Q.D., Yang, Y., Gu, H.Y., Song, G.L., Lu, N., Xin, J., 2007. Anti-hepatitis B virus activity of wogonin *in vitro* and *in vivo*. Antiviral Res. 74 (1), 16–24.

Hernandez-Gea, V., Friedman, S.L., 2011. Pathogenesis of liver fibrosis. Annu. Rev. Pathol. 6, 425–456.

Hessin, A.F., Hegazy, R.R., Hassan, A.A., Yassin, N.Z., Kenawy, S.A., 2017. Resveratrol prevents liver fibrosis via two possible pathways: modulation of α fetoprotein transcriptional levels and normalization of protein kinase C responses. Indian J. Pharm. 49, 282–289.

Hu, Z., Wang, W., 2015. Effect of *Carthamus tinctorius* L. extract on diethylnitrosamine-induced liver cirrhosis in rats. Trop. J. Pharm. Res. 14, 1213–1216.

Ikeda, K., Kawamura, Y., Kobayashi, M., Fukushima, T., Sezaki, H., Hosaka, T., Akuta, N., Saitoh, S., Suzuki, F., Suzuki, Y., Arase, Y., Kumada, H., 2014. Prevention of disease progression with anti-inflammatory therapy in patients with HCV-related cirrhosis: a Markov model. Oncology 86 (5–6), 295–302.

Ip, S.P., Poon, M.K., Che, C.T., Ng, K.H., Kong, Y.C., Ko, K.M., 1996. Schisandrin B protects against carbon tetrachloride toxicity by enhancing the mitochondrial glutathione redox status in mouse liver. Free Radic. Biol. Med. 21 (5), 709–712.

Jenne, C.N., Kubes, P., 2013. Immune surveillance by the liver. Nat. Immunol. 14 (10), 996–1006.

Jiang, S., Shi, Z., Li, C., Ma, C., Bai, X., Wang, C., 2014. Hydroxysafflor yellow A attenuates ischemia/reperfusion-induced liver injury by suppressing macrophage activation. Int. J. Clin. Exp. Pathol. 7 (5), 2595–2608.

Jun, M.S., Ha, Y.M., Kim, H.S., Jang, H.J., Kim, Y.M., Lee, Y.S., Kim, H.J., Seo, H.G., Lee, J.H., Lee, S.H., Chang, K.C., 2011. Anti-inflammatory action of methanol extract of *Carthamus tinctorius* involves in heme oxygenase-1 induction. J. Ethnopharmacol. 133 (2), 524–530.

Jung, U.J., Cho, Y.Y., Choi, M.S., 2016. Apigenin ameliorates dyslipidemia, hepatic steatosis and insulin resistance by modulating metabolic and transcriptional profiles in the liver of high-fat diet-induced obese mice. Nutrients 8 (5), 305.

Juza, R.M., Pauli, E.M., 2014. Clinical and surgical anatomy of the liver: a review for clinicians. Clin. Anat. 27 (5), 764–769.

Kershenobich, D., Vargas, F., Garcia-Tsao, G., Perez Tamayo, R., Gent, M., Rojkind, M., 1988. Colchicine in the treatment of cirrhosis of the liver. N. Engl. J. Med. 318 (26), 1709–1713.

Kew, M.C., 2002. Epidemiology of hepatocellular carcinoma. Toxicology 181–182, 35–38.

Krithika, R., Jyothilakshmi, V., Prashantha, K., Verma, R.J., 2015. Mechanism of protective effect of phyllanthin against carbon tetrachloride-induced hepatotoxicity and experimental liver fibrosis in mice. Toxicol. Mech. Methods 25 (9), 708–717.

Krithika, R., Jyothilakshmi, V., Verma, R.J., 2016. Phyllanthin inhibits CCl_4-mediated oxidative stress and hepatic fibrosis by down-regulating TNF-α/NF-κB, and pro-fibrotic factor TGF-β1 mediating inflammatory signaling. Toxicol. Ind. Health 32 (5), 953–960.

Kumada, H., 2002. Long-term treatment of chronic hepatitis C with glycyrrhizin [stronger neo-minophagen C (SNMC)] for preventing liver cirrhosis and hepatocellular carcinoma. Oncology 62, 94–100.

Lee, E.S., Shin, M.O., Yoon, S., Moon, J.O., 2010. Resveratrol inhibits dimethylnitrosamine-induced hepatic fibrosis in rats. Arch. Pharm. Res. 33 (6), 925–932.

Li, H.D., Chen, X., Yang, Y., Huang, H.M., Zhang, L., Zhang, X., Zhang, L., Huang, C., Meng, X.M., Li, J., 2017. Wogonin attenuates inflammation by activating PPAR-γ in alcoholic liver disease. Int. Immunopharmacol. 50, 95–106.

Li, S., Xu, Y., Guo, W., Chen, F., Zhang, C., Tan, H.Y., Wang, N., Feng, Y., 2020. The impacts of herbal medicines and natural products on regulating the hepatic lipid metabolism. Front. Pharmacol. 11, 351.

Lian, L.H., Jin, X., Wu, Y.L., Cai, X.F., Lee, J.J., Nan, J.X., 2010. Hepatoprotective effects of *Sedum sarmentosum* on D-galactosamine/lipopolysaccharide-induced murine fulminant hepatic failure. J. Pharmacol. Sci. 114 (2), 147–157.

Liang, B., Guo, X.L., Jin, J., Ma, Y.C., Feng, Z.Q., 2015. Glycyrrhizic acid inhibits apoptosis and fibrosis in carbon-tetrachloride-induced rat liver injury. World J. Gastroenterol. 21 (17), 5271–5280.

Liu, P., Hu, Y.Y., Liu, C., Zhu, D.Y., Xue, H.M., Xu, Z.Q., Xu, L.M., Liu, C.H., Gu, H.T., Zhang, Z.Q., 2002. Clinical observation of salvianolic acid B in treatment of liver fibrosis in chronic hepatitis B. World J. Gastroenterol. 8 (4), 679–685.

Luersen, G.F., Bhosale, P., Szklaruk, J., 2015. State-of-the-art cross-sectional liver imaging: beyond lesion detection and characterization. J. Hepatocell. Carcinoma 2, 101–117.

Luo, D.Z., Vermijlen, D., Ahishali, B., Triantis, V., Plakoutsi, G., Braet, F., Vanderkerken, K., Wisse, E., 2000. On the cell biology of pit cells, the liver-specific NK cells. World J. Gastroenterol. 6 (1), 1–11.

Ma, T.T., Huang, C., Zong, G.J., Zha, D.J., Meng, X.M., Li, J., Tang, W.J., 2011. Hepatoprotective effects of geniposide in a rat model of nonalcoholic steatohepatitis. J. Pharm. Pharmacol. 63 (4), 587–593.

Malawista, S.E., 1968. Colchicine: a common mechanism for its anti-inflammatory and anti-mitotic effects. Arthritis Rheum. 11 (2), 191–198.

Molloy, J.W., Calcagno, C.J., Williams, C.D., Jones, F.J., Torres, D.M., Harrison, S.A., 2012. Association of coffee and caffeine consumption with fatty liver disease, nonalcoholic steatohepatitis, and degree of hepatic fibrosis. Hepatology 55 (2), 429–436.

Mourelle, M., Meza, M.A., 1989. Colchicine prevents D-galactosamine-induced hepatitis. J. Hepatol. 8 (2), 165–172.

Muriel, P., Moreno, M.G., Hernandez Mdel, C., Chavez, E., Alcantar, L.K., 2005. Resolution of liver fibrosis in chronic CCl_4 administration in the rat after discontinuation of treatment: effect of silymarin, silibinin, colchicine and trimethylcolchicinic acid. Basic Clin. Pharmacol. Toxicol. 96 (5), 375–380.

Naito, M., Hasegawa, G., Ebe, Y., Yamamoto, T., 2004. Differentiation and function of Kupffer cells. Med. Electron Microsc. 37 (1), 16–28.

Nemeth, E., Baird, A.W., O'Farrelly, C., 2009. Microanatomy of the liver immune system. Semin. Immunopathol. 31 (3), 333–343.

Okuno, M., Tanaka, T., Komaki, C., Nagase, S., Shiratori, Y., Muto, Y., Kajiwara, K., Maki, T., Moriwaki, H., 1998. Suppressive effect of low amounts of safflower and perilla oils on diethylnitrosamine-induced hepatocarcinogenesis in male F344 rats. Nutr. Cancer 30 (3), 186–193.

Pan, C.W., Zhou, G.Y., Chen, W.L., Zhuge, L., Jin, L.X., Zheng, Y., Lin, W., Pan, Z.Z., 2015. Protective effect of forsythiaside A on lipopolysaccharide/D-galactosamine-induced liver injury. Int. Immunopharmacol. 26 (1), 80–85.

Panahi, Y., Kianpour, P., Mohtashami, R., Jafari, R., Simental-Mendia, L.E., Sahebkar, A., 2017. Efficacy and safety of phytosomal curcumin in non-alcoholic fatty liver disease: a randomized controlled trial. Drug Res. (Stuttg) 67 (4), 244–251.

Park, H.J., Lee, S.J., Song, Y., Jang, S.H., Ko, Y.G., Kang, S.N., Chung, B.Y., Kim, H.D., Kim, G.S., Cho, J.H., 2014. *Schisandra chinensis* prevents alcohol-induced fatty liver disease in rats. J. Med. Food 17 (1), 103–110.

Qin, L.F., Qin, J.M., Zhen, X.M., Yang, Q., Huang, L.Y., 2018. Curcumin protects against hepatic stellate cells activation and migration by inhibiting the CXCL12/CXCR4 biological axis in liver fibrosis: a study *in vitro* and *in vivo*. Biomed. Pharmacother. 101, 599–607.

Qu, Y., Chen, W.H., Zong, L., Xu, M.Y., Lu, L.G., 2012. 18α-Glycyrrhizin induces apoptosis and suppresses activation of rat hepatic stellate cells. Med. Sci. Monit. 18 (1), Br24–Br32.

Qu, Y., Zong, L., Xu, M., Dong, Y., Lu, L., 2015. Effects of 18α-glycyrrhizin on TGF-β1/Smad signaling pathway in rats with carbon tetrachloride-induced liver fibrosis. Int. J. Clin. Exp. Pathol. 8 (2), 1292–1301.

Ramadori, G., Moriconi, F., Malik, I., Dudas, J., 2008. Physiology and pathophysiology of liver inflammation, damage and repair. J. Physiol. Pharmacol. 59 (1), 107–117.

Rotman, Y., 2015. Comment on "Resveratrol improves insulin resistance, glucose and lipid metabolism in patients with non-alcoholic fatty liver disease: a randomized controlled trial" by Shihui Chen et al. [Dig. Liver Dis. 2015;47:226-32]. Dig. Liver Dis. 47 (12), 1090.

Sahebkar, A., 2011. Potential efficacy of ginger as a natural supplement for nonalcoholic fatty liver disease. World J. Gastroenterol. 17 (2), 271–272.

Sakata, R., Nakamura, T., Torimura, T., Ueno, T., Sata, M., 2013. Green tea with high-density catechins improves liver function and fat infiltration in non-alcoholic fatty liver disease (NAFLD) patients: a double-blind placebo-controlled study. Int. J. Mol. Med. 32 (5), 989–994.

Selmanovic, S., Beganlic, A., Salihefendic, N., Ljuca, F., Softic, A., Smajic, E., 2017. Therapeutic effects of curcumin on ultrasonic morphological characteristics of liver in patients with metabolic syndrome. Acta Inform. Med. 25 (3), 169–174.

She, L.L., Xu, D., Wang, Z.X., Zhang, Y.R., Wei, Q.L., Aa, J.Y., Wang, G.J., Liu, B.L., Xie, Y., 2018. Curcumin inhibits hepatic stellate cell activation via suppression of succinate-associated HIF-1 α induction. Mol. Cell. Endocrinol. 476, 129–138.

Shim, S.G., Jun, D.W., Kim, E.K., Saeed, W.K., Lee, K.N., Lee, H.L., Lee, O.Y., Choi, H.S., Yoon, B.C., 2013. Caffeine attenuates liver fibrosis via defective adhesion of hepatic stellate cells in cirrhotic model. J. Gastroenterol. Hepatol. 28 (12), 1877–1884.

Si-Tayeb, K., Lemaigre, F.P., Duncan, S.A., 2010. Organogenesis and development of the liver. Dev. Cell 18 (2), 175–189.

Soleimanpour, H., Safari, S., Rahmani, F., Ameli, H., Alavian, S.M., 2015. The role of inhalational anesthetic drugs in patients with hepatic dysfunction: a review article. Anesth. Pain Med. 5 (1), e23409.

Souza, I.C., Martins, L.A., Coelho, B.P., Grivicich, I., Guaragna, R.M., Gottfried, C., Borojevic, R., Guma, F.C., 2008. Resveratrol inhibits cell growth by inducing cell cycle arrest in activated hepatic stellate cells. Mol. Cell. Biochem. 315 (1–2), 1–7.

Stickel, F., Schuppan, D., 2007. Herbal medicine in the treatment of liver diseases. Dig. Liver Dis. 39 (4), 293–304.

Sun, X., Zhang, X., Hu, H., Lu, Y., Chen, J., Yasuda, K., Wang, H., 2009. Berberine inhibits hepatic stellate cell proliferation and prevents experimental liver fibrosis. Biol. Pharm. Bull. 32 (9), 1533–1537.

Sun, H., Liu, Q., Hu, H., Jiang, Y., Shao, W., Wang, Q., Jiang, Z., Gu, A., 2018. Berberine ameliorates blockade of autophagic flux in the liver by regulating cholesterol metabolism and inhibiting COX2-prostaglandin synthesis. Cell Death Dis. 9 (8), 824.

Tahir, M.A., Cheema, A., Tareen, S., 2015. Frequency of hepatitis-B and C in patients undergoing cataract surgery in a tertiary care centre. Pak. J. Med. Sci. 31 (4), 895–898.

Tao, Y.Y., Wang, Q.L., Shen, L., Fu, W.W., Liu, C.H., 2013. Salvianolic acid B inhibits hepatic stellate cell activation through transforming growth factor β-1 signal transduction pathway *in vivo* and *in vitro*. Exp. Biol. Med. 238 (11), 1284–1296.

Thresiamma, K.C., Kuttan, R., 1996. Inhibition of liver fibrosis by ellagic acid. Indian J. Physiol. Pharmacol. 40 (4), 363–366.

Trappoliere, M., Caligiuri, A., Schmid, M., Bertolani, C., Failli, P., Vizzutti, F., Novo, E., di Manzano, C., Marra, F., Loguercio, C., Pinzani, M., 2009. Silybin, a component of sylimarin, exerts anti-inflammatory and anti-fibrogenic effects on human hepatic stellate cells. J. Hepatol. 50 (6), 1102–1111.

Tu, C.T., Li, J., Wang, F.P., Li, L., Wang, J.Y., Jiang, W., 2012. Glycyrrhizin regulates CD4+ T cell response during liver fibrogenesis via JNK, ERK and PI3K/AKT pathway. Int. Immunopharmacol. 14 (4), 410–421.

Tung, Y.T., Wu, J.H., Huang, C.C., Peng, H.C., Chen, Y.L., Yang, S.C., Chang, S.T., 2009. Protective effect of *Acacia confusa* bark extract and its active compound gallic acid against carbon tetrachloride-induced chronic liver injury in rats. Food Chem. Toxicol. 47 (6), 1385–1392.

Tzeng, T.F., Liou, S.S., Chang, C.J., Liu, I.M., 2015. 6-Gingerol protects against nutritional steatohepatitis by regulating key genes related to inflammation and lipid metabolism. Nutrients 7 (2), 999–1020.

Vidya, S.M., Krishna, V., Manjunatha, B.K., Mankani, K.L., Ahmed, M., Singh, S.D., 2007. Evaluation of hepatoprotective activity of *Clerodendrum serratum* L. Indian J. Exp. Biol. 45 (6), 538–542.

Wallace, D.F., Pedersen, P., Dixon, J.L., Stephenson, P., Searle, J.W., Powell, L.W., Subramaniam, V.N., 2002. Novel mutation in ferroportin1 is associated with autosomal dominant hemochromatosis. Blood 100 (2), 692–694.

Wang, Q., Dai, X., Yang, W., Wang, H., Zhao, H., Yang, F., Yang, Y., Li, J., Lv, X., 2015a. Caffeine protects against alcohol-induced liver fibrosis by dampening the cAMP/PKA/CREB pathway in rat hepatic stellate cells. Int. Immunopharmacol. 25 (2), 340–352.

Wang, Y., Tang, C., Zhang, H., 2015b. Hepatoprotective effects of kaempferol 3-*O*-rutinoside and kaempferol 3-*O*-glucoside from *Carthamus tinctorius* L. on CCl4-induced oxidative liver injury in mice. J. Food Drug Anal. 23 (2), 310–317.

Wang, F., Liu, J.C., Zhou, R.J., Zhao, X., Liu, M., Ye, H., Xie, M.L., 2017. Apigenin protects against alcohol-induced liver injury in mice by regulating hepatic CYP2E1-mediated oxidative stress and PPARα-mediated lipogenic gene expression. Chem. Biol. Interact. 275, 171–177.

Xiang, C., Cao, M., Miao, A., Gao, F., Li, X., Pan, G., Zhang, W., Zhang, Y., Yu, P., Teng, Y., 2020. Antioxidant activities of anastatin A & B derivatives and compound 38c's protective effect in a mouse model of CCl4-induced acute liver injury. RSC Adv. 10 (24), 14337–14346.

Xin-Hua, W., Chang-Qing, L., Xing-Bo, G., Lin-Chun, F., 2001. A comparative study of *Phyllanthus amarus* compound and interferon in the treatment of chronic viral hepatitis B. Southeast Asian J. Trop. Med. Public Health 32 (1), 140–142.

Xu, H., Zhou, Y., Lu, C., Ping, J., Xu, L.M., 2012. Salvianolic acid B lowers portal pressure in cirrhotic rats and attenuates contraction of rat hepatic stellate cells by inhibiting RhoA signaling pathway. Lab. Invest. 92 (12), 1738–1748.

Yagihashi, S., Miura, Y., Yagasaki, K., 2008. Inhibitory effect of gingerol on the proliferation and invasion of hepatoma cells in culture. Cytotechnology 57 (2), 129–136.

Yan, H.M., Xia, M.F., Wang, Y., Chang, X.X., Yao, X.Z., Rao, S.X., Zeng, M.S., Tu, Y.F., Feng, R., Jia, W.P., Liu, J., Deng, W., Jiang, J.D., Gao, X., 2015. Efficacy of berberine in patients with non-alcoholic fatty liver disease. PLoS One 10 (8).

Yao, H., Qiao, Y.J., Zhao, Y.L., Tao, X.F., Xu, L.N., Yin, L.H., Qi, Y., Peng, J.Y., 2016. Herbal medicines and nonalcoholic fatty liver disease. World J. Gastroenterol. 22 (30), 6890–6905.

Ying, L., Yan, F., Zhao, Y., Gao, H., Williams, B.R., Hu, Y., Li, X., Tian, R., Xu, P., Wang, Y., 2017. (−)-Epigallocatechin-3-gallate and atorvastatin treatment down-regulates liver fibrosis-related genes in non-alcoholic fatty liver disease. Clin. Exp. Pharmacol. Physiol. 44 (12), 1180–1191.

Yoshikawa, M., Xu, F., Morikawa, T., Ninomiya, K., Matsuda, H., 2003. Anastatins A and B, new skeletal flavonoids with hepatoprotective activities from the desert plant *Anastatica hierochuntica*. Bioorg. Med. Chem. Lett. 13 (6), 1045–1049.

Yu, H.B., Zhang, H.F., Li, D.Y., Zhang, X., Xue, H.Z., Zhao, S.H., 2011. Matrine inhibits matrix metalloproteinase-9 expression and invasion of human hepatocellular carcinoma cells. J. Asian Nat. Prod. Res. 13 (3), 242–250.

Yu, D.K., Zhang, C.X., Zhao, S.S., Zhang, S.H., Zhang, H., Cai, S.Y., Shao, R.G., He, H.W., 2015. The anti-fibrotic effects of epigallocatechin-*3*-gallate in bile duct-ligated cholestatic rats and human hepatic stellate LX-2 cells are mediated by the PI3K/Akt/Smad pathway. Acta Pharmacol. Sin. 36 (4), 473–482.

Zhang, F., Wang, X., Tong, L., Qiao, H., Li, X., You, L., Jiang, H., Sun, X., 2011a. Matrine attenuates endotoxin-induced acute liver injury after hepatic ischemia/reperfusion in rats. Surg. Today 41 (8), 1075–1084.

Zhang, Y., Guo, J., Dong, H., Zhao, X., Zhou, L., Li, X., Liu, J., Niu, Y., 2011b. Hydroxysafflor yellow A protects against chronic carbon tetrachloride-induced liver fibrosis. Eur. J. Pharmacol. 660 (2–3), 438–444.

Zhang, D.Q., Sun, P., Jin, Q., Li, X., Zhang, Y., Zhang, Y.J., Wu, Y.L., Nan, J.X., Lian, L.H., 2016. Resveratrol regulates activated hepatic stellate cells by modulating NF-κB and the PI3K/Akt signaling pathway. J. Food Sci. 81 (1), H240–H245.

Zhou, W.C., Zhang, Q.B., Qiao, L., 2014. Pathogenesis of liver cirrhosis. World J. Gastroenterol. 20 (23), 7312–7324.

Hepatoprotective activity of natural compounds and plant extracts in liver diseases

CHAPTER 2

Hepatitis B

Umair Younas[a], Sana Tehseen[b], Fazlullah Khan[c], and Kamal Niaz[d]

[a]Department of Livestock Management, Faculty of Animal Production and Technology, Cholistan University of Veterinary and Animal Sciences, Bahawalpur, Pakistan [b]Department of Botany, Government College Women University Faisalabad, Faisalabad, Pakistan [c]Department of Allied Health Sciences, Bashir Institute of Health Sciences, Bhara Kahu, Islamabad, Pakistan [d]Department of Pharmacology and Toxicology, Faculty of Bio-Sciences, Cholistan University of Veterinary and Animal Sciences (CUVAS), Bahawalpur, Pakistan

2.1 Introduction

The liver is not only a vital organ of the human body, but also the largest gland. Various physiological functions such as metabolism, secretion, and storage are the foremost responsibilities of the liver. Similarly, the detoxification of various drugs and xenobiotics is also performed by the liver. In the digestion process, without bile secretion digestion cannot be completed; this is also attributed to the functioning of the liver (Govind and Pandey, 2011).

However, the liver is prone to various infections from various foreign invading particles that start with inflammation of the liver; further complications will follow if this is not treated well. It is roughly estimated that almost 90% of hepatitis is a viral type, including hepatitis B, A, C, D (delta agents), E, and G. Of all these types of viral agents, hepatitis B is of primary importance as it often causes chronic liver disease as well as liver cirrhosis (Kumar et al., 2011). The hepatitis B virus (HBV) belongs to the Hepadnaviridae family.

Sarpel et al. (2017) stated that of the many leading causes of morbidity and mortality related to the liver, chronic hepatitis B is the one that is a blood-borne virus. It may be spread through blood-to-blood contact, leading to serious infective complications such as hepatocellular carcinoma.

More than 257 million people suffer from HBV (chronic type), while 887,000 deaths occurred due to primary liver cancer according to the World Health Organization (WHO) 2015 (Montuclard et al., 2015; Terrault et al., 2016; WHO, 2017).

According to another study, among individuals affected by HBV that are untreated, about 15%–40% of the cases become cirrhosis, which ultimately becomes liver cancer as well as liver failure (Tang et al., 2018). Infants are more prone to develop a chronic HBV

Influence of Nutrients, Bioactive Compounds, and Plant Extracts in Liver Diseases. https://doi.org/10.1016/B978-0-12-816488-4.00012-7

infection after an acute attack of HBV infection. In fact, 90% of infants may progress from acute to chronic infection as compared to adults, where the number is 5%–10% (WHO, 2017).

Regarding the life cycle of HBV, in the nucleus of the hepatocyte, the DNA of HBV is transformed to stable and circular DNA called covalently closed circular DNA (CCC DNA). Therefore, the DNA from HBV is joined with the DNA of the host cell. The CCC DNA acts as a model viral RNA transcription that is likely to persist inside the long-lived hepatocyte nucleus so that it may act as a resource for virus replication (Tang et al., 2018).

Individuals suffering from chronic HBV infection are not likely to show any symptoms and are often diagnosed during screening or a routine health checkup (for example, a checkup for an increased level of liver enzymes or a blood donation). Adults facing acute infection for HBV may progress to a chronic infection; however, that number is not alarming as it is only 5%–10%. Symptoms such as fatigue, fever, abdominal pain, malaise, and jaundice are developed by one-third of adults after an acute HBV infection while the other two-thirds undergo an asymptomatic and subclinical illness (Liang et al., 2009).

For the treatment of virus-related diseases (including HBV), there are several plants that prevent or decrease infection via various biological mechanisms. Medicinal plant extracts are very effective in counteracting the HBV issue. Medicinal plants serve crucial roles in maintaining the health and survival of humans and animals. They contribute to the treatment of nontoxic liver disease (Pandey and Madhuri, 2008, 2010; Madhuri and Pandey, 2009; Madhuri, 2008). The purpose of this article is to investigate and identify effective medicinal plants for the prevention and treatment of viral diseases, especially hepatitis B, and the involved various therapeutic mechanisms.

2.2 Rheum palmatum L.

Regarding HBV treatment, two antiviral drugs—lamivudine and interferon—are famous and their efficiency is acceptable to inhibit HBV replication (Maddrey, 2000; Humphries and Dixon, 2003) as biochemical and virological remission may be induced by these drugs against HBV infection. However, it was noted that the clinical effects are inadequate as the mutation occurred in the virus genome, that shows adverse effects, which is ultimately costly to treat. Another factor is that the percentage of patients who benefitted from the combination therapy of lamivudine and interferon is only 20%.

In the pursuit of an effective anti-HBV agent, the traditional Chinese herbal plant *Rheum palmatum* L. is a good choice, as shown in Fig. 2.1. The distribution of this herbal plant in China is widespread, and it carries quite a long history regarding the treatment of viral diseases and gastroenteritis problems (Sun et al., 2007).

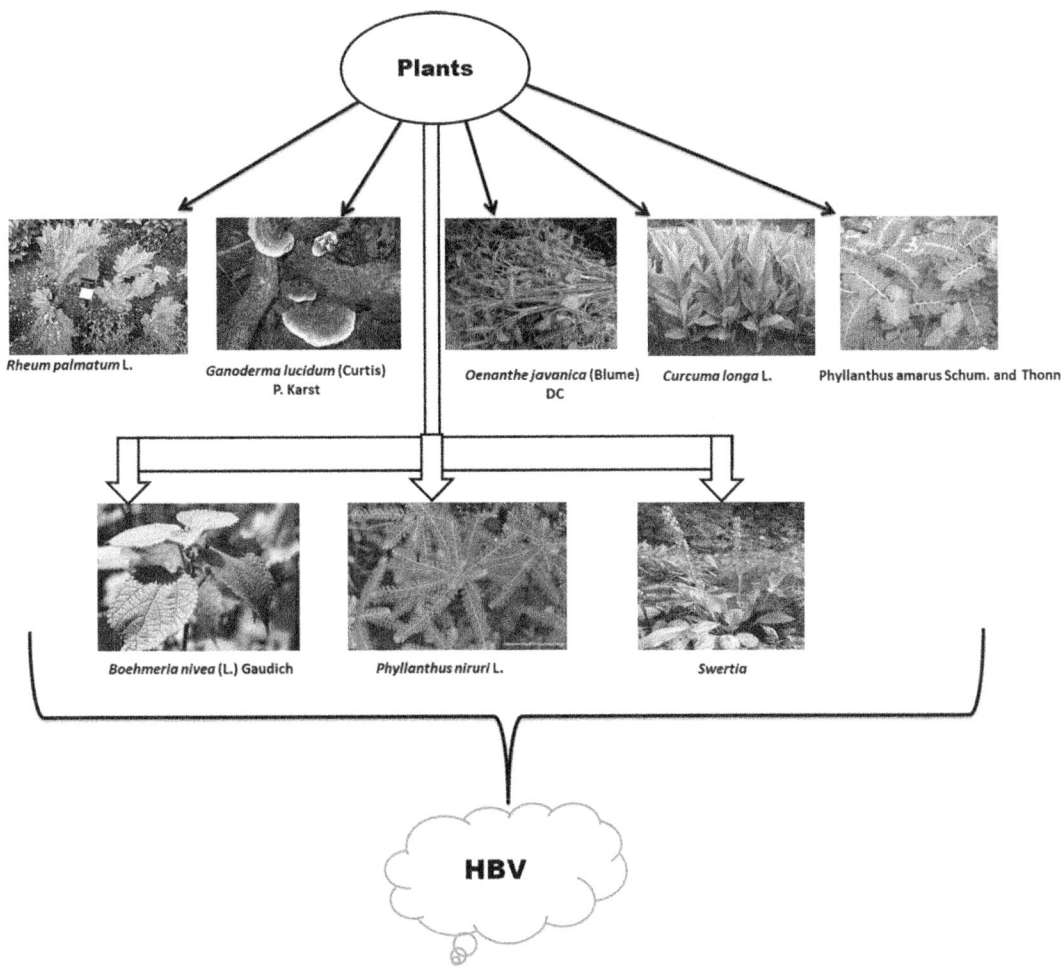

Fig. 2.1
Plants possesing anti-HBV activities.

Several anthraquinone derivates are contained in *Rheum palmatum* L. that are shown to have antiviral activities, specifically against the polio virus, the vesicular stomatitis virus, human cytomegalovirus, and the herpes simplex type 1 and 2 viruses (Sun et al., 2007; Semple et al., 2001).

To find a novel anti-HBV agent having high biological activity and a lower incidence of side effects, Sun et al. (2007) investigated the counteractive activity of the herbal plant *Rheum palmatum* L. The real-time quantitative polymerase chain reaction (PCR) was considered in their study to evaluate the counteractive activity of RPS against the DNA replication of HBV in a stable HBV-producing cell line.

Sun et al., (2007) reported that in comparison to two different anthraquinone derivatives, rhein and emodin, the *Rheum palmatum* L. ethanol extract (RPE) showed good efficacy against HBV as well as less cytotoxicity.

In another study, Li et al. (2007) reported that *Rheum palmatum* extract was able to show good efficacy to inhibit HBV. It is noted that combined anthraquinone chrysophanol 8-*O*-D-glucoside is mainly responsible for anti-HBV activity in RPE and is a capable agent in the treatment of HBV infection.

2.3 Ganoderma lucidum *(Curtis) P. Karst.*

The famous medicinal plant *Ganoderma*, also known as Linghzi, is regarded as a marvelous herb plant that is widely used in the United States, Korea, Japan, China, and other countries (Meng et al., 2011). The use of *Ganoderma* is well established. It is used against natural antifungal-associated diseases (Cao et al., 2018) and is also effective against HBV (Li and Wang, 2006). Various researchers have reported the *Ganoderma* plant to have medicinal properties such as a mechanism of immunity regulation (Zhang et al., 2002a,b). Furthermore, it possesses antiviral (Sahar et al., 1998; Kim et al., 2000) and anticarcinogenic (Wang et al., 1997) as well as liver protective characteristics (Back et al., 1999), as shown in Fig. 2.1. The chief bioactive ingredients in *G. lucidum* include polysaccharides, triterpenes, and sterols (Min et al., 1998, 2000, 2001; Oh et al., 2000). Another researcher reported that ganodermic acid extracted from *Ganoderma* plant lessen the liver injury in mice caused by the *Mycobacterium bovis* bacillus Calmette-Guerin (BCG) along lipo-polysaccharide (Zhang et al., 2002a,b).

Polysaccharides, triterpenes, and peptidoglycans are the main physiologically active components in *G. lucidum* (Zhou et al., 2007; Boh et al., 2007). Polysaccharides are considered to be vital biological macromolecules in diversity, which has long-range physiochemical properties (Zhou et al., 2007). *G. lucidum* is enriched with triterpenes, a class of compounds that gives a bitter taste to herbs. This is believed to confer different health-related benefits, including antioxidant and lipid-lowering effects. Almost 100 triterpenes with known molecular configurations and chemical compositions are known to be present in *G. lucidum*. Triterpenes may also be used as a measure of quality of different *Ganoderma* samples (Chen et al., 1999; Su et al., 2001).

Similarly, the isolation of various bioactive peptidoglycans from the *G. lucidum* peptidoglycan shows antiviral activity (GLPG) (Li et al., 2005), including a *G. lucdum* immunomodulating substance (GLIS) (Ji et al., 2007), PGY (a water-soluble glycol-peptide) (Wu and Wang, 2009), GL-PS peptide (glucagon like peptides) (Ho et al., 2007), and fucose-containing glycoprotein fraction (F3) (Chien et al., 2004).

2.4 Oenanthe javanica *(Blume) DC.*

O. javanica, commonly known as the water dropwort plant, has been used in various ethnomedical systems for a long time in various Asian countries. The plant is famous for treating acute and chronic hepatitis, jaundice, and inflammatory conditions, among others (Lu and Li, 2019). It is a small perennial herb plant that has been cultivated in tropical and temperate regions of Asia for a very long time. It is used to alleviate a broad spectrum of diseases. Ali et al., (2016) and Yang et al., (2014) reported its hepatoprotective properties, as illustrated in Fig. 2.1. An enhancement in immunity was described by Liu and Zhang (2016) while its antioxidant and antiviral characteristics were shown by Kongkachuichai et al. (2015) and Han et al. (2008). Chen et al. (2016) found out that phenylpropanoids, phenolic acids, flavonoids, isorhamnetin, and persicarin are the constituents of the dropwort plant.

Huang et al. (2001) reported that *O. javanica* has benefits for the treatment of hepatitis B infection by inhibiting HBsAg and HBeAg secretion in vitro.

According to another study by Chen et al. (2016), the water dropwort plant has a long list of medicinal properties other than hepatoprotective, anti-HBV, and antiinflammatory such as antidiabetes, antioxidant, alcohol detoxification, neurogenesis, antiquorum sensing, melanogenic, neuroprotective, and antiarryhythmic, among others.

Many biological activities are carried out by *O. javanica* including hepatoprotective (Ai et al., 2016; Yang et al., 2014), immune enhancement (Liu and Li, 2016), antiviral (Han et al., 2008), antiinflammatory (Ahn and Lee, 2017; Yang et al., 2013), and ethanol elimination (Kim et al., 2009a,b). As a result of phytochemical assessment, it was noted that *O. javanica* contains natural compounds such as flavonoids, flavonoid glycosides (Wang et al., 2005), coumarins (Kim et al., 2016), and polyphenols (Ai et al., 2016). Moreover, toxicity studies revealed that *O. javanica* did not show genetic and acute toxicity (Yu et al., 2017; Wang et al., 2016).

2.5 Curcuma longa *L.*

The common name of *Curcuma longa* L. is turmeric. *C. longa* is a perennial herb and it has widespread distribution in the tropics of Asia, Africa, and Australia with more than 80 species (Ashraf, 2018). In vitro and in vivo studies of turmeric have indicated that this plant is efficient in suppressing the activity of common mutagens in a variety of cell types. Turmeric is also shown to have the ability to increase glutathione levels and thereby promote hepatic detoxifications of mutagens. Wei et al. (2017) reported that *C. longa* inhibits HBV by the downregulation of CCC DNA bound histone acetylation, as shown in Fig. 2.1.

The pharmacological activities of *C. longa* include antimicrobial, antiinflammatory, and antioxidant effects (Maheshwari et al., 2006). There is also evidence that the development of liver cirrhosis can be counteracted by the action of curcumin (Bruck et al., 2007). Kim et al. (2009a,b) reported that *C. longa* has long been used as a traditional Asian remedy to alleviate liver ailments caused by HBV infection. However, it is not fully understood why *C. longa* has antiviral activity against HBV replication. The general markers for HBV replication are the HBV antigen (HBsAg) and the DNA of HBV. Therefore, the removal of HBsAg is considered an indication toward the complete treated condition of HBV epidemiology accompanying the eradication of HBV DNA.

2.6 Phyllanthus amarus Schum. and Thonn.

P. amarus is a plant that has been used as traditional medicine for more than 3000 years. It is commonly known as carry me seed, stone breaker, gala of wind, etc. It is widely distributed in the tropics and subtropics throughout China, India, and South America (Meena et al., 2018).

P. amarus is gaining popularity for its hepatoprotective property and is a good choice of anti-HBV, as shown in Fig. 2.1. Various other health-related positive marks include antiinflammatory, antibacterial, anticarcinogenic, and antiviral activity as a result of various combinations of secondary metabolites present that render medicinal properties (Meena et al., 2018). In another study, it was reported that the *Phyllanthus* species contains lignans that possess cytotoxic activity that helps in suppressing HBV antigen secretion (Gittings and Hume, 2014). The major classes of bioactive compounds of *P. amarus* have been isolated, and they include sterols, flavonoids, alkaloids, lignans, tannins, triterpenes, and volatile oils. Lignans such as phyllanthin and hypophyllanthin and flavonoids such as quercetin were isolated from the leaves of *P. amarus* (Meena et al., 2018).

Data were evaluated in 1326 patients in 16 trials regarding the effectiveness of the *Phyllanthus* species in chronic HBV infection. Three different species of *Phyllanthus* were used, including *P. amarus*. *Phyllanthus* was used in combination with standard antiviral therapy compared with standard antiviral therapy alone (Fig. 2.2). As a result of these trials, the *Phyllanthus* significantly reduced serum HBV DNA (a marker of efficacy) as well as HBeAg (a marker of viral replication) when combined with antiviral therapy (Gittings and Hume, 2014). Similarly, in another study, Leelarasamee et al. (1990) reported that a trial using *Phyllanthus* in chronic hepatitis cases was not successful. The HBeAg level was significantly decreased at day 30 of the trial in patients receiving *P. amarus* treatment ($P < 0.01$) but not at day 60. Patients felt that their clinical status had not changed. However, no toxic effects were observed or detected.

2.7 Phyllanthus niruri L.

P. niruri is an annual small herb available in the subtropical and tropical parts of world. The use of the genus *Phyllanthus* in traditional remedies as a hepatoprotective is common.

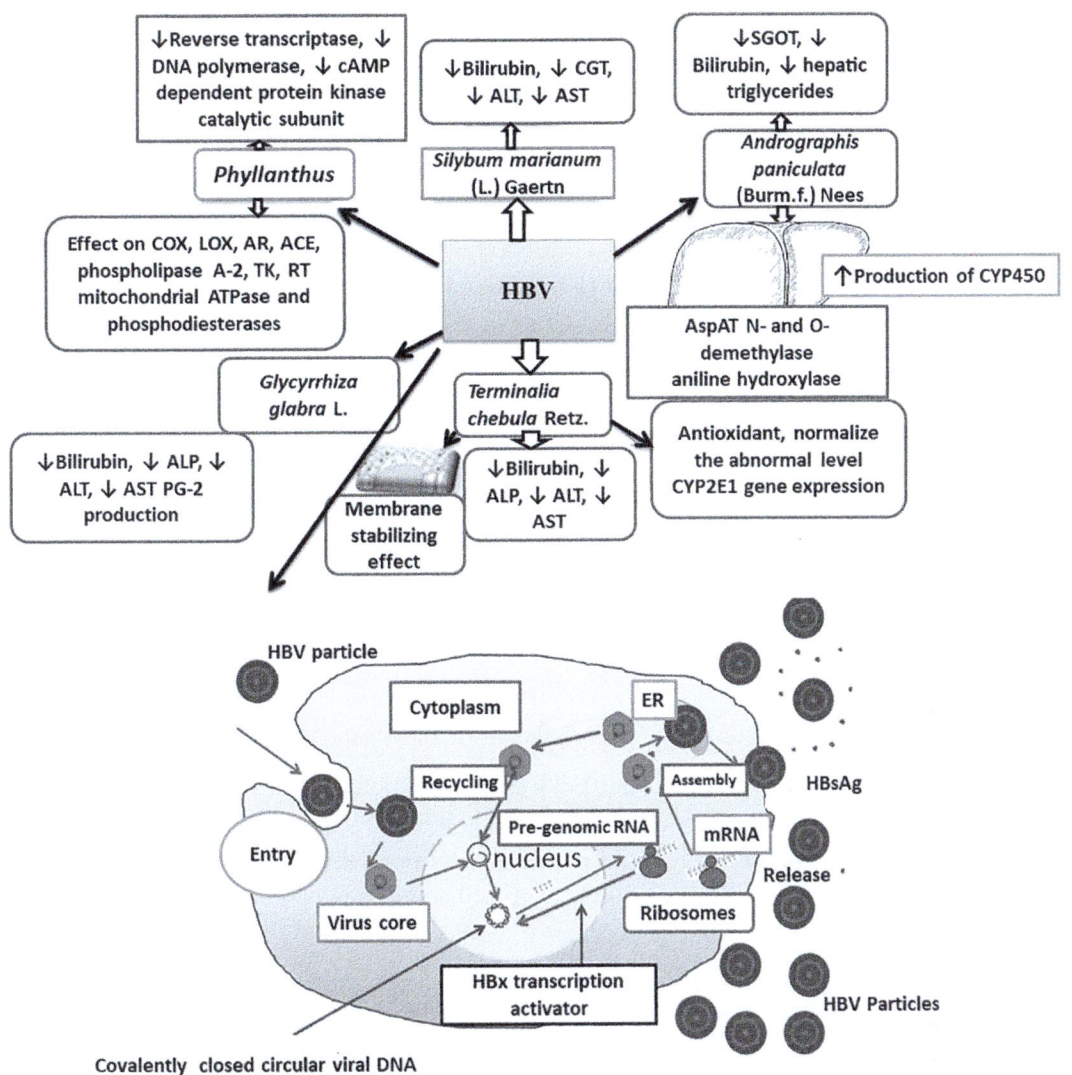

Fig. 2.2
Hepatoprotective effect of various plants and the mechanism of HBV degradation.

According to scientists, *P. amarus* and *P. niruri* are often confused and many of the plant experts have used both names interchangeably or as a synonym. The origin of the taxonomic confusion is mainly because of the use of the same common name as well as the use of vernacular names among various Indian languages (Patel et al., 2011).

A wide diversity of bioactive components is present in *P. niruri* (tannins, alkaloids, anthocyanins, chlorogenic acid, phenolic acids, flavonoids, coumarins, lignans, glycosidic consitutents, and terpenoids) (Bagalkotkar et al., 2006). Baiguera et al. (2018) investigated the efficacy and safety of using *P. niruri* for a period of 12 months as a treatment for patients suffering from chronic HBV infection, as shown in Fig. 2.1. It is concluded that the trial did not support the use of *P. niruri* for the treatment of chronic hepatitis B. There was no fruitful evidence that, compared to placebo benefits, the use of *Phyllanthus* was beneficial to patients with chronic HBV infections to check the hypothesis. Xia et al. (2011) conducted a study on HBV patients and concluded that no results were found in favor of the *Phyllanthus* species, including *P. niruni,* compared to a placebo regarding chronic HBV infection. However, it was noted that an antiviral drug (interferon alpha, lamivudine, adefovir dipivoxil, thymosin, and vidarabine) along with *Phyllanthus* may give positive results over that drug alone.

2.8 Swertia patens Burkill

The *Swetia patens* plant is commonly distributed in the Yunnan and Sichuan provinces of China and it has been used as a traditional remedy to treat hepatitis (Geng and Chen, 2018), as shown in Fig. 2.1. He et al. (2016) and Zhou et al. (2015) reported the antihepatitis activity of the *Swertia patens* plant, specifically against HBV. However, the chemical constituents and bioactivities of this plant are rarely reported. There are two known compounds, (+)-dehydrodiconiferyl alcohol and dehydrozingerone, that have been shown to moderately inhibit the secretion of HBsAg (Geng and Chen, 2018).

The continuous efforts to discover the anti-HBV active compounds from *Swertia patens* led to secoiridois swerpatic acid and swerpalactone, along with 10 known compounds (He et al., 2016). However, a C-8 skeleton was noted in a new secoirdoid, that is, swerpatic acid. It was reported that more than 200 secoiridoids were isolated in this plant and that they mainly existed with the C10 skeleton while fewer than 10 carbons were rarely reported. Compounds such as 3–6, 8–10, and 12 have shown effective anti-HBV activity as compared with Tenofovir as a positive control variable.

2.9 Boehmeria nivea (L.) Gaudich.

Ramie or *Boehmeria nivea* is one of the most important crops that may be used in various fields. *Bohmeria nivea* is a perennial and herbaceous plant that belongs to the *Urticaceae* family. Generally, most subtropic and tropic regions such as the Philippines, India, China, and some other Asian countries are good for the adaptation and growth of this plant (Liu et al., 2001). *Boehmeria nivea,* also known as Chinese grass, in addition to its high-quality fiber also has several other uses such as biocompost, green fodder, medicinal, and geo-tactile (Sharma et al., 2014).

A reduction in soil nutrients may happen due to the rapid growth of ramie; therefore, its normal growth and sustainable yield may be impaired. Therefore, a regular supply is quite important for this crop (Subandi, 2012; Huang et al., 2014a,b). Chang et al. (2010) reported that a reduction in supernatant HBV DNA in HBV-producing cells (HepG2.2.15) may be reduced by using *Boehmeria nivea* extract, which has shown anti-HBV properties, as represented in Fig. 2.1. Li et al., (2017) demonstrated that without any cytotoxicity, the secretion of HBeAg and HBsAg may be reduced in HepG2.2.15 cells when treated with *Boehmeria nivea* leaves extract. In another study, *Boehmeria nivea* shows no harmful effect on intracellular DNA; however, infected virus was suppressed in HepG2.2.15 cells transfected with human HBV DNA (Wei et al., 2014). So, a synergistic effect may be achieved when *Boehmeria nivea* extract works with other antivirus compounds (Chang et al., 2010). It was reported that anti-HBV activity was exhibited (in vivo and in vitro) with the use of 20% ethanol *Boehmeria nivea* root extract (BNE) in the HepG2 2.2.15 cell model system while BNE lessened HBV, which differs from the nucleoside analogues. BNE suppressed the 78-kDa glucose-regulated protein (GRP78) and the potential inhibitory effect of BNE on blocking the assembled virion secretion is due to the reduction of GRP78 (Huang et al., 2006, 2009; Chang et al., 2010).

2.10 Role of natural compounds in ameliorating hepatitis B

Several natural products found in plants are quite helpful in ameliorating HBV infection. Natural products will be discussed with respect to their chemical classification.

2.10.1 Terpenoids

Singh and Sharma (2015) reported that terpenoids are the largest group with respect to natural products that is extensively applied as spices, fragrances, and flavors. They are also used in perfumes and cosmetics in the industrial sector. Many terpenoids have biological activities and are also used for medical purposes.

Due to definite numbers of 5-C in terpene units, the terpenoids are considered the biggest class of natural products. Terpenoids play many functions in regulating the antagonistic interactions, specifically in traditional herbal medicines. Various naturally occurring terpenes are well known for their anti-HBV activity. Some of these terpenoid compounds are betulinic acid, asiatocoside, astataricusones, sweriyunnangenin-A, 3-epitaraxerol, epishionol, dehydroandrographolide, pumilaside-A, 24-acetate, alisol F 24-acetate, hemslecin A, perovskatone-A, andrographolide, demethylsalvicanol, caudatin, phyllanthacidoid acid methyl ester, alisol F, and methyl helicterate (Wu, 2016).

Yao et al. (2009) reported that the inhibitory effect of betulinic acid on HBV replication as the expression of SOD2 (manganese superoxide dismutase) was downregulated in transgenic mice for HBV trailed by ROS (reactive oxygen species) of mitochondria. *Pulsatilla chinensis* was used for the isolation of betulinic acid.

Asiaticoside derived from hydrocotyle sibthorpioids effectively inhibit the surface antigen of HBV (HBsAg). HBV DNA and the CCC DNA level act in a dose-dependent way. Besides this, asiaticoside lessened the replication and transcription of viral DNA via a counteractive mechanism on the X, S1, and S2 gene promoter activities. Moreover, a marked reduction in hepatitis was noted by asiaticoside (Huang et al., 2013). Similarly, glycyrrhetinic acid is a five cyclic triterpenoid compound that is related to β-amyrin, possessing a skeletal structure of dodecahydropicene that occurs in nature chiefly in the form of glycyrrhizic acid (a saponin glycoside along with two molecules of glucuronic acid) (Shegokar, 2016).

The chief and effective constituents of *Glycyrrhizae glabra* (Licorice root) are glycyrrhizin with its metabolite glycyrrhetinic acid (GA). Wu (2016) reported that glycyrrhetinic acid (GA) showed a counteractive mechanism against the DNA replication of HBV replication. Similarly, caudatin derived from the *Cynanchum auriculatum* showed an antagonistic effect against the secretion of HbsAg and the DNA replication of HBV.

2.10.2 Lignans

Lignans belong to phenylpropanoid derivates and they are widely distributed in medicinal plants. Their classification is made into five different structure types, that is, hybrid lignans, oligomeric lignans, lignans, and neo- and nor-lignans. Lignans are considered important natural anti-HBV components (Wu, 2016). Helioxanthine (HE-145) is a nonnucleoside lignan compound that was extracted from the *Taiwania cryptomerioides* Hayata. This compound is noted for inhibiting the replication of HBV and gene expression (Tseng et al., 2008).

A lignan glycoside (+)-cycloolivil-4′-*O*-β-D glucopyranoside extracted from *Swertia chiravita* showed antagonistic activity against the secretion of HBeAg and HBsAg. Also, it showed a counteractive effect on the DNA replication of HBV (Kanchanapoom et al., 2006; Zhou et al., 2015).

The dried fruits from the medicinal plant *Schisandra chinensis* Turcz. (Baill.) are indexed as a traditional Chinese herb that has been used for more than 2000 years to cure hepatitis. The plant species is also present in other countries such as Japan, Korea, Russia, etc. The plant is officially part of different editions of the National Pharmacopoeia of the People's Republic of China (Yu and Liu, 2009). Recently, a phytochemical investigation on leaves, fruits, and stems obtained from *Schisandra Chinensis* (Baill.) that were taken from various regions in China led to the identification of different dibenzyl butane lignans and tetrahydrofuran (Xue et al., 2010) along with different nortriterpenoids with several medical effects (Huang et al., 2007a,b,c, 2008; Shi et al., 2011).

A new lignan was reported as nirtetralin B that was extracted from *Phyllanthus niruni* L. Among folk medicines, this plant has been used for a long time as a useful remedy against chronic liver disease and against HBV in different countries of Asia. Research was carried out to understand the effectiveness of anti-HBV for nitetralin B using HepG 2.2.15 cells and duck HBV (DHBV) infected ducks in in vitro and in vivo models. It was noted from experimental data that anti-HBV activity was exhibited both in vitro and in vivo by the action of nirtetralin (Liu et al., 2014a).

Two more lignan compounds, lignan helioxanthin and helioxanthin analogs, were shown to be an effective mechanism for anti-HBV holding a unique pattern (Tseng et al., 2008; Yeo et al., 2005). The inhibition of gene expression was shown as well as the replication of DNA from HBV in wild-type resistant mutants for lamivudine. The two lignans extracted from *Phyllanthus niruni* L., niranthin and nirtetralin B, were reported to have anti-HBV activity both in vivo and in vitro (Liu et al., 2014a,b).

Currently, various issues are related to anti-HBV drugs such as a slow response rate, drug resistance, and harmful effects. Therefore it is evident that there is a need to explore effective anti-HBV agents with different antiviral targets and mechanisms. A number of nonnucleoside HBV inhibitor agents are found to offer effective and potent inhibitory effects ameliorating HBV; however, less attention is paid to their mechanism of action and respective targets. Therefore, for further clinical investigation, attention must be paid in order to promote the new anti-HBV affect, drug discovery, and the development of treatment procedures.

2.10.3 Phenolic acids

Phenolic acids contain a phenol ring and carboxylic acid functions, therefore they exist as different types of naturally occurring aromatic compounds. Antiviral effects are reported from phenolic acids. From *Laggera alata*, 3,4-*O*-dicaffeoylquinic acid and 3,5-*O*-dicaffeoylquinic acid were extracted that led to a decrease in the production of HBsAg and HbeAg with the help of their inhibitory rates (Wu, 2016).

Moreover, it was noted that 3,4-*O*-dicaffeoylquinic acid noticeably lowered the contents of HBV CCC DNA and markedly increased the HO-1 expression in HepG2.2.15 cells and HBV in transgenic mice. A similar effect was shown by 3,5-*O*-dicaffeoylquinic acid. Because HO-1 has the ability to undermine the HBV core protein, this observation suggested that HO-1 overexpression may help in the antiviral activity of 3,5-*O*-dicaffeoylquinic acid and 3,4-*O*-dicaffeoylquinic acid, lowering the HBV core protein stability (Hao et al., 2012).

Some other types of phenolic acids include 3,5-*O*-dicaffeoyl-muco-quinic acid, 5-*O*-(*E*)-*p*-coumaroylquinic acid, caffeic acid, and chlorogenic acid (Wu, 2016). Geng et al. (2015) reported that past investigations led to phenolic acids and chlorogenic acid analogs as two main constituents present in *Artemisia capillaris*. However, there is no investigation concerned with the anti-HBV components of *A. scoparia*.

Wang et al. (2009) stated that the distribution of chlorogenic acid along associated compounds present in dicotyledonous plants (fruits and leaves) possesses a wide spectrum of antiviral activity. The inhibition of HBsAg production along with the replication of hepatitis B viral DNA in Hep.G2.2.15 cells was noted by the action of quinic acid, chlorogenic acid, and caffeic acid. Caffeic acid and chlorogenic acid also lower the serum duck HBV level in a duck HBV (DHBV) infected duckling model (Wang et al., 2009).

2.10.4 Polyphenols

Regarding chronic hepatitis treatment, there are two main agents that are used at present, nucleus[t]ide analogues and interferon α. Interferon α carries antiviral activity as an immunomodulator. The selective inhibition of viral polymerase with reverse transcriptase activity by nucleus[t]ide analogues was reported. However, interferon α is less effective and expensive. It also possesses harmful side effects as well as invasive administration (Merle and Trepo, 2001). Moreover, the induction of replication of resistant HBV strains may happen if a long exposure of nucleus[t]ide is done as a treatment in patients suffering from chronic hepatitis with chronic infection (Benhamou et al., 2001; Manesis and Hadziyannis, 2001). In this regard, it would be beneficial to look for antiviral agents with high efficacy and fewer adverse effects.

Green tea (*Camellia sinensis* L.) polyphenols are generally known as catechins that may include (−)-epicatechin (EC), (−)-epigallocatechin-3-gallate (EGCG), (−)-epicatechin-3-gallate (ECG), and (−)-epigallatecatechin (EGC). However, (−)-epigallocatechin-3-gallate (EGCG) is most active and the chief catechin present in the green tea (Yang et al., 2006). Kawai et al. (2003) reported the anti-HIV activity of epigallocatechin gallate (EGCG), which is a major constituent of tea polyphenol. The EGCG extracted from green tea was shown to have counteractive characteristics against HBV entry inside hepatocytes with a concentration of 50 μmol/L for more than 80% (Huang et al., 2014a,b). Several other characteristics of green tea include immunoregulation (Katiyar, 2007) and antitumor action (Lambert et al., 2005). Green tea polyphenols possessing a low level of toxicity are considered highly safe agents (Chen et al., 2007). Pang et al., (2014) also reported that EGCG significantly lowered the extracellular DNA levels of HBV for 6 and 9 days as well as the intracellular HBV DNA level for 9 days. Therefore, it may be concluded that EGCG activity not only blocks the secretion but also the overall production of viral genomic replication.

Li et al. (2018) reported that natural polyphenols are secondary metabolites of plants that have emerged as suitable agents regarding prevention as well as treatment for various disease conditions. Li et al. (2014) and Domitrovic and Potocnjak (2016) stated that polyphenols possess a wide variety of pharmacological characteristics on lipid metabolism, oxidative stress, insulin resistance, and inflammation. These pharmacological effects are very important in the pathological processes of liver diseases.

Arbab et al. (2015) investigated the leaf extracts of *Acacia mellifera* for hepatoprotective and anti-HBV efficacy as polyphenols are found to be present in these leaf extracts. The result showed positive effects of the *A. mellifera* leaf fraction in both in vivo and in vitro experimental conditions. Lactone contains a cyclic ester of hydrocarboxylic acid that acts as an antiviral natural component (Wu, 2016). Chen et al. (1995) reported that dehydrocostus and costunolide lactone extracted from the roots of *Saussurea lappa* Clarks showed a counteracting effect on HBeAg and HBsAg expression in Hep3B cells (IC_{50} values = 2.0 and 1.0 µmol/L, respectively).

The various naturally occurring lactones are clausenidin, nordentatin, herpetosperin, swerilactones, swerilactones, swerilactones, swerilactones, swerilactones, swerilactones, etc. (Wu et al., 2016).

Geng et al. (2011) stated that four novel lactones were isolated from *Swertia mileensis*, which has been used as a Chinese herb with respect to the treatment of viral hepatitis. An effective anti-HBV action against DNA replication in HBV was noted by the swerilactones H-K while the IC_{50} value ranged within 1.53–5.34 µM. The herpetosperin B isolated from *Herpetospermum caudigerum* (seeds) expressed anti-HBV activity with HbsAg secretion with a rate of 33% at 200 µg/mL (Xu et al., 2015). Nordentatin and pyranocoumarins clausenidin from *Clausena excavata* counteract the HbsAg in HepA2 cells (Su et al., 2009).

Artemisinin (*Artemisia annua*) caused suppression in the secretion of HBsAg and HBV DNA replication while the IC_{50} values were 55 and > 100 mmol/L, respectively (Romero et al., 2005). Lactones containing a phenyl group such as swerilactones E and F (*Swertia mileensis*) were reported to have major suppressive activity on HbsAg secretions (IC_{50} = 0.22 and 0.70 mM) as well as HbeAg (IC_{50} = 0.52 and > 6.78 mmol/L in HepG2.2.15, respectively) (Geng et al., 2010).

According to Zhou et al. (2012), cepharanthine is a natural alkaloid derived compound extracted from the plant *Stephania cepharantha* (Hayata). This alkaloid counteracts the production of HBeAg and HBV DNA replication. Squalamine extracted from *Petromyzon marinus* (lamprey) has an antiviral broad spectrum on HBV. The basis for the antiviral effect of squalamine is its efficacy for neutralizing the negative electrostatic charge on the surface of intracellular membranes that makes host cells less effective during viral replication (Zasloff et al., 2011). Wang et al. (2011) reported a decrease in the blood HBeAg (70%) and HBV DNA (96%) by using the monotherapy with oxymatrine (oral use for 12 months) in patients suffering from chronic hepatitis B that were lamivudine resistant (*n* = 17). *Evodia fargesii* Dode (Rutaceae) is a liver protective medicinal plant from which the extracted compound *N,N*-dimethyltryptamine N12-oxide expressed counteractive action on hepatitis B viral DNA replication (Qu et al., 2011).

Dehygroisoapocavadine, dehydrocavidine, and dehydroapocavidine extracted from Papaveraceae (*Corydalis saxicola* Bunting) showed antagonistic effects against HbsAg and HbeAg secretion in Hep2.2.15 cells (Li et al., 2008). Du et al. (2011) reported the significant downregulation of mRNA expression by the act of oxymatrine. The expression of host cognat 70 (Hsc70) was also downregulated at the level of posttranscription, whereas Hsc70 mRNA is destabilized. As a consequence of this, HBV replication was inhibited and the efficacy of anti-HBV was noted.

The IC_{50} value of 0.450 mM (SI=4.13) was expressed in response to dauricumidine (extracted from *Hypserpa nitida* Miers) with respect to HBsAg secretion in HepG2.2.15 cells. Dihydrochelerythrine isolated from *Corydalis saxicola* Bunting exhibited the strongest effect on HBsAg and HBeAg secretion with IC_{50} values < 0.05 mM and SI > 3.5, respectively (Wu et al., 2007).

Flavonoids belong to the group of polyphenolic compounds. They have a vast range of pharmacological effects, including antiviral activity (Wu et al., 2016). However, Shimizu et al. (2017) aimed his study at estimating the antiviral effects of two flavonoids from pterogyne nitrens, that is, pedalitin and sorbifolin, on the HCV replication cycle. These flavonoid compounds were evaluated for their anti-HCV viral activity and they found an inhibitory effect on HCV.

Similarly, in another study Pang et al. (2014) reported the effective suppression of HBeAg and the inhibition of HBsAg and HBeAg by the action of EGCG in HepG2 2.2.15 cells in a time- and dose-dependent manner, whereas its effect was stronger than that of lamivudine. EGCG also decreased the level of HBV DNA.

Wogonin, a flavonoid extracted from *Scutellaria radix,* counteracts the secretion of HBV antigen with an IC_{50} value of 4 mg/mL regarding HBeAg and HbsAg, thereby the concentration of HBV DNA was reduced in HepG2.2.15 cells. DNA polymerase in DHBV was subjected to dramatic suppression by the action of wogonin while the IC_{50} value was 0.57 mg/mL (Guo et al., 2007).

2.10.5 Alkaloids

Alkaloids are a class of naturally occurring compounds carrying a basic nitrogen atom along with related neutral and in some cases weakly acidic compounds. Various potent pharmacological characteristics are exhibited by alkaloids such as atropine, pilocarpine, and quinine (Wu et al., 2016). An alkaloid, oxymatrine extracted from *Sophora japonica* (Kushen), is famous for its use in patients suffering from hepatitis B in China for many years. So, it is reported to be a safer remedy and would replace nucleoside analogues to lessen the rising issue of a mutant form of HBV that is resistant to conventional treatment (Chen et al., 2012).

2.11 Conclusion

Natural products have been applied for thousands of years to treat liver disorders and have now become a promising therapy in this regard. There are numerous herbal species that have hepato-protective properties. They serve as vital new and potential therapeutic drugs that contain a wide range of phtyochemical molecules with a role in protecting against hepatic disorders. The active phytochemicals demonstrating hepatoprotective potential have been isolated from several species. Various plants such as *Rheum palmatum, Ganoderma lucidum, Oenanthe javanica, C. longa, P. amarus*, and *P. niruri*, with natural products such as terpenoids, lignans, phenolic acids, and polyphenols, work effectively against HBV. These phytochemicals can be purified and developed into drugs with the standards and quality of modern developed medicine. Several serious challenges are faced by the pharmaceutical industry because the drug discovery procedure is becoming costly, riskier, and seriously ineffective. These products have served for centuries as a basis of drugs, with about half the drugs in use these days of natural origin. Natural products possess a prime role in our life and presently serve globally as a promising therapy for several hepatitis ailments.

Acknowledgments

All the authors of the manuscript thank and acknowledge their respective universities and institutes.

Conflict of interest

There is no conflict of interest.

References

Ahn, H., Lee, G.-S., 2017. Isorhamnetin and hyperoside derived from water dropwort inhibits inflammasome activation. Phytomedicine 24, 77–86.

Ai, G., Huang, Z.M., Liu, Q.C., Han, Y.Q., Chen, X., 2016. The protective effect of total phenolics from *Oenanthe javanica* on acute liver failure induced by D-galactosamine. J. Ethnopharmacol. 186, 53–60.

Ali, A., Badshah, L., Hussain, F., Shinwari, Z.K., 2016. Floristic composition and ecological characteristics of plants of Chail valley, district Swat, Pakistan. Pak. J. Bot. 48 (3), 1013–1026.

Arbab, A.H., Parvez, M.K., Dosari, M.S., Al-Rehaily, A.J., Al-Sohaibani, M., Zaroug, E.E., AlSaid, M.S., Rafatullah, S., 2015. Hepatoprotective and antiviral efficacy of *Acacia mellifera* leaves fractions against hepatitis B virus. BioMed Res. Int., 1–10. https://doi.org/10.1155/2015/929131. Article ID 929131, 10 pages.

Ashraf, K., 2018. A comprehensive review on *Curcuma longa* Linn.: phytochemical, pharmacological, and molecular study. Inter. J. Green Pharmacy 11 (4), S671–S685.

Back, S.J., Jung, W.T., Kim, D.Y., Cho, K.D., 1999. G009: hepatoprotectant, immunostimulant. Drugs Future 24, 1068–1071.

Bagalkotkar, G., Sagineedu, S.R., Saad, M.S., Stanslas, J., 2006. Phytochemicals from *Phyllanthus niruri* Linn. and theirpharmacological properties: a review. J. Pharm. Pharmacol. 58, 1559–1570.

Baiguera, C., Boschetti, A., Raffetti, E., Zanini, B., Puoti, M., Donato, F., 2018. *Phyllanthus niruri* versus placebo for chronic HBV Infection: a randomized controlled trial. Complement. Med. Res., 1–7. https://doi.org/10.1159/000484927.

Benhamou, Y., Bochet, M., Thibault, V., 2001. Safety and efficacy of adefovir dipivoxil in patents co-infected with HIV and lamivudine-resistant HBV: an open label pilot study. Lancet 358 (9283), 718–723.

Boh, B., Berovic, M., Zhang, J., Zhi-Bin, L., 2007. *Ganoderma lucidum* and its pharmaceutically active compounds. Biotechnol. Annu. Rev. 13, 265–301. https://doi.org/10.1016/S1387-2656(07)13010-6.

Bruck, R., Ashkenazi, M., Weiss, S., Goldiner, I., Shapiro, H., Aeed, H., Genina, O., Helpern, Z., Pines, M., 2007. Prevention of liver cirrhosis in rats by curcumin. Liver Int. 27, 373–383.

Cao, Y., Xu, X., Liu, S., Huang, L., Gu, J., 2018. *Ganoderma*: a cancer immunotherapy review. Front. Pharmacol. 9, 1217.

Chang, J.M., Huang, K.L., Yuan, T.T., 2010. The anti-HBV activity of *Boehmeria nivea* extract in HBV-viremia SCID mice. Evid. Based Complement. Alternat. Med. 7, 189–195.

Chen, H.C., Chou, C.K., Lee, S.D., Wang, J.C., Yeh, S.F., 1995. Active compounds from *Saussurea lappa* Clarks that suppress HBV surface antigen gene expression in human hepatoma cells. Antiviral Res. 27, 99–109.

Chen, D.H., Shiou, W.Y., Wang, K.C., 1999. Chemotaxonomy of triterpenoid pattern of HPLC of *Ganoderma lucidum* and *Ganoderma tsugae*. J. Chin. Chem. Soc. 46, 47–51.

Chen, H., Zhang, M., Qu, Z., 2007. Compositional analysis and preliminary toxicological evaluation of a tea polysaccharide conjugate. J. Agric. Food Chem. 55 (6), 2256–2260.

Chen, Y.X., Mao, B.Y., Jiang, J.H., 2012. Relationship between serum load of HBV-DNA and therapeutic effect of oxymatrine in patients with chronic hepatitis B. Zhongguo Zhong Xi Yi Jie He Za Zhi 22, 335–336. 12584828.

Chen, C.-M., Chen, I.-C., Chen, Y.L., 2016. Medicinal herbs *Oenanthe javanica* (Blume) DC., *Casuarina equisetifolia* L. and *Sorghum bicolor* (L.) Moench protect human cells from MPP+ damage via inducing FBXO7 expression. Phytomedicine 23 (12), 1422–1433.

Chien, C.M., Cheng, J.L., Chang, W.T., 2004. Polysaccharides of *Ganoderma lucidum* alter cell immunophenotypic expression and enhance CD56+ NK-cell cytotoxicity in cord blood. Bioorg. Med. Chem. 12, 5603–5609.

Domitrovic, R., Potocnjak, I., 2016. A comprehensive overview of hepatoprotective natural compounds: mechanism of action and clinical perspectives. Arch. Toxicol. 90 (1), 39–79.

Du, N.N., Li, X., Wang, Y.P., Liu, F., Liu, Y.X., Li, C.X., Peng, Z.G., Gao, L.M., Jiang, J.D., Song, D.Q., 2011. Synthesis, structure-activity relationship and biological evaluation of novel N-substituted matrinic acid derivatives as host heat-stress cognate 70 (Hsc70) down-regulators. Bioorg. Med. Chem. Lett. 21, 4732–4735. https://doi.org/10.1016/j.bmcl.2011.06.071. 21757347.

Geng, C.-A., Chen, J.-J., 2018. The progress of anti-HBV constituents from medicinal plants in China. Nat. Prod. Bioprospect. 8 (4), 227–244. https://doi.org/10.1007/s13659-018-0178-6.

Geng, C.A., Zhang, X.M., Ma, Y.B., Jiang, Z.Y., Luo, J., Zhou, J., Wang, H.L., Chen, J.J., 2010. Swerilactones E-G, three unusual lactones from *Swertia mileensis*. Tetrahedron Lett. 51, 2483–2485. https://doi.org/10.1016/j.tetlet.2010.02.156.

Geng, C.A., Wang, L.J., Zhang, X.M., Ma, Y.B., Huang, X.Y., Luo, J., Guo, R.H., Zhou, J., Shen, Y., Zuo, A.X., Jiang, Z.Y., Chen, J.J., 2011. Anti-HBV active lactones from the traditional Chinese herb: *Swertia mileensis*. Chemistry 17, 3893–3903. https://doi.org/10.1002/chem.201003180. 21365705.

Geng, C.A., Huang, X.Y., Chen, X.L., Ma, Y.B., Rong, G.Q., Zhao, Y., Zhang, X.M., Chen, J.J., 2015. Three new anti-HBV active constituents from the traditional. Chinese Herb of Yin-Chen (*Artemisia scoparia*) 24 (176), 109–117. https://doi.org/10.1016/j.jep.2015.10.032.

Gittings, K., Hume, A.L., 2014. Phyllanthus for chronic HBV infection. J. Viral Hepat. 8, 358–366. https://doi.org/10.1002/14651858.CD008960.pub2.

Govind, P., Pandey, S.P., 2011. Phytochemical and toxicity study of *Emblica officinalis* (Amla). Int. Res. J. Pharm. 2 (3), 270–272.

Guo, Q., Zhao, L., You, Q., Yang, Y., Gu, H., Song, G., Lu, N., Xin, J., 2007. Anti-HBV activity of wogonin in vitro and in vivo. Antiviral Res. 74, 16–24. https://doi.org/10.1016/j.antiviral.2007.01.002. 17280723.

Han, Y.-Q., Huang, Z.-M., Yang, X.-B., Liu, H.-Z., Wu, G.-X., 2008. In vivo and in vitro anti-HBV activity of total phenolics from *Oenanthe javanica*. J. Ethnopharmacol. 118 (1), 148–153.

Hao, B.J., Wu, Y.H., Wang, J.G., Hu, S.Q., Keil, D.J., Hu, H.J., Lou, J.D., Zhao, Y., 2012. Hepatoprotective and antiviral properties of isochlorogenic acid A from *Laggera alata* against HBV infection. J. Ethnopharmacol. 144, 190–194. https://doi.org/10.1016/j.jep.2012.09.003. 22982394.

He, K., Geng, C.A., Cao, T.W., 2016. Two new secoiridoids and other anti-HBV active constituents from *Swertia patens*. J. Asian Nat. Prod. Res. 18 (6), 528–534.

Ho, Y.W., Yeung, J.S., Chiu, P.K., Tang, W.M., Lin, Z.B., Man, R.Y., Lau, C.S., 2007. *Ganoderma lucidum* polysaccharide peptide reduced the production of proinflammatory cytokines in activated rheumatoid synovial fibroblast. Mol. Cell. Biochem. 301, 173–179.

Huang, Z.M., Yang, X.B., Cao, W.B., 2001. Textual study on *Oenanthe javanica* documented in ancient Chinese medicinal literatures. Chin. Tradit. Herb. Drug 32 (1), 59–62.

Huang, K.L., Lai, Y.K., Lin, C.C., 2006. Inhibition of HBV production by *Boehmeria nivea* root extract in HepG2 2.2.15 cells. World J. Gastroenterol. 12, 5721–5725.

Huang, S.X., Yang, L.B., Xiao, W.L., Lei, C., Liu, J.P., Lu, Y., Weng, Z.Y., Li, L.M., Li, R.T., Yu, J.L., Zheng, Q.T., Sun, H.D., 2007a. Wuweizidilactones A–F: highly oxygenated nortriterpenoids with unusual skeletons isolated from *Schisandra chinensis*. Chem. A Eur. J. 13, 4816–4822.

Huang, S.X., Li, R.T., Liu, J.P., Lu, Y., Chang, Y., Lei, C., Xiao, W.L., Yang, L.B., Zheng, Q.T., Sun, H.D., 2007b. Isolation and characterization of biogenetically related highly oxygenated nortriterpenoids from *Schisandra chinensis*. Org. Lett. 9, 2079–2082.

Huang, S.X., Yang, J., Huang, H., Li, L.M., Xiao, W.L., Li, R.T., Sun, H.D., 2007c. Structural characterization of schintrilactone, a new class of nortriterpenoids from *Schisandra chinensis*. Org. Lett. 9, 4175–4178.

Huang, S.X., Han, Q.B., Lei, C., Pu, J.X., Xiao, W.L., Yu, J.L., Yang, L.M., Xu, H.X., Zheng, Y.T., Sun, H.D., 2008. Isolation and characterization of miscellaneous terpenoids of *Schisandra chinensis*. Tetrahedron 64, 4260–4267.

Huang, K.L., Lai, Y.K., Lin, C.C., 2009. Involvement of GRP78 in inhibition of HBV secretion by *Boehmeria nivea* extract in human HepG2 2.2.15 cells. J. Viral Hepat. 16, 367–375.

Huang, Q., Zhang, S., Huang, R., Wei, L., Chen, Y., Lv, S., Liang, C., Tan, S., Liang, S., Zhuo, L., Lin, X., 2013. Isolation and identification of an antiHBV compound from *Hydrocotyle sibthorpioides* Lam. J. Ethnopharmacol. 150, 56–575.

Huang, C., Wei, G., Luo, Z., Xu, J., Zhao, S., Wang, L., Jie, Y., 2014a. Effects of nitrogen on ramie (*Boehmeria nivea*) hybrid and its parents grown under field conditions. J. Agric. Sci. 6, 230–243.

Huang, H.C., Tao, M.H., Hung, T.M., Chen, J.C., Lin, Z.J., Huang, C., 2014b. (−)-Epigallocatechin-3-gallate inhibits entry of HBV into hepatocytes. Antiviral Res. 111, 100–111. https://doi.org/10.1016/j.antiviral.2014.09.009. 25260897.

Humphries, J.C., Dixon, J.S., 2003. Antivirals for the treatment of chronic hepatitis B: current and future options. Intervirology 46, 413–420.

Ji, Z., Tang, Q., Zhang, J., Yang, Y., Jia, W., Pan, Y., 2007. Immunomodulation of RAW264.7 macrophages by GLIS, a proteopolysaccharide from *Ganoderma lucidum*. J. Ethnopharmacol. 112, 445–450.

Kanchanapoom, T., Noiarsa, P., Otsuka, H., Ruchirawat, S., 2006. Phenolic and iridoid glycosides from *Stereospermum cylindricum*. Phytochemistry 67, 516–520. https://doi.org/10.1016/j.phytochem.2005.10.009. 16310232.

Katiyar, S.K., 2007. UV-induced immune suppression and photocarcinogenesis: chemoprevention by dietary botanical agents. Cancer Lett. 255 (1), 1–11.

Kawai, K., Tsuno, N.H., Kitayama, J., 2003. Epigallocatechin gallate, the main component of tea polyphenol, binds to CD4 and interferes with gp120 binding. J. Allergy Clin. Immunol. 112 (5), 951–957.

Kim, Y.S., Eo, S.K., Oh, K.W., Lee, C.k., Han, S.S., 2000. Antiherpetic activities of acidic protein bound polysaccharide isolated from *Ganoderma lucidum* alone and in combinations with interferons. J. Ethnopharmacol. 72, 451–458.

Kim, H.J., Yoo, H.S., Kim, J.C., Park, C.S., Choi, M.S., Kim, M., Choi, H., Min, J.S., Kim, Y.S., Yoon, S.W., Ahn, J.K., 2009a. Antiviral effect of *Curcuma longa* Linn extract against HBV replication. J. Ethnopharmacol. 124, 189–196.

Kim, J.Y., Kim, K.-H., Lee, Y.J., Lee, S.H., Park, J.C., Nam, D.H., 2009b. *Oenanthe javanica* extract accelerates ethanol metabolism in ethanol-treated animals. BMB Rep. 42 (8), 482–485.

Kim, J.K., Shin, E.-C., Park, G.G., Kim, Y.-J., Shin, D.-H., 2016. Root extract of water dropwort, *Oenanthe javanica* (Blume) DC, induces protein and gene expression of phase I carcinogen-metabolizing enzymes in HepG2 cells. SpringerPlus 5 (1), 413–418.

Kongkachuichai, R., Charoensiri, R., Yakoh, K., Kringkasemsee, A., Insung, P., 2015. Nutrients value and antioxidant content of indigenous vegetables from Southern Thailand. Food Chem. 173, 836–846.

Kumar, C.H., Ramesh, A., Kumar, S.J.N., Ishaq, M.B., 2011. A review on hepatoprotective activity of medicinal plants. Int. J. Pharm. Sci. Res. 2 (3), 501–515.

Lambert, J.D., Hong, J., Yang, G.Y., 2005. Inhibition of carcinogenesis by polyphenols: evidence from laboratory investigations. Am. J. Clin. Nutr. 81 (1), 284–291.

Leelarasamee, A., Trakulsomboon, S., Maunwongyathi, P., Somanabandhu, A., Pidetcha, P., Matrakool, B., Lebnak, T., Ridthimat, W., Chandanayingyong, D., 1990. Failure of *Phyllanthus amarus* to eradicate the hepatitis B surface antigen from symptomless carrier. Lancet 335, 1600–1601.

Li, Y.-Q., Wang, S.-F., 2006. Anti-hepatitis B activities of ganoderic acid from *Ganoderma lucidum*. Biotechnol. Lett. 28, 837–841. https://doi.org/10.1007/s10529-006-9007-9. 123 Original Paper Received: 28 September 2005/Accepted: 20 February.

Li, Z., Liu, J., Zhao, Y., 2005. Possible mechanism underlying the antiherpetic activity of a proteoglycan isolated from the mycelia of *Ganoderma lucidum* in vitro. J. Biochem. Mol. Biol. 38 (1), 34–40.

Li, Z., Li, L., Sun, Y., Li, J., 2007. Identification of natural compounds with anti-HBV activity from *Rheum palmatum* L. ethanol extract. Chemotherapy 53, 320–326.

Li, H.L., Han, T., Liu, R.H., Zhang, C., Chen, H.S., Zhang, W.D., 2008. Alkaloids from *Corydalis saxicola* and their anti-HBV activity. Chem. Biodivers. 5, 777–783. https://doi.org/10.1002/cbdv.200890074. 18493964.

Li, A.N., Li, S., Zhang, Y.J., Xu, X.R., Chen, Y.M., Li, H.B., 2014. Resources and biological activities of natural polyphenols. Nutrients 6 (12), 6020–6047.

Li, Y., Cai, Q., Xie, Q., Zhang, Y., Meng, X., Zhang, Z., 2017. Different mechanisms may exist for HBsAg synthesis and secretion during various phases of chronic hepatitis B virus infection. Med. Sci. Monit. Inter. Med. J. Exp. Clin. Res. 23, 1385.

Li, S., Tan, H.Y., Wang, N., Cheung, F., Hong, M., Feng, Y., 2018. The potential and action mechanism of polyphenols in the treatment of liver diseases. Oxid. Med. Cell. Longev. 1–25. https://doi.org/10.1155/2018/8394818.

Liang, X., Bi, S., Yang, W., Wang, L., Cui, G., Cui, F., Zhang, Y., Liu, J., Gong, X., Chen, Y., et al., 2009. Epidemiological serosurvey of hepatitis B in China—declining HBV prevalence due to hepatitis B vaccination. Vaccine 27, 6550–6557.

Liu, S., Li, Y., 2016. A review of novel non-nucleoside anti-HBV agents and their mechanism of action. Med. Chem. (Los Angeles) 6 (7), 21–24. ISSN: 2161-0444.

Liu, Z.H., Zhang, L., 2016. Effects of total flavone extract from shuiqin (*Oenanthe javanica*) on immune function of immunosuppression mice. Chin. J. Tradit. Med. Sci. Technol. 23 (4), 423–425.

Liu, F., Liang, X., Zhang, N., Huang, Y., Zhang, S., 2001. Effect of growth regulators on yield and fibre quality in ramie (*Boemheria nivea* L. Gaud.) China grass. Field Crop Res. 69, 41–46.

Liu, S., Wei, W.X., Li, Y.B., Lin, X., Shi, K.C., 2014a. In vitro and in vivo anti-HBV activities of the lignan nirtetralin B isolated from *Phyllanthus niruri* L. J. Ethnopharmacol. 157, 62–68.

Liu, S., Wei, W.X., Shi, K.C., Cao, X., Zhou, M., 2014b. In vitro and in vivo antiHBV activities of the lignan niranthin isolated from *Phyllanthus niruri* L. J. Ethnopharmacol. 155, 1061–1067.

Lu, C., Li, X.F., 2019. A review of *Oenanthe javanica* (Blume) DC. as traditional medicinal plant and its therapeutic potential. Evid. Based Complement. Alternat. Med., 1–17. https://doi.org/10.1155/2019/6495819 (Review Article).

Maddrey, W.C., 2000. Hepatitis B: an important public health issue. J. Med. Virol. 61, 362–366.

Madhuri, S., 2008. Studies on Oestrogen Induced Uterine and Ovarian Carcinogenesis and Effect of ProImmu in Rats (Ph.D. Thesis). RDVV, Jabalpur, MP, India.

Madhuri, S., Pandey, G., 2009. Some anticancer medicinal plants of foreign origin. Curr. Sci. 96 (6), 779–783.

Maheshwari, R.K., Singh, A.K., Gaddipati, J., Srimal, R.C., 2006. Multiple biological activities of curcumin: a short review. Life Sci. 78, 2081–2087.

Manesis, E.K., Hadziyannis, S.J., 2001. Interferon α treatment and retreatment of hepatitis be antigen-negative chronic hepatitis B. Gastroenterology 121 (1), 101–109.

Meena, J., Sharma, R.A., Rolania, R., 2018. A review on phytochemical and pharmacological properties of *Phyllanthus amarus* Schum. and Thonn. Int. J. Pharm. Sci. Res. 9 (4), 1377–1386. https://doi.org/10.13040/IJPSR.0975-8232.9(4).1377-86.

Meng, J., Hu, X., Shan, F., Hua, H., Lu, C., Wang, E., 2011. Analysis of maturation of murine dendritic cells (DCs) induced by purified *Ganoderma lucidum* polysaccharides (GLPs). Int. J. Biol. Macromol. 49, 93–699. https://doi.org/10.1016/j.ijbiomac.2011.06.029.

Merle, P., Trepo, C., 2001. Therapeutic management of hepatitis B-related cirrhosis. J. Viral Hepat. 8 (6), 391–399.

Min, B.S., Nakamura, N., Hattori, M., 1998. Triterpenes from the spores of *Ganoderma lucidum* and their inhibitory activity against HIV-1 protease. Chem. Pharm. Bull. 46, 1607–1612.

Min, B.S., Gao, J.J., Nakamura, N., Hattori, M., 2000. Triterpenes from the spores of *Ganoderma lucidum* and their cytotoxicity against meth-A and LLC tumor cells. Chem. Pharm. Bull. 48, 1026–1033.

Min, B.S., Gao, J.J., Hattori, M., Lei, H.K., Kim, Y.H., 2001. Anticomplement activity of terpenoids from the spores of *Ganoderma lucidum*. Planta Med. 67, 811–814.

Montuclard, C., Hamza, S., Rollot, F., 2015. Causes of death in people with chronic HBV infection: a population-based cohort study. J. Hepatol. 62 (6), 1265–1271. https://doi.org/10.1016/j.jhep.2015.01.020.

Oh, K.W., Lee, C.K., Kim, Y.S., Eo, S.K., Han, S.S., 2000. Antiherpetic activities of acidic protein bound polysacchride isolated from *Ganoderma lucidum* alone and in combinations with acyclovir and vidarabine. J. Ethnopharmacol. 72, 221–227.

Pandey, G., Madhuri, S., 2008. Some anticancer agents from plant origin. Pl. Arch. 8 (2), 527–532.

Pandey, G., Madhuri, S., 2010. Significance of fruits and vegetables in malnutrition cancer. Pl. Arch. 10 (2), 517–522.

Pang, J.Y., Zhao, K.J., Wang, J.b., Ma, Z.J., Xiao, X.H., 2014. Green tea polyphenol, epigallocatechin-3-gallate, possesses the antiviral activity necessary to fight against the hepatitis B virus replication in vitro. J. Zhejiang Univ. Sci. B 15 (6), 533–539. https://doi.org/10.1631/jzus.B1300307. 24903990.

Patel, J.R., Tripathi, P., Sharma, V., Chauhan, N.S., Dixit, V.K., 2011. *Phyllanthus amarus*: ethnomedicinal uses, phytochemistry and pharmacology: a review. J. Ethnopharmacol. 138, 286–313.

Qu, S.J., Wang, G.F., Duan, W.H., Yao, S.Y., Zuo, J.P., Tan, C.H., Zhu, D.Y., 2011. Tryptamine derivatives as novel non-nucleosidic inhibitors against HBV. Bioorg. Med. Chem. 19, 3120–3127. https://doi.org/10.1016/j.bmc.2011.04.004. 21524588.

Romero, M.R., Efferth, T., Serrano, M.A., Castaño, B., Macias, R.I., Briz, O., Marin, J.J., 2005. Effect of artemisinin/artesunate as inhibitors of HBV production in an "in vitro" replicative system. Antiviral Res. 68, 75–83.

Sahar, E.M., Meselhy, M.R., Nakamura, N., Tezuka, Y., Hattori, M., Kakiuchi, N., Shimotohno, K., Kawahata, T., Otake, T., 1998. Anti-HIV-1 and anti-HIV-1-protease substances from *Ganoderma lucidum*. Phytochemistry 49, 1651–1657.

Sarpel, D., Carter, D., Wasserman, I., Oxnard, M., Dieterich, D.T., 2017. An update on the management of chronic hepatitis B and C infection. Clin. Pharm. 9 (8).

Semple, S.J., Pyke, S.M., Reynolds, G.D., 2001. In vitro antiviral activity of the anthraquinone chrysophanic acid against poliovirus. Antiviral Res. 49, 169–178.

Sharma, A.K., Gawande, S.P., Satpathy, S., 2014. Ramie (*Boehmeria nivea* L.): recent technologies for commercialization of its cultivation in North east. Biotech Today 4 (2), 48–54. https://doi.org/10.5958/2322-0996.2014.00029.5.

Shegokar, A., 2016. What nanocrystals can offer to cosmetic and dermal formulations. In: Nanobiomaterials. Galenic Formulations and Cosmetics, pp. 69–91, https://doi.org/10.1016/B978-0-323-42868-2.00004-8.

Shi, Y.M., Li, X.Y., Li, X.N., Luo, X., Xue, Y.B., Liang, C.Q., Zou, J., Kong, L.M., Li, Y., Pu, J.X., Xiao, W.L., Sun, H.D., 2011. Schicagenins A–C: three cagelike nortriterpenoids from leaves and stems of *Schisandra chinensis*. Org. Lett. 13, 3848–3851.

Shimizu, J.F., Lima, C.S., Pereira, C.M., Bittar, C., Batista, M.N., Nazaré, A.C., Polaquini, C.R., Zothner, C., Harris, M., Rahal, P., Regasini, L.O., Jardim, A.C.G., 2017. Flavonoids from *Pterogyne nitens* inhibit hepatitis C virus entry. Sci. Rep. 7 (1), 16127. https://doi.org/10.1038/s41598-017-16336-y.

Singh, B., Sharma, R.A., 2015. Plant terpenes: defense responses, phylogenetic analysis, regulation and clinical applications. 3 Biotech 5 (2), 129–151.

Su, C.H., Yang, Y.Z., Ho, H., Hu, C.H., Sheu, M.T., 2001. High-performance liquid chromatographic analysis for the characterization of triterpenoids from *Ganoderma*. J. Chromatogr. Sci. 39, 93–100.

Su, C.R., Yeh, S.F., Liu, C.M., Damu, A.G., Kuo, T.H., Chiang, P.C., Bastow, K.F., Lee, K.H., Wu, T.S., 2009. Anti-HBV and cytotoxic activities of pyranocoumarin derivatives. Bioorg. Med. Chem. 17, 6137–6143. https://doi.org/10.1016/j.bmc.2008.12.007. 19635670.

Subandi, M., 2012. The effect of fertilizers on the growth and the yield of ramie (*Boehmeria nivea* L. Gaud). Asian J. Agric. Rural Dev. 2, 126–135.

Sun, Y., Li, L., Li, J., Li, Z., 2007. Inhibition of HBV replication by *Rheum palmatum* L. ethanol extract in a stable HBV-producing cell line. Virol. Sin. 22 (1), 14–20.

Tang, L.S.Y., Covert, E., Wilson, E., Kottilil, S., 2018. Chronic hepatitis B infection. Clin. Rev. Educ. 319 (17), 1802–1813.

Terrault, N.A., Bzowej, N.H., Chang, K.-M., 2016. AASLD guidelines for treatment of chronic hepatitis B. Hepatology 63 (1), 261–283. https://doi.org/10.1002/hep.28156.

Tseng, Y.P., Kuo, Y.H., Hu, C.P., Jeng, K.S., Janmanchi, D., Lin, C.H., Chou, C.K., Yeh, S.F., 2008. The role of helioxanthin in inhibiting human hepatitis B viral replication and gene expression by interfering with the host transcriptional machinery of viral promoters. Antiviral Res. 77, 206–214. https://doi.org/10.1016/j.antiviral.2007.12.011. 18249449.

Wang, S.Y., Hsu, H.H., Tzeng, C.H., Lee, S.S., Shiao, M.S., Ho, C.K., 1997. The antitumor effect of *Ganoderma lucidum* is mediated by cytokines released from activated macrophages and T lymphocytes. Int. J. Cancer 70, 699–705.

Wang, W.-N., Yang, X.-B., Liu, H.-Z., Huang, Z.-M., Wu, G.-X., 2005. Effect of *Oenanthe javanica* flavone on human and duck HBV infection. Acta Pharmacol. Sin. 26 (5), 587–592.

Wang, G.F., Shi, L.P., Ren, Y.D., Liu, Q.F., Liu, H.F., Zhang, R.J., Li, Z., Zhu, F.H., He, P.L., Tang, W., Tao, P.Z., Li, C., Zhao, W.M., Zuo, J.P., 2009. AntiHBV activity of chlorogenic acid, quinic acid and caffeic acid in vivo and in vitro. Antiviral Res. 83, 186–190. https://doi.org/10.1016/j.antiviral.2009.05.002. 19463857.

Wang, Y.P., Zhao, W., Xue, R., Zhou, Z.X., Liu, F., Han, Y.X., Ren, G., Peng, Z.G., Cen, S., Chen, H.S., Li, Y.H., Jiang, J.D., 2011. Oxymatrine inhibits hepatitis B infection with an advantage of overcoming drug resistance. Antiviral Res. 89, 227–231. 21277330.

Wang, Y., Wu, K.F., Yu, H., Gao, M., Liu, J., Zhang, R.H., 2016. Toxicological security evaluation of *Oenanthe javanica*. Food Res. Dev. 37 (22), 196–201.

Wei, J., Lin, L., Su, X., Qin, S., Xu, Q., Tang, Z., Deng, Y., Zhou, Y., He, S., 2014. Anti-HBV activity of *Boehmeria nivea* leaf extracts in human HepG2.2.15 cells. Biomed. Rep. 2 (1), 147–151.

Wei, Z.Q., Zhang, Y.H., Ke, C.Z., Chen, H.X., Ren, P., He, Y.L., Hu, P., Ma, D., Luo, J., Meng, Z.J., 2017. Curcumin inhibits HBV infection by down-regulating cccDNA-bound histone acetylation. World J. Gastroenterol. 23 (34), 6252–6260.

WHO, 2017. Global Hepatitis Report., ISBN: 978-92-4-156545-5, pp. 1–83.

Wu, Y.H., 2016. Naturally derived anti-HBV agents and their mechanism of action. World J. Gastroenterol. 22 (1), 188–204. ISSN 1007-9327 (print) ISSN 2219-2840 (online).

Wu, Y.R., Ma, Y.B., Zhao, Y.X., Yao, S.Y., Zhou, J., Zhou, Y., Chen, J.J., 2007. Two new quaternary alkaloids and anti-HBV active constituents from *Corydalis saxicola*. Planta Med. 73, 787–791. https://doi.org/10.1055/s-2007-981549. 17611928.

Wu, Y., Wang, D., 2009. A new class of natural glycopeptides with sugar moiety-dependent antioxidant activities derived from *Ganoderma lucidum* fruiting bodies. J. Proteome Res. 8 (2), 436–442.

Wu, H.B., Wu, H.B., Wang, W.S., Liu, T.T., Qi, M.G., Feng, J.C., Li, X.Y., Liu, Y., 2016. Insecticidal activity of sesquiterpene lactones and monoterpenoid from the fruits of *Carpesium abrotanoides*. Ind. Crops Prod. 92, 77–83.

Xia, Y., Luo, H., Liu, J.P., Gluud, C., 2011. Phyllanthus species for chronic HBV infection. Cochrane Database Syst. Rev. 4, CD008960.

Xu, B., Liu, S., Fan, X.D., Deng, L.Q., Ma, W.H., Chen, M., 2015. Two new coumarin glycosides from *Herpetospermum caudigerum*. J. Asian Nat. Prod. Res. 17, 738–743. https://doi.org/10.1080/10286020.2014. 996137. 25559035.

Xue, Y.B., Zhang, Y.L., Yang, J.H., Du, X., Pu, J.X., Zhao, W., Li, X.N., Xiao, W.L., Sun, H.D., 2010. Nortriterpenoids and lignans from the fruit of *Schisandra chinensis*. Chem. Pharm. Bull. 58, 1606–1611.

Yang, C.S., Lambert, J.D., Hou, Z., 2006. Molecular targets for the cancer preventive activity of tea polyphenols. Mol. Carcinog. 45 (6), 431–435.

Yang, J.H., Kim, S.C., Shin, B.Y., 2013. O-Methylated flavonol isorhamnetin prevents acute inflammation through blocking of NF-κB activation. Food Chem. Toxicol. 59, 362–372.

Yang, S.-A., Jung, Y.-S., Lee, S.-J., Park, S.C., Kim, M.J., Lee, E.J., Byun, H.J., Jhee, K.H., Lee, S.P., 2014. Hepatoprotective effects of fermented field water-dropwort (*Oenanthe javanica*) extract and its major constituents. Food Chem. Toxicol. 67, 154–160.

Yao, D., Li, H., Gou, Y., Zhang, H., Vlessidis, A.G., Zhou, H., Evmiridis, N.P., Liu, Z., 2009. Betulinic acid-mediated inhibitory effect on HBV by suppression of manganese superoxide dismutase expression. FEBS J. 276, 2599–2614.

Yeo, H., Li, Y., Fu, L., Zhu, J.L., Gullen, E.A., 2005. Synthesis and antiviral activity of helioxanthin analogues. J. Med. Chem. 48, 534–546.

Yu, L.H., Liu, G.T., 2009. The structure–activity relationship of dibenzo(a,c) cyclooctene lignans isolated from fructus schizandrae and innovation of anti-hepatitis drugs. Huaxue Jinzhan 21, 66–76.

Yu, Z.X., Wei, L.H., Gao, Y., Guo, X.Q., 2017. Study on acute toxicity of *Oenanthe javanica*. J. Anhui Agric. Sci. 45 (2), 106–107.

Zasloff, M., Adams, A.P., Beckerman, B., Campbell, A., Han, Z., Luijten, E., Meza, I., Julander, J., Mishra, A., Qu, W., Taylor, J.M., Weaver, S.C., Wong, G.C., 2011. Squalamine as a broad-spectrum systemic antiviral agent with therapeutic potential. Proc. Natl. Acad. Sci. U. S. A. 108, 15978–15983. https://doi.org/10.1073/pnas.1108558108. 21930925.

Zhang, J.S., Tang, Q.J., Martin, Z.K., Reutter, W., Fan, H., 2002a. Activation of B lymphocytes by GLIS, a bioactive proteoglycan from *Ganoderma lucidum*. Life Sci. 71, 623–638.

Zhang, G.L., Wang, Y.H., Ni, W., Teng, H.L., Lin, Z.B., 2002b. Hepatoprotective role of *Ganoderma lucidum* polysaccharide against BCG-induced immune liver injury in mice. World J. Gastroenterol. 8 (4), 728.

Zhou, X., Lin, J., Yin, Y., Zhao, J., Sun, X., Tang, K., 2007. Ganodermataceae: natural products and their related pharmacological functions. Am. J. Chin. Med. 35, 559–574.

Zhou, Y.B., Wang, Y.F., Zhang, Y., Zheng, L.Y., Yang, X.A., Wang, N., Jiang, J.H., Ma, F., Yin, D.T., Sun, C.Y., Wang, Q.D., 2012. In vitro activity of cepharanthine hydrochloride against clinical wild-type and lamivudine-resistant HBV isolates. Eur. J. Pharmacol. 683, 10–15. https://doi.org/10.1016/j.ejphar.2012.02.030. 22387093.

Zhou, N.J., Geng, C.A., Huang, X.Y., Ma, Y.B., Zhang, X.M., Wang, J.L., Chen, J.J., 2015. Anti-HBV active constituents from *Swertia chirayita*. Fitoterapia 100, 27–34. https://doi.org/10.1016/j.fitote.2014.11.011. 25447162.

Further reading

Cheng, P., Ma, Y.B., Yao, S.Y., Zhang, Q., Wang, E.J., Yan, M.H., Zhang, X.M., Zhang, F.X., Chen, J.J., 2007. Two new alkaloids and active antiHBV constituents from *Hypserpa nitida*. Bioorg. Med. Chem. Lett. 17, 5316–5320. https://doi.org/10.1016/j.bmcl.2007.08.027. 17723297.

Hepatitis C

Abdullah[a], Kamal Niaz[b], and Fazlullah Khan[c]

[a]Department of Pharmacy, University of Malakand, Chakdara, Pakistan [b]Department of Pharmacology and Toxicology, Faculty of Bio-Sciences, Cholistan University of Veterinary and Animal Sciences (CUVAS), Bahawalpur, Pakistan [c]Department of Toxicology and Pharmacology, The Institute of Pharmaceutical Sciences, School of Pharmacy, Tehran University of Medical Sciences, Tehran, Iran

3.1 Introduction

Hepatitis C, one of the major health issues across the globe, has great potential to become chronic. Liver cirrhosis and hepatocellular carcinoma are the complications of chronic hepatitis C (Choo et al., 1989). According to a research study, about 200 million individuals are infected with hepatitis C (3.3% of the world population), which results in about 350,000 deaths per annum (Lavanchy, 2011; Mohd Hanafiah et al., 2013). Hepatitis C is a contagious hepatic illness caused by infection by the hepatitis C virus (HCV). In Europe, there are more than 25 million HCV patients. Worldwide, HCV prevalence is highest in Egypt (15%). Annually, about one million new cases are reported across the globe (Kamal and Nasser, 2008; Rockstroh et al., 2012). Similarly, the frequency of hepatitis C is higher in certain countries such as Pakistan, where 5% of the population is infected; in the Khyber Pakhtunkhwa province of Pakistan, the prevalence is 5%–9% (Afridi et al., 2013; Khan et al., 2014).

HCV transmission occurs by the parenteral route via using contaminated syringes by drug abusers and inadequate medical equipment sterilization (Nelson et al., 2011; World Health Organization, 2015). The virus, after transmission, may remain in the latent phase due to suppression by the immune system of the host. HCV replication is very robust during the infectious phase and about 1 trillion virion particles may be generated in a single day (Neumann et al., 1998). Although several drugs are available for HCV treatment, unfortunately no vaccine is currently available for the prevention of infection. The standard therapy until recently included interferon and ribavirin (Manns et al., 2001; Fried et al., 2002). Antiviral drugs are used for the eradication of HCV from chronically infected patients. The outcome of standard HCV therapy (ribavirin and pegylated interferon alpha, IFN-α) is variable and very costly while the adverse effects are unendurable for patients (McHutchison et al., 1998; Di Bisceglie and Hoofnagle, 2002).

Influence of Nutrients, Bioactive Compounds, and Plant Extracts in Liver Diseases. https://doi.org/10.1016/B978-0-12-816488-4.00014-0

The development of new, directly acting antiviral drugs (DAAs) that target NS3/4A protease, NS5B polymerase, and NS5A has remarkably improved treatment outcomes for HCV genotype 1 (Pawlotsky, 2014). Clinical trials are in progress to develop new drugs that target other viral proteins, which will help improve response to HCV treatment (Poordad and Dieterich, 2012; Wartelle-Bladou et al., 2012). The escape risk of virus mutants will be decreased by the combination of DAAs. Without the use of interferon, the DAA combination will reduce side effects to a great level because many of the adverse effects are associated with interferon, which contributes to the treatment failure (Wartelle-Bladou et al., 2012).

With the increase of available techniques to grow HCV in cell cultures, the search for DAAs has been greatly stimulated. This has led to increased research on natural compounds/compounds from plants exhibiting anti-HCV activity. Medicinal plants and their bioactive compounds are increasingly being used for the treatment of several diseases. Between 2000 and 2010, about 40 new drugs were launched into the market based on plants, microorganisms, and animals (Brahmachari, 2012; Khan et al., 2017; Abdullah et al., 2020). Traditional medicine can be an important source of new drugs that may be used for therapeutic or prophylactic purposes (Balick and Cox, 1997; Samuelsson and Bohlin, 1999). The main advantage of natural compounds from plants is their low cost and no need for chemical synthesis. A large number of medicinal plants have shown antiviral activities against hepatitis B, hepatitis C (Kitazato et al., 2007), the influenza virus (Hudson, 1989), HIV (Chang and Yeung, 1988), and the herpes simplex virus (Samuelsson and Bohlin, 1999). Natural product screening has resulted in the development of more effective inhibitors of in vitro virus growth (Baker et al., 1995). Moreover, several plant extracts and natural compounds have exhibited hepatoprotective activity (Khan et al., 2017; Abdullah et al., 2020). In the last decades, scientists have analyzed the active compounds used in traditional medicine for the treatment of hepatitis (Kong et al., 2007). This chapter aims to give insight into the hepatoprotective activity of natural compounds and plant extracts in HCV infection.

3.2 Etiology

Hepatitis C is caused by HCV, which was disclosed in 1989 by Choo et al. HCV is the main cause of chronic hepatic illness that ends in hepatocellular carcinoma and liver cirrhosis. HCV is a small circular (50 nm diameter), positive-sense, enveloped single-stranded RNA virus that belongs to the genus *Hepacivirus* of the *Flaviviridae* family (Choo et al., 1989).

3.3 Signs and symptoms

The majority of patients suffering from HCV have either no symptoms or mild symptoms. Symptoms may appear at any time from 2 weeks to 6 months after exposure to the virus. The symptoms of HCV are jaundice, fatigue, gray-colored stool, joint pain, dark urine, anorexia, weakness, belly pain, malaise, and nausea (Wang et al., 2016). In most cases, the infection becomes chronic where the patient experiences no symptoms. Most of the chronic infections lead to hepatitis and fibrosis, which may result in cirrhosis in 15%–20% of the infected cases (Chen and Morgan, 2006).

3.4 Genotypes and serotypes of HCV

Based on phylogenetic and sequence analysis, strains of HCV are classified into seven genotypes (1–7) (Simmonds et al., 1994). Different strains of HCV differ at 30%–35% nucleotide sites from each other. The 67 confirmed HCV strain subtypes differ < 15% of nucleotide sites (Smith et al., 2014). Globally, the most prevalent type of HCV is genotype 1, which accounts for 46.2% of all HCV cases (Magiorkinis et al., 2009). The second most prevalent type of genotype is 3. The endemic strains from HCV genotype 1 and 2 are mainly in West Africa, 3 in South Asia, 4 in the Middle East and Central Africa, 5 in Southern Africa, and 6 in Southeast Asia (Simmonds, 2001; Pybus et al., 2009). A single infection of genotype 7 was reported in Canada from an African patient (Murphy et al., 2007).

3.5 Diagnosis (serology, biopsy, and screening)

Extensive studies for about two decades on viral RNA, proteins, and HCV life cycles have resulted in a better understanding of HCV with consequent sensitive diagnostic tools and effective therapeutic options. Currently, in high-risk individuals, serologic screening is recommended while for the confirmation of active HCV infections, nucleic acid testing is performed. To determine the treatment duration and to predict the response, the quantification and genotyping of HCV RNAs are recommended.

The main purpose of the diagnosis of HCV is to identify and treat infected individuals. This helps in the prevention of disease progression and the spreading of the virus. As most HCV patients are asymptomatic and despite the normal ALT levels, viremia could still exist. Therefore, it is recommended to use virological techniques instead of SGPT levels for the diagnosis of HCV (Chevaliez and Pawlotsky, 2009).

3.6 Serology

HCV can be diagnosed by anti-HCV antibody detection in the plasma or serum. An accurate HCV diagnosis is required before therapy initiation. It is crucial to determine the HCV infection stage because in 15%–45% of the infected patients, the infection gets clear in 6–12 months. These individuals react positively to the anti-HCV antibody test without detectable viremia. Therefore, physicians should differentiate between recovered and infected individuals. Nowadays, nucleic acid testing (NAT) is the most commonly used technique for HCV RNA detection (Dow et al., 1996; Micallef et al., 2006). Screening tests and confirmatory tests are carried out for the detection of anti-HCV antibodies. To screen the antibody-positive specimens, the screening is first done, which is then verified by the confirmatory test.

3.7 Screening tests

3.7.1 Enzyme immunosorbent assay (EIA)

In the diagnostic laboratory, the third-generation EIA is commonly used to detect the anti-HCV antibody. NS3, NS4, NS5, and HCV core antigens are employed to detect antibodies against HCV. This test is inexpensive and easy to use while it may also be fully automated and accustomed to testing on a large scale. Therefore, it is commonly employed for the screening of HCV infections (Colin et al., 2001; Campos-Outcalt, 2012). However, EIA should not be used for screening patients less than 18 months of age due to reactivity with maternal antibodies (Mack et al., 2012). The time between the appearance of detectable antibodies and HCV infection (serologic window period) is about 40 days for third-generation EIAs. However, a fourth-generation EIA is available now that can detect antibodies earlier. For the fourth-generation EIAs, antigens are derived from the core, NS3, NS4A, NS4B, and NS5 regions (Barrera et al., 1995).

3.7.2 The rapid test (point of care test)

This is a highly sensitive and specific test done outside the laboratory (de Paula Scalioni et al., 2014; Saludes et al., 2014). The FDA-approved point-of-care test is the OraQuick HCV Rapid Antibody Test, recommended for patients more than 15 years old who are more susceptible to HCV infection. This test is used to detect anti-HCV antibodies in serum, plasma, whole blood, or oral fluid. The immobilization of the synthetic peptides of the NS3, NS4, and core antigens or recombinant proteins is done on a membrane made of nitrocellulose to carry out the lateral flow immunoassay indirectly. The result is observed directly through colloidal gold-labeled protein A. If anti-HCV antibodies are present in the specimens, within 20–40 min, the protein A results in the formation of a reddish-purple line. This test is fast, cheap, and simple to perform (Lee et al., 2011).

3.7.2.1 Confirmatory tests
I.   **Recombinant immunoblot assays (RIBA)**

These are employed for the confirmation of anti-HCV antibodies in patients who have already exhibited a positive EIA test. It is a highly specific assay because an antibody against each HCV protein is determined as an individual band on a membrane strip (Martin et al., 1998). Anti-HCV EIAs are highly specific and sensitive; therefore, there is no need for RIBA to be performed for verification (Alborino et al., 2011).

II. **Qualitative HCV RNA detection**

This works on the assumption of target amplification by RT-PCR or transcription-mediated amplification (TMA). After the extraction of HCV RNA, it is converted by reverse transcriptase into complementary DNA (cDNA). This is followed by processing through cyclic enzymatic reactions resulting in the formation of a huge count of double-stranded DNAs in a PCR-based assay or a single-stranded RNA in TMA. The amplified DNA/RNA is then detected via hybridization of the resulting amplicons on distinct probes. Usually, among different genotypes, the most conserved 5′UTR region is the target area for HCV genomic RNA detection (Mack et al., 2012; Saludes et al., 2014).

III. **Quantitative HCV RNA detection**

HCV RNA quantification is done by target amplification (RT-PCR or TMA) or signal amplification (branched DNA or bDNA). For RNA quantification, the method of choice is real-time RT-PCR in clinical settings, although several FDA-approved assays are available. RT-PCR is a highly sensitive test with a wide quantification range, and it can halt hangover contamination (Mack et al., 2012).

3.8 Biopsy

A liver biopsy is an important tool in the diagnosis of the severity of a hepatic disease. But it is invasive, costly, and in some patients, may result in complications including hematoma formation, biliary leakage, infection, and internal bleeding (Mazhar et al., 2009). A liver biopsy is rarely done for acute hepatitis because clinical testing provides diagnostic information. It is done in those cases of acute hepatitis where the liver enzymes are elevated due to unknown/unidentified etiology. Moreover, it is done for chronic hepatitis (Brunt, 2010).

Chronic hepatitis C is characterized by lymphoid aggregates and mild to moderate foci of interface activity. Spotty necrosis with 1–2 mononuclear cells with occasional acidophil is/are noted in lobules. Macrovesicular steatosis is observed in 30%–66% of cases of a biopsy in genotype 3. In nongenotype 3, macrovesicular steatosis may be present in various zones in varying amounts that represent predisposing conditions (alcohol use, diabetes, obesity) (Paradis and Bedossa, 2008). The grading of steatosis is done according to the percent acinus filled or the surface area of biopsy filled; it is reported as 0%–5%, 5%–33%, 33%–66%, and > 66%.

Moreover, Poulsen lesions have been reported in HCV in which the bile duct is infiltrated by lymphocytes and eosinophils in the portal infiltrate while portal venous endothelium is found in some cases. Hepatic fibrosis in HCV originates from portal tracts (Ferrell et al., 2007).

3.9 Screening

One of the barriers to the elimination of HCV is that a substantial proportion of patients are unaware of their infection. To analyze the magnitude of the HCV pandemic in different regions and to design public health interventions, accurate prevalence and incidence data are required. Hence, HCV screening is required for the identification and treatment of infected individuals. Based on local epidemiology, different screening strategies have been implemented in different regions of the world. People at high risk can be identified and must be tested (Chhatwal et al., 2016; Pawlotsky, 2016).

3.10 Prevention

As one of the modes of HCV transmission is through blood, therefore blood screening must be done before donation. The use of second- and third-generation enzyme immunoassays has significantly reduced the transmission of HCV (Kamal, 2008). In developed countries, intravenous drug use still is the major reason for HCV. However, avoiding syringe exchange and the single use of disposable syringes is needed for the prevention of HCV (Hutchinson et al., 2000; Maher et al., 2007). All individuals in general and HCV-positive patients in particular should not share razors, toothbrushes, or other articles of personal use that might have blood on them (Alter, 2002). Although HCV transmission via the sexual route is controversial, studies have shown a slight increase in risk between monogamous spouses (Tahan et al., 2005). Many hard-to-reach communities and the general public should be made aware of HCV, and the advantages of prevention (Ward et al., 2012). Without effective antiviral treatment, > 75% of the acute HCV infections may become chronic, often causing progressive, serious, and fatal liver disease. The development of a vaccine for HCV is direly needed (Ward et al., 2012).

3.11 Treatment

Initially, HCV was treated with IFN-α, but the frequency of adverse effects, the low rate of sustained response, and the increased duration of treatment for genotype 1 led to the need for another antiviral agent that may be added to or replace IFN-alpha (Poynard et al., 1998; Hoofnagle, 1999). Therefore ribavirin, a guanosine analog, was used in combination with IFN-alpha (van der Meer et al., 2012). IFN-alpha was administered thrice weekly, and the frequency could be reduced to once weekly by generating pegylated IFN-alpha (attaching IFN-alpha to polyethylene glycol moiety, PEG) (Pawlotsky et al., 2004).

IFN-α2a was developed and coupled to a branched PEG molecule (40-kD) while IFN-α2b was coupled to a linear PEG molecule (12-kD) with 75 and 30 h elimination half-lives, respectively. The dose of PegIFN-α2a was 180 µg per week as a single weekly injection while the dose of PegIFN-α2b was 1.5 µg/kg per week. Both the pegylated IFNs were found to be more effective than their unpegylated counterparts when given as monotherapy for 48 weeks (Lindsay et al., 2001; Zeuzem et al., 2001).

Table 3.1: Direct-acting antiviral (DAAs) drugs (World Health Organization, 2018).

S. no.	DAA class	Examples of drugs
1	NS3/4A inhibitors	Glecaprevir, Grazoprevir, Paritaprevir, Voxilaprevir, Simeprevir
2	NS5A inhibitors	Velpatasvir, Daclatasvir, Ombitasvir, Ledipasvir, Elbasvir, Pibrentasvir
3	NS5B polymerase inhibitor (nucleotide analogue)	Sofosbuvir
4	NS5B polymerase inhibitor (nonnucleoside analogue)	Dasabuvir

With the advancement in the understanding of molecular virology, directly acting antivirals (DAAs) were developed (Table 3.1). In this connection, NS3-4A was developed. In 2011, the first-generation HCV NS3-4A protease inhibitors (Bocepriver, telaprevir) were approved for use in combination with PegIFN-α and ribavirin for the treatment of chronic HCV genotype 1 (Ghany et al., 2011; Liver, 2014).

3.12 Hepatoprotective activity of natural compounds and plant extracts in Hepatitis C

3.12.1 Silymarin

This is extracted from milk thistle seeds found across the globe. Seed extracts of this plant have been used as a hepatoprotective since ancient times. It contains flavonolignans and a flavonoid including silybin A, isosilybin A, silybin B, isosilybin B, silydianin, isosilychristin, silychristin, and taxifolin. Polyphenols have a subclass called flavonolignans, which consist of lignan and flavonoid. Silibinin (a main constituent of silymarin) is a mixture of silybin A and silybin B (the two diastereoisomers) and possesses an anti-HCV effect. Moreover, silymarin exerts anti-HCV activity by blocking virus replication while also having immunomodulatory and antiinflammatory activities that contribute to its hepatoprotective activity (Table 3.2) (Polyak et al., 2007; Morishima et al., 2010).

HCV replication is inhibited by silibinin via the inhibition of NS5B RNA-dependant RNA polymerase (Ahmed-Belkacem et al., 2010; Wagoner et al., 2011). Another study reported that silymarin causes the inhibition of NS5B-independent HCV genotype 3a core expression (Ashfaq et al., 2011). But the problem with silymarin is its low bioavailability. This may be the reason for the unsuccessful treatment of patients suffering from HCV after oral administration of silymarin (Hawke et al., 2010; Fried et al., 2012). Therefore, the intravenous administration of more water-soluble formulations of silymarin may be more effective.

Table 3.2: Natural compounds used in hepatitis C treatment.

S. no.	Name of compound	Source	Mechanism of action	Reference(s)
1	Silymarin extract	*Silybum marianum*	Entry/replication	Wagoner et al. (2010) and Blaising et al. (2013)
2	Epigallocatechin-3-gallate	*Camellia sinensis*	Entry/replication	Calland et al. (2012a) and Chen et al. (2012)
3	Plambagin	*Plumbago indica*	Replication	Hassan et al. (2016)
4	Apigenin	*Matricaria chamomilla*	Replication	Shibata et al. (2014)
5	Ladanein	*Marrubium peregrinum*	Entry	Haid et al. (2012)
6	Naringenin	*Citrus paradisi*	Assembly/release	Nahmias et al. (2008)
7	Quercetin	Embelia ribes	Replication	Bachmetov et al. (2012)
8	Honokiol	*Magnolia grandiflora*	Entry/replication	Lan et al. (2012)
9	3-Hydroxy caruilignan C	*Swietenia macrophylla*	Replication	Wu et al. (2012)
10	Corilagin	*Excoecaria agallocha*	Replication	Hanna et al. (2012)

3.12.2 Naringenin

This is a flavanone found in grapefruit that exhibits antiinflammatory, antioxidant, and anticarcinogenic activities. It is responsible for the bitter taste of grapes. In one study, naringenin exhibited an anti-HCV effect by decreasing HCV-positive strand RNA, core protein, infectious particles, and ApoB in the infected Huh-7 cell supernatant (Nahmias et al., 2008). While in another study, the blockage of the assembly of intracellular viral particles was observed in the primary hepatocyte culture. There was no effect on the intracellular levels of viral proteins or RNA (Nahmias et al., 2008).

3.12.3 Quercetin

This is a flavanol found in onions, asparagus, broccoli, cherries, green peppers, tomatoes, potatoes, spinach, apple, and pears (Nishimuro et al., 2015). In a research study, the interactions between heat shock proteins (HSP) HSP40 and HSP70 and viral NS5A (from HCV genotype 1a) were observed. Quercetin reduced the activity of the internal ribosome entry site (IRES) in the presence or absence of NS5A (Gonzalez et al., 2009). In the cell culture, quercetin (at 50 µM) resulted in the inhibition of HCV production. Quercetin may exert its anti-HCV activity by the inhibition of virus secretion or morphogenesis (Gonzalez et al., 2009).

3.12.4 (−)-Epigallocatechin-3-gallate (EGCG)

EGCG is catechin (flavonoid) present in green tea. One cup of tea contains about 150 mg of EGCG (Chow et al., 2003). It inhibits the entry of HCV into the cells (Ciesek et al., 2011; Chen et al., 2012). It does not affect the replication of HCV RNA and the HCV particle release (Calland et al., 2012a), despite the inhibitory effect of EGCG on NS5B and NS3 in the in vitro studies (Zuo et al., 2007; Roh and Jo, 2011).

EGCG has some interesting properties, including the inhibition of transmission from one cell to another, which is the main route of spreading infection in hepatic tissues of infected patients. It directly inactivates the virus and is not genotype-specific. These properties lead to EGCG preventing HCV recurrence and spread in liver transplant patients who are chronically infected (Calland et al., 2012b).

3.12.5 Luteolin and apigenin

These are natural flavones with anti-HCV potential. In a cell-based antiviral assay, apigenin and luteolin exhibited an anti-HCV effect with EC50 values of 4.3 and 7.9 µM, respectively. Luteolin displayed inhibition of NS5B polymerase (Luo et al., 2000).

3.12.6 Honokiol

This belongs to the lignans group of phytochemicals, which is a class of phytoestrogens (estrogen-like chemical) that acts as antioxidants. Honokiol is obtained from the bark, leaves, and cones of *Magnolia officinalis.* It has been found to inhibit HCVpp entry from genotypes 1a, 1b, and 2a. It inhibited the expression of NS5A, NS5B, and NS3 in a dose-dependent manner. The replication inhibition of genotype 1a and 2a is also done in a dose-dependent fashion (Lan et al., 2012).

3.12.7 3-Hydroxy caruilignan C (3-HCL-C)

3-HCL-C is a lignan obtained from the stem of *Swietenia macrophylla.* In the subgenomic replicon system, 3-HCL-C caused a reduction in the HCV RNA level and NS3 proteins. The fruits of *Swietenia macrophylla* are used in folk medicine in different countries, including Malaysia. Furthermore, the combination of 3-HCL-C with IFN-α, telaprevir (NS3/4A protease inhibitor), or 2′-C-methylcytidine (NS5B polymerase inhibitor) enhanced HCV RNA replication inhibition. It also interferes with the replication of HCV by inducing IFN-stimulated response element transcription and IFN-dependent antiviral gene expression. Therefore, 3-HCL-C can be developed as an adjuvant for anti-HCV therapy (Wu et al., 2012).

3.12.8 Ladanein

This is a flavone obtained from *Marrubium peregrinum.* Ladanein causes the inhibition of the entry of HCV into cells in a genotype-independent manner. Ladanein acts synergistically with cyclosporine A (HCV replication inhibitor) in HCV infection. It also displayed an antiviral effect in the primary hepatocytes of humans. Most importantly, Ladanein exhibited good oral bioavailability in mice. These facts show the potential of Ladanein as an anti-HCV compound in patients (Haid et al., 2012) (Fig. 3.1).

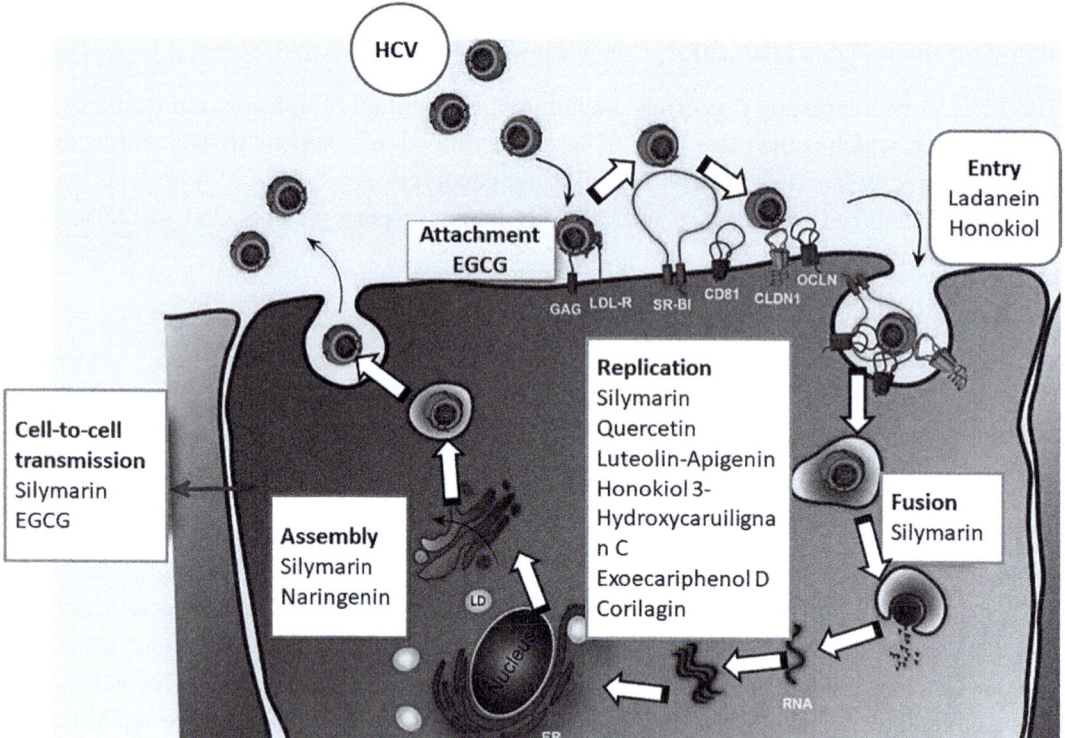

Fig. 3.1

Blocking step of Hepatitis C by natural compounds (Calland et al., 2012b).

3.12.9 Plumbagin

Plumbagin is 5-hydroxy-2-methyl-1,4-naphthoquinone that is isolated from *Plumbago indica* roots. Its activity on the life cycle of HCV was studied by infecting Huh-7.5 cells with HCV FL-J6/JFH/JC1 for 6 h and then plumbagin application for 96 h. The inhibition of HCV RNA was observed after the quantification of intracellular HCV RNA by RT-PCR (Hassan et al., 2016). In another study, it was found that plumbagin decreased the expression of NS3 protein while the expression of hA3G (a histidine deaminase) was increased in a dose-dependent manner (Zhu et al., 2015).

3.12.10 Corilagin

Corilagin is an ellagitannin isolated from *P. amarus*. It significantly inhibited NS3 protease and NS5B RNA-dependent RNA polymerase. In the infectious cell culture system, corilagin displayed significant viral inhibition and good antioxidant potential via a blockade of HCV-induced ROS generation while inhibiting the upregulation of TGF-β mRNA and NOX4.

Moreover, corilagin exhibited better oral bioavailability in mice. Furthermore, it reduced collagen deposition, the HCV RNA level, and the denaturation of liver cells in mice that accommodate human hepatocytes (Reddy et al., 2018).

3.13 Conclusion

Hepatitis C is a major health problem all over the world that affects millions of people. Due to the mutation and route of infection, the prevalence of HCV genotypes varies in different regions of the world. HCV carries a high risk of becoming chronic, causing liver cirrhosis and liver failure. As most patients are asymptomatic, therefore blood tests should be performed on a monthly or annual basis. New drugs for the treatment of HCV must be introduced that have minimum/no side effects and are cheaper. In recent years, several natural compounds having anti-HCV activities have been identified, but still many aspects related to their mechanisms of action have to be unveiled. In most cases, the only step that was investigated was the replication of the viral life cycle and NS3 protease assay-based conclusions were made in several older reports. However, EGCG and ladanein are proved to be potent entry inhibitors. Moreover, studies on the anti-HCV activity of quercetin demonstrated that it is a more active inhibitor of assembly, rather than the replication step of the viral life cycle. Therefore, it is recommended to carry out further animal studies in ideal models and well-designed clinical trials with larger sample sizes and a longer duration of treatment to further assess the efficacy and safety of plant-based medicines for HCV infection. Therefore, the journey toward treating HCV infections with natural compounds, from bench to bedside, still has a long way to go.

Conflict of interest

The authors declare that there is no conflict of interest.

References

Abdullah, Khan, M.A., et al., 2020. Exploration of hepatoprotective potential and phytochemicals of *Ziziphus oxyphylla* Edgew. Pakistan Vet. J. https://doi.org/10.29261/pakvetj/2020.054.

Afridi, S.Q., et al., 2013. Prevalence of HCV genotypes in district Mardan. Virol. J. 10 (1), 90.

Ahmed-Belkacem, A., et al., 2010. Silibinin and related compounds are direct inhibitors of hepatitis C virus RNA-dependent RNA polymerase. Gastroenterology 138 (3), 1112–1122.

Alborino, F., et al., 2011. Multicenter evaluation of a fully automated third-generation anti-HCV antibody screening test with excellent sensitivity and specificity. Med. Microbiol. Immunol. 200 (2), 77–83.

Alter, M.J., 2002. Prevention of spread of hepatitis C. Hepatology 36 (5B), s93–s98.

Ashfaq, U.A., et al., 2011. Inhibition of HCV 3a core gene through silymarin and its fractions. Virol. J. 8 (1), 153.

Bachmetov, L., et al., 2012. Suppression of hepatitis C virus by the flavonoid quercetin is mediated by inhibition of NS3 protease activity. J. Viral Hepat. 19 (2), e81–e88.

Baker, J.T., et al., 1995. Natural product drug discovery and development: new perspectives on international collaboration. J. Nat. Prod. 58 (9), 1325–1357.

Balick, M.J., Cox, P.A., 1997. Ethnobotanical research and traditional health care in developing countries. In: Medicinal Plants for Forest Conservation and Health Care. vol. 92, pp. 12–23.

Barrera, J., et al., 1995. Improved detection of anti-HCV in post-transfusion hepatitis by a third-generation ELISA. Vox Sang. 68 (1), 15–18.

Blaising, J., et al., 2013. Silibinin inhibits hepatitis C virus entry into hepatocytes by hindering clathrin-dependent trafficking. Cell. Microbiol. 15 (11), 1866–1882.

Brahmachari, G., 2012. Natural products in drug discovery: impacts and opportunities—an assessment. In: Bioactive Natural Products: Opportunities and Challenges in Medicinal Chemistry. World Scientific, pp. 1–199.

Brunt, E.M., 2010. Liver biopsy diagnosis of hepatitis: clues to clinically-meaningful reporting. Mo. Med. 107 (2), 113.

Calland, N., et al., 2012a. (−)-Epigallocatechin-3-gallate is a new inhibitor of hepatitis C virus entry. Hepatology 55 (3), 720–729.

Calland, N., et al., 2012b. Hepatitis C virus and natural compounds: a new antiviral approach? Viruses 4 (10), 2197–2217.

Campos-Outcalt, D., 2012. Hepatitis C: new CDC screening recommendations: screen everyone born between 1945 and 1965-regardless of risk level. J. Fam. Practice 61 (12), 744–747.

Chang, R.S., Yeung, H., 1988. Inhibition of growth of human immunodeficiency virus in vitro by crude extracts of Chinese medicinal herbs. Antiviral Res. 9 (3), 163–175.

Chen, S.L., Morgan, T.R., 2006. The natural history of hepatitis C virus (HCV) infection. Int. J. Med. Sci. 3 (2), 47.

Chen, C., et al., 2012. (−)-Epigallocatechin-3-gallate inhibits the replication cycle of hepatitis C virus. Arch. Virol. 157 (7), 1301–1312.

Chevaliez, S., Pawlotsky, J.M., 2009. How to use virological tools for optimal management of chronic hepatitis C. Liver Int. 29, 9–14.

Chhatwal, J., et al., 2016. Hepatitis C disease burden in the United States in the era of oral direct-acting antivirals. Hepatology 64 (5), 1442–1450.

Choo, Q.-L., et al., 1989. Isolation of a cDNA clone derived from a blood-borne non-A, non-B viral hepatitis genome. Science 244 (4902), 359–362.

Chow, H.S., et al., 2003. Pharmacokinetics and safety of green tea polyphenols after multiple-dose administration of epigallocatechin gallate and polyphenon E in healthy individuals. Clin. Cancer Res. 9 (9), 3312–3319.

Ciesek, S., et al., 2011. The green tea polyphenol, epigallocatechin-3-gallate, inhibits hepatitis C virus entry. Hepatology 54 (6), 1947–1955.

Colin, C., et al., 2001. Sensitivity and specificity of third-generation hepatitis C virus antibody detection assays: an analysis of the literature. J. Viral Hepat. 8 (2), 87–95.

de Paula Scalioni, L., et al., 2014. Performance of rapid hepatitis C virus antibody assays among high-and low-risk populations. J. Clin. Virol. 60 (3), 200–205.

Di Bisceglie, A.M., Hoofnagle, J.H., 2002. Optimal therapy of hepatitis C. Hepatology 36 (S1), S121–S127.

Dow, B., et al., 1996. Relevance of RIBA-3 supplementary test to HCV PCR positivity and genotypes for HCV confirmation of blood donors. J. Med. Virol. 49 (2), 132–136.

European Association for Study of Liver, 2014. EASL Clinical Practice Guidelines: management of hepatitis C virus infection. J. Hepatol. 60 (2), 392.

Ferrell, L.D., et al., 2007. Arterialization of central zones in nonalcoholic steatohepatitis (NASH). In: Hepatology. John Wiley & Sons Inc., Hoboken, NJ.

Fried, M.W., et al., 2002. Peginterferon alfa-2a plus ribavirin for chronic hepatitis C virus infection. N. Engl. J. Med. 347 (13), 975–982.

Fried, M.W., et al., 2012. Effect of silymarin (milk thistle) on liver disease in patients with chronic hepatitis C unsuccessfully treated with interferon therapy: a randomized controlled trial. JAMA 308 (3), 274–282.

Ghany, M.G., et al., 2011. An update on treatment of genotype 1 chronic hepatitis C virus infection: 2011 practice guideline by the American Association for the Study of Liver Diseases. Hepatology (Baltimore, Md.) 54 (4), 1433.

Gonzalez, O., et al., 2009. The heat shock protein inhibitor quercetin attenuates hepatitis C virus production. Hepatology 50 (6), 1756–1764.

Haid, S., et al., 2012. A plant-derived flavonoid inhibits entry of all HCV genotypes into human hepatocytes. Gastroenterology 143 (1), 213–222. e215.

Hanna, C.W., et al., 2012. DNA methylation changes in whole blood is associated with exposure to the environmental contaminants, mercury, lead, cadmium and bisphenol A, in women undergoing ovarian stimulation for IVF. Hum. Reprod. 27 (5), 1401–1410.

Hassan, S.T., et al., 2016. Plumbagin, a plant-derived compound, exhibits antifungal combinatory effect with amphotericin B against *Candida albicans* clinical isolates and anti-hepatitis C virus activity. Phytother. Res. 30 (9), 1487–1492.

Hawke, R.L., et al., 2010. Silymarin ascending multiple oral dosing phase I study in noncirrhotic patients with chronic hepatitis C. J. Clin. Pharmacol. 50 (4), 434–449.

Hoofnagle, J.H., 1999. Management of hepatitis C: current and future perspectives. J. Hepatol. 31, 264–268.

Hudson, J., 1989. Plant photosensitizers with antiviral properties. Antiviral Res. 12 (2), 55–74.

Hutchinson, S.J., et al., 2000. Factors associated with injecting risk behaviour among serial community-wide samples of injecting drug users in Glasgow 1990–94: implications for control and prevention of blood-borne viruses. Addiction 95 (6), 931–940.

Kamal, S.M., 2008. Acute hepatitis C: a systematic review. Am. J. Gastroenterol. 103 (5), 1283–1297.

Kamal, S.M., Nasser, I.A., 2008. Hepatitis C genotype 4: what we know and what we don't yet know. Hepatology 47 (4), 1371–1383.

Khan, N., et al., 2014. Geographic distribution of hepatitis C virus genotypes in pakistan. Hepat. Mon. 14 (10).

Khan, M.A., et al., 2017. Hepatoprotective effect of the solvent extracts of *Viola canescens* Wall. ex. Roxb. against CCl_4 induced toxicity through antioxidant and membrane stabilizing activity. BMC Complement. Altern. Med. 17 (1), 10.

Kitazato, K., et al., 2007. Viral infectious disease and natural products with antiviral activity. Drug Discov. Ther. 1 (1), 14–22.

Kong, L., et al., 2007. Inhibition of HCV RNA-dependent RNA polymerase activity by aqueous extract from Fructus Ligustri Lucidi. Virus Res. 128 (1–2), 9–17.

Lan, K.H., et al., 2012. Multiple effects of Honokiol on the life cycle of hepatitis C virus. Liver Int. 32 (6), 989–997.

Lavanchy, D., 2011. Evolving epidemiology of hepatitis C virus. Clin. Microbiol. Infect. 17 (2), 107–115.

Lee, S.R., et al., 2011. Evaluation of a new, rapid test for detecting HCV infection, suitable for use with blood or oral fluid. J. Virol. Methods 172 (1–2), 27–31.

Lindsay, K.L., et al., 2001. A randomized, double-blind trial comparing pegylated interferon alfa-2b to interferon alfa-2b as initial treatment for chronic hepatitis C. Hepatology 34 (2), 395–403.

Luo, G., et al., 2000. De novo initiation of RNA synthesis by the RNA-dependent RNA polymerase (NS5B) of hepatitis C virus. J. Virol. 74 (2), 851–863.

Mack, C.L., et al., 2012. NASPGHAN practice guidelines: diagnosis and management of hepatitis C infection in infants, children, and adolescents. J. Pediatr. Gastroenterol. Nutr. 54 (6), 838–855.

Magiorkinis, G., et al., 2009. The global spread of hepatitis C virus 1a and 1b: a phylodynamic and phylogeographic analysis. PLoS Med. 6 (12), e1000198.

Maher, L., et al., 2007. High hepatitis C incidence in new injecting drug users: a policy failure? Aust. N. Z. J. Public Health 31 (1), 30–35.

Manns, M.P., et al., 2001. Peginterferon alfa-2b plus ribavirin compared with interferon alfa-2b plus ribavirin for initial treatment of chronic hepatitis C: a randomised trial. Lancet 358 (9286), 958–965.

Martin, P., et al., 1998. Automated RIBA hepatitis C virus (HCV) strip immunoblot assay for reproducible HCV diagnosis. J. Clin. Microbiol. 36 (2), 387–390.

Mazhar, S.M., et al., 2009. Noninvasive assessment of hepatic steatosis. Clin. Gastroenterol. Hepatol. 7 (2), 135–140.

McHutchison, J.G., et al., 1998. Interferon alfa-2b alone or in combination with ribavirin as initial treatment for chronic hepatitis C. N. Engl. J. Med. 339 (21), 1485–1492.

Micallef, J., et al., 2006. Spontaneous viral clearance following acute hepatitis C infection: a systematic review of longitudinal studies. J. Viral Hepat. 13 (1), 34–41.

Mohd Hanafiah, K., et al., 2013. Global epidemiology of hepatitis C virus infection: new estimates of age-specific antibody to HCV seroprevalence. Hepatology 57 (4), 1333–1342.

Morishima, C., et al., 2010. Silymarin inhibits in vitro T-cell proliferation and cytokine production in hepatitis C virus infection. Gastroenterology 138 (2), 671–681. e672.

Murphy, D.G., et al., 2007. Use of sequence analysis of the NS5B region for routine genotyping of hepatitis C virus with reference to C/E1 and 5′ untranslated region sequences. J. Clin. Microbiol. 45 (4), 1102–1112.

Nahmias, Y., et al., 2008. Apolipoprotein B-dependent hepatitis C virus secretion is inhibited by the grapefruit flavonoid naringenin. Hepatology 47 (5), 1437–1445.

Nelson, P.K., et al., 2011. Global epidemiology of hepatitis B and hepatitis C in people who inject drugs: results of systematic reviews. Lancet 378 (9791), 571–583.

Neumann, A.U., et al., 1998. Hepatitis C viral dynamics in vivo and the antiviral efficacy of interferon-α therapy. Science 282 (5386), 103–107.

Nishimuro, H., et al., 2015. Estimated daily intake and seasonal food sources of quercetin in Japan. Nutrients 7 (4), 2345–2358.

Paradis, V., Bedossa, P., 2008. Definition and natural history of metabolic steatosis: histology and cellular aspects. Diabetes Metab. 34 (6), 638–642.

Pawlotsky, J.M., 2014. New hepatitis C therapies: the toolbox, strategies, and challenges. Gastroenterology 146 (5), 1176–1192.

Pawlotsky, J.M., 2016. The end of the hepatitis C burden: R eally? Hepatology 64 (5), 1404–1407.

Pawlotsky, J.-M., et al., 2004. Antiviral action of ribavirin in chronic hepatitis C. Gastroenterology 126 (3), 703–714.

Polyak, S.J., et al., 2007. Inhibition of T-cell inflammatory cytokines, hepatocyte NF-κB signaling, and HCV infection by standardized silymarin. Gastroenterology 132 (5), 1925–1936.

Poordad, F., Dieterich, D., 2012. Treating hepatitis C: current standard of care and emerging direct-acting antiviral agents. J. Viral Hepat. 19 (7), 449–464.

Poynard, T., et al., 1998. Randomised trial of interferon α2b plus ribavirin for 48 weeks or for 24 weeks versus interferon α2b plus placebo for 48 weeks for treatment of chronic infection with hepatitis C virus. Lancet 352 (9138), 1426–1432.

Pybus, O.G., et al., 2009. Genetic history of hepatitis C virus in East Asia. J. Virol. 83 (2), 1071–1082.

Reddy, B.U., et al., 2018. A natural small molecule inhibitor corilagin blocks HCV replication and modulates oxidative stress to reduce liver damage. Antiviral Res. 150, 47–59.

Rockstroh, J., et al., 2012. Increases in acute hepatitis C (HCV) incidence across Europe: which regions and patient groups are affected. In: 11th International Congress on Drug Therapy in HIV Infection (HIV11), Glasgow.

Roh, C., Jo, S.-K., 2011. (−)-Epigallocatechin gallate inhibits hepatitis C virus (HCV) viral protein NS5B. Talanta 85 (5), 2639–2642.

Saludes, V., et al., 2014. Tools for the diagnosis of hepatitis C virus infection and hepatic fibrosis staging. World J. Gastroenterol. 20 (13), 3431.

Samuelsson, G., Bohlin, L., 1999. Drugs of natural origin. In: A Textbook of Pharmacognosy, fourth ed. Swedish Pharmaceutical Press, Sweden.

Shibata, C., et al., 2014. The flavonoid apigenin inhibits hepatitis C virus replication by decreasing mature microRNA122 levels. Virology 462, 42–48.

Simmonds, P., 2001. 2000 Fleming Lecture. The origin and evolution of hepatitis viruses in humans. J. Gen. Virol. 82 (4), 693–712.

Simmonds, P., et al., 1994. A proposed system for the nomenclature of hepatitis C viral genotypes. Hepatology 19 (5), 1321–1324.

Smith, D.B., et al., 2014. Expanded classification of hepatitis C virus into 7 genotypes and 67 subtypes: updated criteria and genotype assignment web resource. Hepatology 59 (1), 318–327.

Tahan, V., et al., 2005. Sexual transmission of HCV between spouses. Am. J. Gastroenterol. 100 (4), 821–824.

van der Meer, A.J., et al., 2012. Association between sustained virological response and all-cause mortality among patients with chronic hepatitis C and advanced hepatic fibrosis. JAMA 308 (24), 2584–2593.

Wagoner, J., et al., 2010. Multiple effects of silymarin on the hepatitis C virus lifecycle. Hepatology 51 (6), 1912–1921.

Wagoner, J., et al., 2011. Differential in vitro effects of intravenous versus oral formulations of silibinin on the HCV life cycle and inflammation. PLoS One 6 (1), e16464.

Wang, L.S., et al., 2016. Hepatitis C—a clinical review. J. Med. Virol. 88 (11), 1844–1855.

Ward, J.W., et al., 2012. Hepatitis C virus prevention, care, and treatment: from policy to practice. Clin. Infect. Dis. 55 (Suppl. 1), S58–S63.

Wartelle-Bladou, C., et al., 2012. Hepatitis C therapy in non-genotype 1 patients: the near future. J. Viral Hepat. 19 (8), 525–536.

World Health Organization, 2015. WHO Guideline on the Use of Safety-Engineered Syringes for Intramuscular, Intradermal and Subcutaneous Injections in Health-Care Settings. World Health Organization.

World Health Organization, 2018. Guidelines for the Care and Treatment of Persons Diagnosed With Chronic Hepatitis C Virus Infection.

Wu, S.F., et al., 2012. Anti-hepatitis C virus activity of 3-hydroxy caruilignan C from *Swietenia macrophylla* stems. J. Viral Hepat. 19 (5), 364–370.

Zeuzem, S., et al., 2001. Viral kinetics in patients with chronic hepatitis C treated with standard or peginterferon α2a. Gastroenterology 120 (6), 1438–1447.

Zhu, Y.-P., et al., 2015. Host APOBEC3G protein inhibits HCV replication through direct binding at NS3. PLoS One 10 (3), e0121608.

Zuo, G., et al., 2007. Activity of compounds from Chinese herbal medicine *Rhodiola kirilowii* (Regel) Maxim against HCV NS3 serine protease. Antiviral Res. 76 (1), 86–92.

CHAPTER 4

Alcoholic liver disease

Anna Blázovics

Department of Pharmacognosy, Semmelweis University, Budapest, Hungary

4.1 Introduction

The direct elimination of alcohol is 2%–10% through the lungs and kidneys. Alcohol is only metabolized in insignificant amounts in the stomach and intestines with the most important site of metabolism being the liver at approximately 90%.

Alcohol is an energy source that represents 29.7 kJ/g of energy. Due to its molecular structure, alcohol solubles both in lipids and water, and it is easily absorbed from the gastrointestinal tract. It displaces the energy from natural nutrition, therefore causing malnutrition.

The amount of alcohol consumed plays a significant role in the development of liver diseases caused by alcohol. Women are significantly more susceptible to alcohol-related oxidative damage. The risk of cirrhosis in women is approximately three times higher than in men (Argawal, 1997; Blázovics, 1999; Bosron et al., 1988; Groenbaeck et al., 1995; Harada, 1990; Mizoi et al., 1994; EASL, 2018). Drinking alcohol is accompanied by the lack of folate, thiamine, and other vitamins. The amount of antioxidant molecules in the body is reduced. Vitamin A stored in the liver or its precursor β-carotene is also damaged. Secondary malabsorption is a consequence of gastrointestinal complications. Such complications are pancreatic insufficiency, an impaired nutritional hepatic metabolism, and the direct nutrient-damaging effect of alcohol itself (Degrell et al., 1980; Lieber, 1990, 1997a; Leo et al., 1993).

As a result of excessive alcoholism, liver changes of varying severity occur, such as alcoholic fatty liver, alcoholic hepatitis, and alcoholic cirrhosis. Symptoms of alcoholic cirrhosis include portal hypertension, varicose bleeding, ascites, spontaneous bacterial peritonitis, hepatic encephalopathy, hepatorenal syndrome, and finally hepatocellular carcinoma.

Alcoholic hepatitis can also cause diffuse interstitial fibrosis. The complete transformation of the liver structure eventually leads to the death of the patient (Koivisto et al., 1996; Meyer, 1996).

There are a number of metabolic abnormalities in the background of histological changes, which occur also in the rough deviation in redox status and are closely related to

Influence of Nutrients, Bioactive Compounds, and Plant Extracts in Liver Diseases. https://doi.org/10.1016/B978-0-12-816488-4.00010-3

alcohol-induced oxidative stress (Horváth and Blázovics, 1992; Horváth et al., 1992; Lewis and Paton, 1992; Lieber, 1997b; Nordmann and Rouach, 1996).

A higher blood alcohol concentration causes neurological symptoms, memory loss, lack of motor coordination, ataxia, mood changes, amnesia, and even aggression. General anesthesia, coma, and hypothermia may occur in alcohol poisoning (Gyires et al., 2017).

Besides the genetic background, the factors that aggravate the disease (obesity, metabolic syndrome, smoking, drug abuse, hepatitis virus infections, other diseases) should also be taken into consideration during treatment. Only 15%–20% of big drinkers will have cirrhosis (Pár and Pár, 2019).

In 2014, according to World Health Organization (WHO) data, the transplantation in cases of alcoholic liver disease ranked second (WHO, 2014).

A multicenter, prospective, national cohort study published in 2019 in JAMA Internal Medicine showed that the indication of alcohol-associated liver disease preceded the hepatitis C virus infection, given the successful treatment of HCV in liver transplantation in the United States. It is especially dangerous that transplantation is taking place at an increasingly young age (Brian et al., 2019).

The aim of this chapter is to summarize the toxic effect of alcohol and the causes and consequences of alcohol toxicity as well as to focus on alcohol-caused oxidative stress. The aim is also to show the genetic alterations in developing alcoholic liver diseases, and the role of cytokines, chemokines, adipocytokines in it and to point to the sex differences in alcohol sensitivity.

The aim is to discuss the problematic nature of alcohol as a depressant and the complex treatment of alcohol disease as well as the treatment of alcoholic liver diseases with vitamin supplements, nutrition, and medicines with natural ingredients to show the favorable and adverse effects.

Finally, we hope to show the use of some traditional herbal medicines in the treatment of alcoholic liver disease, discussing their favorable and adverse effects.

4.2 The cause and consequences of alcohol toxicity

4.2.1 Alcohol metabolism and oxidative stress

Ethanol is converted into acetaldehyde through three major metabolic pathways in the liver: in the cytosol, alcohol dehydrogenase; in the microsome, inducible microsomal ethanol oxidizing enzyme CYP2E1; and in the peroxisomes, the catalase. All these are involved in the transformation (Lieber, 1997b). Severe alcoholic poisoning or alcoholism is also known as a nonspecific metabolic pathway, direct esterification of fatty acids (Dan and Laposata, 1997).

During alcohol metabolism, primary and secondary free radical formations can be observed (Horváth and Blázovics, 1992; Lieber, 1997b; Hagymási et al., 2001).

Gene polymorphism of the encoding alcohol dehydrogenase (ADH) in the cytosol and mitochondrial aldehyde dehydrogenase (ALDH) isoenzymes are responsible for the kinetics of alcohol absorption and elimination. The appearance, activity, or absence of individual isoenzymes cause significant differences in sensitivity to alcohol (Bosron and Li, 1986; Bosron et al., 1988). ALDH activity is significantly reduced in chronic alcoholics. Acetaldehyde toxicity is manifested by the fact that acetaldehyde with proteins produces inactive enzymes, generates autoantibodies, and inhibits the DNA repair mechanism. Acetaldehyde accelerates glutathione (GSH) depletion, free radical mediated toxicity, and lipid peroxidation. Acetyl-CoA is formed from a portion of the acetate that enters the citrate cycle, and participates in lipid formation. Carbon dioxide and water are formed from most of the acetate in peripheral tissues (Dan and Laposata, 1997; Worral et al., 1993). Oxidative stress influences the immune system in several routes, promotes immune responses, and the interplay between oxidative stress and immunity forms autoantibody targeting CYP2E1 and oxidized phospholipids in the progression of alcohol-mediated liver injury (Vidali et al., 2008).

The ADH and ALDH isoenzymes work differently in the gastrointestinal tract (Yoshida, 1994; Wong et al., 2000), therefore several articles and cohort studies deal with the controversial role of alcohol consumption in the development of inflammatory bowel diseases (Yang et al., 2018; Bergmann et al., 2018).

Catalase can oxidize alcohol in vitro in the presence of H_2O_2. Nevertheless, H_2O_2 produced by catalase can contribute to the β-oxidation of fatty acids in peroxisomes. Although the oxidation of short-chain fatty acids in peroxisomes is not possible, octanoate oxidation was observed in the ADH deficiency (Lieber, 1997b).

It has been known that alcohol also inhibits the ω-oxidation degradation of leukotrienes due to increased NADH (nicotinamide adenine dinucleotide) concentration (Baumert et al., 1989).

In alcoholism, microsomal alcohol and acetaldehyde metabolisms also play a significant role. In the oxidation of alcohol and acetaldehyde, cytochrome P450 isoenzyme CYP2EI is involved, which is induced when alcohol is no longer physiologically eliminated due to the high alcohol content or in cases of severe alcoholism (Kunitoh et al., 1997). Genetic polymorphism of CYP2EI is also known (Hu et al., 1997).

Alcohol produces hydroxyl and ethoxyl radicals. The microsomal xenobiotic transformation enhances the free radical production and thus damages the liver's microsomal system. The induction of CYP2EI has an effect on liver oxidative damage because ethanol reacts with H_2O_2 formed by detoxification, forming a 1-hydroxyethyl free radical. Reactions of 1-hydroxyethyl free radicals and malondialdehyde with proteins induce immune reactions.

However, the IgG reactive hydroxyethyl protein adduct does not appear in alcoholics where CYP2EI induction is absent. IgG, produced against the malondialdehyde-protein adduct, also appears even when induced by CYP2EI and even if induction is not present. The formation of a 1-hydroxyethyl free radical contributes to the development of alcoholic liver disease (Dupont et al., 1998; Rao et al., 1996).

The CYP2E1 microsomal enzyme is one of the major ROS generators in the liver. Human CYP2A6 and its mouse analogue CYP2A5 are also induced by alcohol. In mice, the alcohol induction of CYP2A5 is CYP2E1-dependent, although CYP2A5 protects against the development of alcoholic liver disease (Lu and Cederbaum, 2018).

Alcoholism accelerates the hepatocyte absorption of iron. Iron plays a central role in lipid peroxidation and in consequential collagen formation and tissue necrosis (Beilby et al., 1992).

Glutathione, which can inhibit lipid peroxidation, is rapidly eliminated from the liver in alcoholism. This is due to the lack of sufficient methionine for the synthesis of cysteine, the main factor of glutathione synthesis. Because the concentration of *S*-adenosylmethionine (SAM) decreases in the cirrhotic liver considerably, GSH regeneration slows. In the absence of SAM, many other vital metabolic pathways also decrease. Methyl donation is extremely important in protein synthesis as well as the synthesis of catecholamines and nucleic acids, mainly DNA methylation. It influences the formation and fluidity of the membrane structure as it participates in the methylation of phosphatidylethanolamine and phosphatidylcholine (Blázovics and Sárdi, 2018; Blázovics et al., 2019).

Phosphatidylethanolamine methyltransferase activity decreases in alcoholics, affecting liver phospholipid synthesis. The lack of its activity causes membrane damage in alcoholic liver disease (Lieber, 1997b).

Among the methyl donor quaternary ammonium compounds involved in transmethylation that have been examined, the physiological effects of carnitine, choline, and betaine are outstanding.

Choline is an important molecule for acetylcholine, glycerophosphocholins, phosphocholine, and membrane phospholipid (phosphatidylcholine, sphingomyelin) synthesis, taking part in neurotransmission. The methyl group donor betaine is the derivate of cholin. Betain is needed to methionine synthesis from the homocysteine.

Methyl group donor compounds of different nutritional factors support the SAM synthesis. The correlations between redox homeostasis and the body's methyl pool were also justified (Finkelstein et al., 1972; Corbin and Zeisel, 2012; Sun et al., 2015; Blázovics and Sárdi, 2018).

Folic acid plays a catalytic role in transmethylation. Folic acid deficiency is associated with triglyceride accumulation in the liver in fatty liver disease and steatohepatitis. Folic acid intake changes the expression of the genes involved in lipid metabolism and metabolic syndrome (Zeisel et al., 1991; Corbin and Zeisel, 2012; Page and Mann, 2015).

The CYP2E1 gene can be methylated at the TATA box (noncoding DNA sequence) as well as at the first exon and intron at several points. In the embryonic age or during a drastic decline of CYP2E1 transcription, these regions are hypermethylated. The gene's volume and activity are mainly regulated at the translational and posttranslational levels (Ioannides, 1996; Umeno et al., 1988). In neoplasia, a "methylation imbalance" can be observed. Genome-wide hypomethylation can lead to chromosome instability, and hypomethylation leads to elevated mutation rates. Hypomethylation is accompanied by localized hypermethylation and an increased expression of DNA methyltransferase (Baylin et al., 1998; Baylin and Ohm, 2006; Blázovics et al., 2008).

Alcohol reduces DNA methyltransferase activity and reduced DNA methylation modifies the transcription of ADH-regulating genes, changes the expression of fibrosis-controlling genes, and increases the risk of hepatocellular carcinoma (Villanueva et al., 2015).

4.2.2 Genetic alterations in developing of alcoholic liver diseases

This chapter discusses only those genetic differences that are directly involved in the alcohol metabolism and does not address the results of genome-wide association studies and epigenetic alterations caused by alcohol, although the new genome-wide association studies can help in understanding the pathogenesis of alcohol (Pár and Pár, 2019).

The polymorphism of the genes encoding the alcohol dehydrogenase (ADH) and the mitochondrial aldehyde dehydrogenase (ALDH) isozymes is responsible for the absorption and elimination kinetics of the alcohol. The appearance, activity, or absence of individual isoenzymes causes significant differences in sensitivity to alcohol (Bosron and Li, 1986; Bosron et al., 1988; Whitfield, 1997). There are significant differences in the kinetic properties of the enzymes encoded by the ADH2, ADH3, and ALDH2 alleles. There is clear and convincing evidence of ALDH polymorphism and liver disease (Tsuritani et al., 1995).

In the 1990s, 12 aldehyde dehydrogenase genes were identified. These genes are localized on different chromosomes and encode enzymes capable of oxidizing a number of aliphatic and aromatic aldehydes. Metabolic abnormalities, including clinical symptoms, are associated with ALDH1, ALDH2, ALDH4, ALDH10, and SSDH (succinic semialdehyde) genes (Harada, 1990; Tsuritani et al., 1995; Yoshida et al., 1998).

Approximately 50% of the Asian population lacks the ALDH2 isoform. In their case, ALDH1 is expressed. Alcohol causes a disulfiram-like effect that in some sense provides protection against alcoholism. Human Class I ADH can also be detected in the gastrointestinal tract in epithelial cells of mucosa. Upper intestinal section sex and age-related differences can be detected while in the colon, there were no significant differences in ADH and ALDH activities. ADH and ALDH isoenzymes function to varying degrees in the gastrointestinal tract and the mucosa is damaged accordingly (Liao et al., 1991; Smith, 1986; Yin et al., 1993, 1994, 1997; Yoshida, 1994; Wang et al., 1993).

Recent research shows that alcohol dependence and alcoholic cirrhosis can be considered hereditary diseases (Farooq and Bataller, 2016; Stickel et al., 2011, 2017; Anstee et al., 2016) based on metaanalyses.

High alcohol dehydrogenase (ADH1B*2 rs1229984 variant) activity with increased hepatotoxicity provides some protection because of the hangover and bad feeling (Li et al., 2011). Low aldehyde dehydrogenase (ALDH2*2 rs671 variant) activity also protects via poor condition (Li et al., 2012). A low activity P450 CYP2E1 activity means protection. High P450 CYP2E1 (CYP2E1 * 5c2) activity increases liver damage, and it is common in cirrhosis. The occurrence of the CYP2E1 c1 allele and the ADH1C*1 homozygous represents a high risk for cirrhosis (Stickel et al., 2017; Anstee et al., 2016).

4.2.3 The role of cytokines, chemokines, and adipocytokines in alcoholic liver disease

In alcoholic liver disease, the importance of genes regulating immune processes increases. Genes that affect the severity of oxidative stress encode proteins that are responsible for the development of alcoholic liver disease and cirrhosis. There are two polymorphisms in the TNF-α (tumor necrosis factor-α) promoter region. The relationship between the TNF-α A allele and alcoholic hepatitis is significant. Plasma TNF-α, IL-1, and IL-6 (interleukins) concentrations are higher in patients with alcoholic liver disease than in healthy subjects (Baumert et al., 1989; Calabrese et al., 1998; Worral et al., 1991; Worral and Wilce, 1994).

The polymorphism of genes responsible for cytokine production may increase the risk of developing alcoholic liver disease in some cases. IL-10 is a pleiotropic cytokine with either immunosuppressive or immunostimulatory activities.

Gene polymorphism is responsible for the reduced production of cytokine IL-10; the appearance of the -592 A allele can also be associated with increased production of certain cytokines (IL-1, TNF-α, IL-6, IL-8, IL-12).

The IL-10 enhances the proliferation and immunoglobulin secretion of B lymphocytes. Its antiinflammatory effect is achieved by inhibiting the proinflammatory cytokine and chemokine synthesis of endotoxin-activated Kupffer cells and monocytes. Among other things, IL-10 reduces the rate of fibrosis in the liver by inhibiting collagen transcription and by enhancing the expression of the collagenase enzyme. Due to the polymorphism of the IL-10 promoter region, the secretion of IL-10 (627 * A allele/ATA haplotype) is reduced, which also contributes to fibrotic liver formation (Grove et al., 2000; Fiorentino et al., 1991; Taga and Tosato, 1992).

The nonparenchymal cells are only 6.5% of the liver volume. The walls of the hepatic sinusoid are lined by three different cell types: sinusoidal endothelial cells (SEC), Kupffer cells, and hepatic stellate cells (Ito cells). Intrahepatic lymphocytes, including pit cells that are specific natural killer cells, are often present in the sinusoidal lumen.

The sinusoidal SEC performs an important filtration function between the blood and the hepatocyte surface. The SEC may function as antigen-presenting cells (APC) in the context of both MHC-I and MHC-II (major histocompatibility complexes) restriction. The SEC secrete cytokines, eicosanoids, endothelin-1, and NO, among others.

Kupffer cells are hepatic macrophages that secrete potent mediators, reactive oxygen species, eicosanoids, prostaglandins, leukotrienes, NO, carbon monoxide, TNF-α, and other cytokines. High exposure of Kupffer cells can lead to the intensive production of inflammatory mediators, and ultimately to liver injury.

Kupffer cells secrete enzymes and cytokines that may damage hepatocytes, and are active in the remodeling of the extracellular matrix.

Hepatic stellate cells store vitamin A, control the turnover of the extracellular matrix, and regulate the contractility of sinusoids in the normal liver (Elpek, 2014).

During liver injury, resting stellate cells differentiate into myofibroblast-like cells and participate in connective tissue transformation and process maintenance. Myofibroblasts produce collagen, elastin, proteoglycans, glycoproteins, hyaluronic acid, TGF-α and TGF-β cytokines (transforming growth factors), chemokines, endothelin, NO, and matrix metalloproteinases. These cells produce TIMP-1 (tissue inhibitor of metalloproteinases) that regulates the catabolism of collagen (Kmieć, 2001; Gressner et al., 2007; Egresi et al., 2016).

The stellate cells can secrete leptin, which influences their own cell cycle. The leptin is a strong transcriptional stimulus in the activation of $\alpha 1$ and $\alpha 2$ fibrils; stimulates TIMP-1 and MMP-2 (matrix metalloproteinase-2) and the de novo mRNA synthesis of TIMP-1, TIMP-2, and α-SMA (α-smooth muscle actin); and thus plays a central role in fibrosis progression (Saxena and Anania, 2015).

Pit cells are hepatic NK cells that spontaneously kill a variety of tumor cells. This antitumor activity may be enhanced by the secretion of interferon-γ.

Substances released from nonparenchymal cells, prostanoids, nitric oxide, endothelin-1, TNF-α, interleukins, chemokines, and many growth factors, for example, TGF-β, PDGF, IGF-I, HGF, and ROS, are involved in the intercellular communication and regulate several hepatocyte functions.

The expression of cell surface ICAM-1 (intercellular adhesion molecule-1) and VCAM-1 (vascular cell adhesion molecule-1) facilitates the migration and adhesion of lymphocytes (Elpek, 2014).

Portal fibroblasts are transformed into myofibroblasts. Although they exhibit biological similarity to activated Ito cells, they differ significantly in their genetic characteristics and signal transduction responses. Fibrocytes are derived from hemopoietic stem cells. They are also able to transform into myofibroblasts, migrate to injured tissue, and produce growth factors that trigger the extracellular matrix deposition. It also implies the indirect role of dendritic cells in liver damage. It is assumed that these cells regulate the production and activity of CD8+ cells (cytotoxic T cell) (Elpek, 2014).

In advanced liver disease, levels of TNF-α, IL-6, IL-8, and hsCRP are significantly increased. TGF-α and TGF-ß increase liver cell death and fibrogenesis (Hagymási et al., 2013).

IL-8 plays a key role in hepatic neutrophil infiltration. Among alcoholics with higher levels of IL-8, there is a higher mortality rate (Neuman et al., 2015).

The levels of IL-6, inflammatory chemokines CCL2, CCL-5, IL-8, osteoportin, semaphorin 7A, CD-68, and TGF-β1 are higher in advanced liver injury. The mRNA expression of osteopontin, semaphorin 7A, and IL-8 chemokines is associated with severe fatty degeneration (Neuman et al., 2015; Morales-Ibanez et al., 2013).

The adiponectin produced by the white adipose tissue binds to the AdipoR-1 and AdipoR-2 receptor produced by the liver cells, and exerts its antifibrotic effect. It inhibits the activity and proliferation of Ito cells and participates in matrix breakdown. The role of plasminogen activator inhibitor-1 (PAI-1), resistin, apelin, visfatin, etc. currently studied in fibrosis in the area (Saxena and Anania, 2015).

4.2.4 Sex differences in alcohol sensitivity

Epidemiological studies show that women are more sensitive to the toxic effects of alcohol than men (Morgan and Sherlock, 1977). In women, cirrhosis and alcohol-related complications develop over a shorter period of time. The lifespan of alcoholic women is shorter, although the probability of developing primary liver cancer is lower (Stein and Cyr, 1997).

There are gender differences in the pharmacokinetics of alcohol. In women, the maximum alcohol concentration and area under the blood alcohol concentration-time curve are significantly higher than in men. Men's higher body weight or water weight results in higher alcohol distribution and lower blood alcohol levels (Kwo et al., 1998).

Animal studies showed that CYP isozymes of castrated male guinea pigs differed from the noncastrated individuals' isoenzyme profile by alcohol. In castrated animals, the induction of CYP2E1 and CYP2A was observed while in noncastrated animals, CYP2E1 and CYP3A isoenzymes were observed. In noncastrated animals, the expression of CYP isozymes was less pronounced and the concentration of the acetaldehyde protein adducts was associated with these. Thus, gender differences in the microsome also occur in the metabolism of ethanol (Niemelä et al., 1999).

The ADH6 gene contains hormone-sensitive elements. In the rat experiment, it was found that androgen inhibited ADH activity while progestin and estrogen increased ADH activity in the cytosol (Yoshida, 1994; Harada et al., 1998).

The ADH activity of the stomach is lower in women, so "first pass" activity is not sufficient during alcohol drinking (Marshall et al., 1983; Frezza et al., 1990).

Fukunaga and coworkers found significant levels of acetaldehyde in women's blood while acetaldehyde could hardly be detected in men (Fukunaga et al., 1993).

There was a difference between the genders in the immune response. In an animal experiment, it was established that long-term alcohol consumption induces hepatic macrophages, and in females a higher immune response could be found than males (Yamada et al., 1999).

In another study, alcohol increased the proportion of CD4+ (T-helper cells) in male animals while in females, IgM and IgG secretion were increased (Grossman et al., 1993).

There was a difference between genders in fat metabolism due to alcohol consumption. Alcohol acts to reduce the β-oxidation of fatty acids in mitochondria, but increases the compensatory microsomal ω-oxidation and β-oxidation in peroxysomes. In women, these auxiliary mechanisms are not sufficient for fat burning, therefore fat accumulation is increased (Ma et al., 1999).

After 1 month of medically acceptable red wine consumption, TNF at alpha levels in men (3 dL/day) and vascular endothelial (VEGF) and epithelial growth factor (EGF) and IL1a and IL-2 levels in women (2 dL/day) a significant increase by the end of the term was found. In men, VEGF and EGF levels were decreased to detract from wine consumption.

Ca, Sr, and Pb levels decrease significantly during wine consumption in both sexes. A significant decrease in Zn and Mg concentrations was detected in women. In men, VEGF and EGF levels decreased as a result of wine consumption.

At the same time in men, the levels of VEGF and EGF were reduced significantly and Zn and Mg concentrations in women at the end of the study. The Ca, Sr, and Pb levels are significantly reduced during wine consumption in both sexes (Bekő et al., 2007, 2008).

A prospective study was to estimate gender differences in anxiety, depression, and alcohol use severity among patients with alcohol use disorder before and after a detoxification program and within 12 months after discharge.

The predictive value of anxiety and depression for alcohol relapse was analyzed by logistic and linear regression. In both genders, the psychopathological dimension that showed the most significant worsening at the 6-month follow-up, that is, anxiety in males and depression in females, was found to be a significant predictor of relapse at the 12-month follow-up (Oliva et al., 2018).

4.3 Alcohol as a depressant

Alcohol acts on the central nervous system as a depressant, like sedatives. Alcohol disrupts cognitive functions. Dopamine has a prominent role in the reward-driven property. The anatomical basis is primarily the mesolimbic dopaminergic system.

The sensitizing effect of alcohol is likely to be expressed by $GABA_A$ (γ-aminobutyric acid) receptors. It exerts its inhibitory effect via glutamate-NMDA (*N*-methyl-D-aspartate) receptors. The reward route activity is increasing with the activation of nicotinic ACh (acetylcholine) receptors. Alcohol affects the $5-HT_3$ (5-hidroxi-triptamin) receptors of serotonin, the Na^+ channels on Ca^{2+} channels, and Na^+/K^+-ATP-ase (adenosine triphosphatase), especially at toxic concentrations (Gyires et al., 2017).

Dopaminergic modulation of corticostriatal transmission is involved in reward-driven behaviors. Modulation is mainly mediated by dopamine receptors, which are highly expressed in medium spiny neurons of the dorsomedial striatum. This region is essential for behaviors and addiction.

Excessive alcohol intake selectively strengthens glutamatergic transmission at the $D2 \rightarrow D1$ synapse, and it is hypothesized that this circuit may play a critical role in the pathogenesis of alcohol use disorder.

Dopaminergic neurons are associated with the medial cerebral hemisphere, the posterior ventral tegmental area, the medial shell nucleus accumbens, the prefrontal cortex, and the medial olfactory tubercle (Lu et al., 2019).

Addiction is a chronic disease accompanied by frequent relapses. Dependence develops. The rewarding and reinforcing effects of alcohol are comparable to drugs.

Long-term consumption of alcohol leads to a transformation of the dopamine system. Chronic alcohol consumption causes decreasing dopaminergic activity while the response to alcohol is increasing, leading to depression and lack of motivation.

In an experimental study, the gene expression profile of different parts of the brain (prefrontal cortex, ventral-tegmental area, nucleus accumbens) showed that alcohol acted differently on the metabolism of certain brain areas in mice (Broom et al., 2019).

These results will help better understand the effects of alcohol.

4.4 Complex treatment of alcohol disease

Alcohol abuse and alcoholism are significant problems not only from a medical point of view, but also from a social one. Alcohol usage by juveniles and adolescents is common. Alcohol causes severe irreversible neurocognitive damage, behavioral changes, and physiological alterations during early ages (Jain and Balhara, 2010). Alcoholic patient therapy should not be undertaken without a psychological approach.

The complex treatment of alcoholic patients should not only reduce or cure liver damage and damage to other organs (gastrointestinal tract, pancreas, cardiovascular system, kidney), but it is also important, that the nervous system symptoms and cravings for alcohol should be reduced so the treatment could be effective. For the sake of success, full abstinence is needed (Grancini et al., 2015).

Clinical observations confirm that prolonged withdrawal of alcohol can lead to regression of steatohepatitis and fibrosis as well as cirrhosis compensation, and that survival can also increase at an advanced stage (Pár and Pár, 2019).

Alcoholism treatment mostly includes difficult and long-lasting psychotherapy and in some cases, quite controversial pharmacological approaches. Lots of medicinal plants and drugs of natural origin are reported to have preventive and therapeutic effects on alcoholism and alcohol dependence, although in several cases their bioactive components, efficacy, and mechanism of action are mostly unknown so far (Tomczyk et al., 2012).

However, it should be stated that prescription drugs and herbal medications used simultaneously can be dangerous. Medical supervision is required.

4.4.1 Treatment of alcoholic liver diseases with vitamin supplements, nutrition, and medicaments with natural ingredients: Favorable and adverse effects

The treatment of alcoholic liver diseases depends on the severity and stage of the disease. The alcohol-induced mildest and reversible stage of steatosis can be cured with total abstinence, protein, a vitamin-rich diet, and adequate calorie intake in the case of malnourished patients. The healing time is relatively short, a few weeks.

Excessive alcohol intake also causes damage to the intestinal tract, therefore pre- and probiotics are also needed for the optimization of the bowel liver axis (Egresi et al., 2017).

Prebiotics include chicory root, dandelion root, garlic, leek, asparagus, banana, cereals, etc.

The proven effective probiotic bacterial strains include:

Bifidobacterium animalis DN 173 010, Bifidobacterium animalis subsp. lactis BB-12, Bifidobacterium breve Yakult, Bifidobacterium infantis 35624, Bifidobacterium lactis HN019 (DR10), Bifidobacterium longum BB536, Escherichia coli Nissle 1917, Lactobacillus acidophilus LA-5, Lactobacillus acidophilus NCFM, Lactobacillus casei DN114-001, Lactobacillus casei CRL431, Lactobacillus casei F19, Lactobacillus casei Shirota, Lactobacillus casei immunitass, Lactobacillus johnsonnii La1 (= Lactobacillus LC1),

Lactobacillus plantarum 299V, Lactobacillus reuteri ATTC 55730, Lactobacillus reuteri SD2112, Lactobacillus rhamnosus ATCC 53013, Lactobacillus rhamnosus LB21, Lactobacillus salivarius UCC118, Lactococcus lactis L1A, Saccharomyces cerevisiae (boulardii) lyo, and *Streptococcus salivarius ssp. thermophilus* (https://www.tankonyvtar.hu/en/tartalom/tamop412A/2010-0008_farma/adatok.html).

During nutrition, attention should be paid to the formation of a diet containing methyl group donor compounds, considering the replacement of *S*-adenosylmethionine and the restoration of redox homeostasis.

Folate has a significant role as a catalyst in the transmethylation processes. A choline-deficient diet with normal folate and vitamin B12 intake caused liver steatosis. At the same time, folate deficiency increased the demand for choline (Zeisel and Blusztajn, 1994; Kim et al., 1995; Zeisel et al., 2003; Craig, 2004)

Some foods contain high levels of choline and/or betaine (Blázovics and Sárdi, 2018):

- Plant origin: cereals; generally the seeds; dried basil; curry powder; mustard seed, paprika and garlic powder; cloves, ginger (~ 10–50 mg moiety/g food).
- Animal origin: eggs; chicken liver and meat; clam; fish; beef, veal, lamb and turkey meat (~ 50–300 mg moiety/g food).

Vegetables and fruits contain insignificant choline and betaine (~ 0.0–10 mg moiety/g food). The exception is table beet. This vegetable contains betaine at ~ 260 mg/g. Adequate intake: 550 mg/day for adult men and 425 mg/day for adult women (Nutrient Data Laboratory Agricultural Research Service U.S. Department of Agriculture, 2008).

Vitamin supplementation will only be effective if the patients actually avoid drinking alcohol and follow the vitamin supplement instructions prescribed by the doctor. Alcohol, vitamin A, and its precursor beta-carotene, due to the parallel induction of liver microsomes, increase the toxicity of vitamin A. Hypervitaminosis causes severe liver damage. Beta-carotene consumption induces isoenzymes of CYP1A1/2, CYP3A1/2, CYP2E1, CYP2B1/2, and CYP2C19, which cause the excessive production of free radicals (Paolini et al., 2001; Blázovics and Fehér, 1996).

Vitamin E has also been shown to increase free radical production (Witting, 1980). Tocopheroxyl free radicals can be converted to an active antioxidant form by vitamin C and glutathione.

Vitamin C also induces the CYP2E1 isoenzyme. Genotoxicity is attributed to the effect of xanthine oxidase (Herbert, 1993). Vitamins combined with alcohol enhance free radical formations. These antioxidant vitamins, besides their scavenger properties, are signal transducer molecules, so their effect cannot be explained by scavenger ability (Azzi et al., 2004; Lunec et al., 2002).

Alcoholics often suffer from vitamin D deficiency, and therefore supplementation of this vitamin is required (Trépo et al., 2013). It was established that vitamin D3 treatment caused differences in the metal and redox homeostasis. The concentration of Fe, Cr, and Pb significantly increased in the erythrocytes of prostate cancer patients. Therefore, the accumulation of these elements by vitamin D3 supplementation needs to be taken into more serious consideration in set terms of occupational diseases (Süle et al., 2018).

Alcohol-induced, more severe, toxic liver damage can be cured effectively with the active flavanolignane ingredients of *Silybum marianum*. Silibinin and multicomponent silymarin have been shown to effectively reduce the development and progression of liver cirrhosis. Due to the choleretic effect of these molecules are contraindicated in extrahepatic obstruction. The laxative effect should be taken into account for the function of the gut-liver axis (Egresi et al., 2017; Hagymási et al., 2018).

In addition to their antioxidant properties, bioactive polyphenols, including flavonoids, can affect many metabolic and catabolic pathways. They can participate in the regulation of protein synthesis. For example, silibinin enters the nucleus, stimulates the activity of the polymerase A, and enhances the transcription of the ribosomal RNA, enhancing protein synthesis (Sonnenbichler and Zetl, 1984; Sonnenbichler et al., 1986). The ability of silibinin to enhance SOD activity is also acknowledged (Hagymási and Blázovics, 2004).

It is known that silybin, silydianin, and silychristine, the isomers of silibinin, are prostaglandin synthetase inhibitors (Fiebrich and Koch, 1979). Thus, they influence signal transduction by indirect routes (Blázovics, 2007).

It was established that silibinin induced hepatic stellate cell cycle arrest via enhancing p53/p27 and inhibiting Akt downstream signaling protein expression. Sirtuin activity also was correlated to silibinin-inhibited proliferation of LX-2 cells. This study gives an insight into the molecular pathways of the silibinin antifibrogenic effect (Ezhilarasan et al., 2017).

Several mechanisms of *Silybum marianum* flavanolignanes have been demonstrated on cellular and molecular pathways as an apoptotic inducer, autophagy modulator, cell cycle inhibitor, and microRNAs regulator as well as an immunomodulator, which supports the beneficial effect of silibinin on healing alcoholic patients (Horváth et al., 2001; Jahanafrooz et al., 2018; Liu et al., 2019; Verdura et al., 2018; Esmaeil et al., 2017; Byun et al., 2017; Neha Jaggi and Singh, 2016).

BDNF/TrkB (brain-derived neurotrophic factor/tropomyosin receptor kinase B) signaling provides a beneficial microenvironment for neuronal survival, neurodevelopment, and neurogenesis. Li and coworkers hypothetized that silibinin may exert antidepressant effects through neurogenesis and/or a BDNF/TrkB signaling transduction signaling pathway to improve neural stem cell proliferation in acute depression. They did not exclude the possibility that silibinin may undergo antioxidation and/or antiinflammation activities through other pathways (Li et al., 2018).

The active ingredients in methadoxine are the pyridoxine (vitamin B6) and pyrrolidone-carboxylate ion pairs, which increase the activity of alcohol and acetaldehyde dehydrogenase enzymes and the degradation of ethanol, thus reducing the damaging effect of acetaldehyde on mitochondria. Metadoxine increases the concentration of glutathione, NADH, and ATP and reduces lipid peroxidation. It has an antifibrotic effect and it is favorable in reducing alcohol-induced mental decline. In manifested hepatic encephalopathy Metadoxine is contraindicated. It causes hypersensitivity in atopic patients. It antagonizes the effect of L-DOPA (L-3,4-dihydroxyphenylalanine) so it is not recommended in Parkinson's disease (Annoni et al., 1988; Caballeria et al., 1998; Jacob and Burri, 1996; Hagymási et al., 2000; Pár, 2000).

In order to prevent free radical damage in alcoholic liver disease, Slater and Eakins (1983) and his research group studied the antioxidant effect of polyphenols.

The (+)-cyanidanol-3, the active ingredient of (Catergen/ZYMA), was used for many years in the treatment of liver disease in alcoholics due to its antioxidant property, but the medicine caused hemolytic anemia (assuming alcohol consumption) and the death of several Italian patients; Catergen was withdrawn from pharmacies. In our own early studies, we also demonstrated the antioxidant activity of the compound and at the same time its inhibitory effects on $Na^+ K^+$-ATPase and Mg^{++}-ATPase activities (Slater and Eakins, 1983; Blázovics et al., 1989).

Based on a number of research findings, resveratrol would be expected to provide protection against alcoholic liver damage. Recently, however, contradictory research results have emerged. Based on the small number of clinical studies, the effect is controversial as well. There is a problem with the limitation of the application, the dose, and the time of therapy (McGill et al., 2015). New research findings confirmed that antioxidants of red wine do not protect against the harmful effects of alcohol in alcoholism (Chachay et al., 2014)

Resveratrol is not considered a panacea, so there is no positive effect on the treatment of alcoholics. This is because resveratrol can bind methyl groups, reducing the role of S-adenosylmethionine in transmethylation (Blázovics et al., 2019; Molnár et al., 2008; Tyihák et al., 1998).

Resveratrol impairs redox homeostasis at high concentrations (12.03 mg/L of red wine), reduces the activity of natural antioxidant protection (GSHPx), and increases lipid peroxidation (diene conjugates) (Blázovics et al., 2019).

Resveratrol can act on multiple molecular targets. It can inhibit the activity of various CYP enzymes and their expression through various nuclear factors, and can influence Phase II enzymes, enhancing fibrosis. Resveratrol along with alcohol consumption enhances autophagy (Wu et al., 2012; McGill et al., 2015).

4.4.2 Some traditional herbal medicines in complex treatment of alcoholists: Favorable and adverse effects

The efficacy of herbal preparations used to combat alcoholism for centuries has recently been confirmed in animal experiments. The active ingredients of these plants help relieve the consequences of alcohol abuse syndrome and maintain abstinence (Abenavoli et al., 2009). Multiple herbal drugs and herbal preparations can be incorporated into the therapy of alcoholic patients. One important area of research is understanding the chemistry of craving, and the cure for this pathologic condition.

4.4.2.1 Hypericum perforatum L. (St. John's wort)

The beneficial effects of *Hypericum perforatum* leaves and flowers, known from the literature, which contain the phloroglucinol derivatives hyperforin, adhyperforin and antraquinone derivatives such as hypercine, pseudohypericin, flavonol glycosides, biflavones, phenylpropanes, proanthocyanidins, tannins, xanthones, and some amino acids such as gamma-amminobutyric acid (Barnes et al., 2001).

The main active component of *Hypericum perforatum* is hyperforin, which has an antidepressant property. This molecule inhibits the uptake of serotonin and noradrenaline into synaptic nerve endings and increases the extracellular concentration of acetylcholine, glutamate, and gamma-aminobutyric acid. It also influences the intracellular sodium concentration and interacts with several receptors and ion channels (Abenavoli et al., 2009).

St. John's wort is known for having many interactions with drugs and foods, therefore the secure application must be in abstinence.

4.4.2.2 Pueraria lobate Willd. (Ohwi kudzu)

Kudzu has been widely used in the treatment of cardiovascular diseases, diabetes, osteonecrosis, and neurodegradation diseases in traditional Chinese medicine. The active ingredients of the *Pueraria lobata* flowers and root are the isoflavon derivatives puerarin, daidzin, and daidzein. In an experimental study during the intraperitoneal administration of a crude extract of the *Pueraria lobate* root, the alcohol intake diminished (Keung and Vallee, 1993). Daidzin inhibits the aldehyde dehydrogenase (ALDH-2) selectively. Direct correlation was demonstrated between ALDH-2 inhibition and suppression (Keung, 2003). Puerarin has an anticarcerogenic property as well (Rezvani et al., 2003). The isoflavonoid-rich extract prepared from kudzu root has potential action as a protector for vascular endothelial cells against intracellular ROS-mediated apoptosis and mitochondrial damage (Gao et al., 2016).

In a study on alcohol-preferring rats, the kudzu root extract contained 150 mg/g of puerarin, 13 mg/g of daidzin, 4 mg/g of daidzein, 3 mg/g of genistin, 0.2 mg/g of genistein, and 1 mg/g of glycetin. Blood and liver samples contained mostly puerarin and a trace amount of daidzein derivative that may have been formed by the hydrolysis of daidzin by liver enzymes. An important observation was that brain samples of treated rats did not contain any of the kudzu root isoflavones. Thus, these isoflavones suppressed alcohol drinking and withdrawal symptoms without entering the brain (Benlhabib et al., 2004).

4.4.2.3 Salvia miltiorrhiza *Bge. (Danshen)*

Tanshinone and miltirone diterpene derivatives from the *Salvia miltiorrhiza* root reduced the alcohol intake or suppressed the desire for alcohol in animal models. Miltirone failed to affect the severity of alcohol withdrawal syndrome. The positive effects of miltirone are explained with the anxiolytic effect (Carai et al., 2000; Colombo et al., 2006; Lee et al., 1991).

In a Wistar rat experiment, the effect of *Salvia miltiorrhiza* extracts with different miltirone content was assessed. It was found that the reducing effect of different extracts on alcohol intake was positively and significantly correlated with their miltirone content. Miltirone as a control markedly reduced blood alcohol levels when alcohol was administered i.g., suggesting that miltirone hampered alcohol absorption from the gastrointestinal system. Miltirone reduced the alcohol intake in alcohol-experienced rats and delayed acquisition of alcohol-drinking behavior in alcohol-naive rats. It was also documented that miltirone failed to affect the severity of alcohol withdrawal syndrome in alcohol-dependent rats (Colombo et al., 2006).

4.4.2.4 Tabernanthe iboga *H. Bn. (Ibogaine)*

It has been hypothesized that derivate of ibogaine, a psychoactive indole alkaloid, stimulates dopaminergic and serotonergic systems (Glick et al., 1991; Rezvani et al., 1995). Animal experiments strengthen that the iboganine reduces the desire for alcohol in intraperitoneal or intragastrical treatment (Rezvani et al., 2003).

4.4.2.5 Panax ginseng *C. A. Mey. (Ginseng)*

Data in the literature confirm that saponines of red ginseng increase the rate of ethanol oxidation, accelerate alcohol clearance, accelerate the removal of acetaldehyde, and prevent memory failure (Saito et al., 1984; Lee et al., 1987; Kwak and Joo, 1988).

Water extracts of *Panax ginseng* and *Hippophae rhamnoides* have long been used in the treatment of acute alcohol intoxication with great confidence as complementary therapeutic agents. The beneficial effects of aqueous solutions of these two drugs were demonstrated in animal experiments. As a result of the treatments, the activity of the liver alcohol dehydrogenase and aldehyde dehydrogenase enzymes increased and the activity of the microsomal ethanol oxidase was decreased in the *male Kunming mice* liver. The aqueous extract strongly reduced β-endorphin and leucine-enkephalin concentrations in the brain and increased survival in acute toxicosis (Wen et al., 2016).

4.4.2.6 Piper methysticum *G. Forst. (Kava)*

Several studies have investigated whether the anxiolytic or antipsychotic properties of Kava pyrones and kava juice can be attributed to an alternative of alcoholism. In an investigation, the patients reported a reduction in their desire for their drug of choice. In another investigation, a standardized amount of kavapyrones led to an apparent difference in abstinence between the experimental and placebo groups for alcohol. Therefore, it was assumed that the neurological process of craving can be interrupted, and the addiction can be successfully treated by kavapyrones. These pyrones have been found to bind to many sites in the brain that are associated with addiction and craving (Cawte, 1986; Steiner, 2001).

However, the hepatotoxicity of kava is reported, including cases of liver transplantation and death. Kava has had its use prohibited or restricted in several countries. Toxicity may be related to overdosage. However, factors such as the botanical characteristics of the plant as well as the harvesting, storage, and production process may be associated with the development of hepatotoxic substances, such as triggering idiosyncratic reactions (Becker et al., 2019).

4.4.2.7 Morus nigra *L. (mulberry)* and Taraxacum coreanum *Nakai (dandelion)*

Recently, it was reported that water extracts of mulberry and white flower dandelion had beneficial effects on chronic ethanol-induced hepatic steatosis in male Sprague Dawley rats. In this study, it was demonstrated that aqueous extracts protected rats against ethanol-induced losses in lean body and bone masses, improved glucose tolerance, and partially normalized gut bacterial populations. The mulberry extract was generally more effective. These results are encouraging to carry out clinical trials (Park et al., 2018).

4.4.2.8 Hovenia dulcis *Thunb. (Japanese raisin tree)*

It was observed that the aqueous extract of *Hovenia dulcis* reduced the blood alcohol concentration and increased the activity of ADH after given alcohol. It means the extract has the effect of relieving alcohol toxicity, restraining the absorption of alcohol from the gastrointestinal tract, and promoting the metabolism of alcohol in the liver (Chen et al., 2006).

In a human study, male adults with heterozygous ALDH2 consumed Korean Soju (50 g alcohol) together with *Hovenia dulcis* fruit extract (HDE/2460 mg) or a matched placebo with subsequent crossover. Declines in hangover symptom scores were significant in the HDE group compared to the placebo group. Significant differences between groups were also observed on interleukin (IL-6, IL-10, IL-10/IL-6 ratio) and aspartate aminotransferase levels. There were positive correlations between total hangover symptom scores and IL-6 and IL-10 levels. Further analyses by CYP2E1 polymorphism at rs10776687, rs2031920, rs3813867, and rs4838767 alleles showed a reversed association, suggesting that CYP2E1 polymorphism might be an effect modifier (Kim et al., 2017).

Table 4.1: Some traditional herbal medicines and their effects in alcoholism.

Plants	Main bioactive agents	Main effects
Hypericum perforatum L. (*St. John's wort*)	Phloroglucinol derivatives hypercine	Antidepressant, inhibits the uptake of serotonin and noradrenaline in human study
Pueraria lobate Willd. (Ohwi kudzu)	Isoflavon derivatives daidzin	ALDH-2 inhibition, suppression in animal experiment
Salvia miltiorrhiza Bge. (Danshen)	Diterpene derivatives tanshinone, miltirone	Reduces alcohol intake or suppresses desire in animal experiment
Tabernanthe iboga H. Bn. (Ibogaine)	Ibogaine	Stimulates dopaminergic and serotonergic systems in animal experiment
Panax ginseng C. A. Mey. (Ginseng) with *Hippophae rhamnoides* L. (sea-buckthorn) water extract	Saponines the active compound not determined	Accelerates alcohol clearance reduce β-endorphin and leucine-enkephalin concentrations increase survival in acute toxicosis in animal experiment
Piper methysticum G. Forst. (Kava)	Kavapyrones	Anxiolytic or antipsychotic properties in human study side effect: hepatotoxicity
Morus nigra L. (mulberry) with *Taraxacum coreanum* Nakai (dandelion) water extract	Flavonoids the active compound not determined	Moderates hepatic steatosis Improves glucose tolerance Protects bone masses Partially normalizes gut bacterial populations in animal experiment
Hovenia dulcis Thunb. (Japanese raisin tree)	The active compound not determined	Reduces the blood alcohol concentration and increases the activity of ADH CYP2E1 polymorphism might be an effect modifier Improves hangover symptoms in a human study

Another research team confirmed that in a randomized, double-blind, placebo-controlled study involving healthy young men with the ALDH2*1/2 genotype, the acute alcohol consumption does not seem to cause dysfunction of intestine permeability leading to endotoxemia. Also, the *H. dulcis* fruit extract may have the potential to improve hangover symptoms and alcohol-induced hepatic damage (Kim et al., 2016) (Table 4.1).

4.5 Conclusions

The treatment of alcoholic individuals depends on the severity and stage of their disease. First and foremost, to be successful, drinking alcohol must be avoided. In the mildest and reversible stages, for example vitamin D, folate, adequate calorie intake, and pre- and probiotics as well as a diet containing methyl group donor compounds are needed.

Alcohol-induced free radical toxicity can be cured with the flavanolignanes of *Silybum marianum* by their scavenger properties, and the pyridoxine (vitamin B6) and pyrrolidone-carboxylate ion pairs of metadoxine because these molecules increase the concentration of glutathione, therefore improving the antioxidant capacity of the liver.

Alcohol as a depressant disrupts the cognitive functions. Therefore, some traditional herbal medicines *such as Hypericum perforatum, Pueraria lobate, Salvia miltiorrhiza, Tabernanthe iboga, Panax ginseng, Hippophae rhamnoides, Morus nigra, Taraxacum coreanum,* and *Hovenia dulcis* are used or recommended to combat alcoholism.

The various active ingredients of these herbs, such as phloroglucinol, isoflavone, diterpene derivatives, saponins or flavonoids are capable of acting through a variety of mechanisms of action.

Some molecules inhibit the uptake of serotonin and noradrenaline or stimulate dopaminergic and other serotonergic systems as well as suppress the desire for alcohol. They, respectively, accelerate alcohol clearance, reduce β-endorphin and leucine-enkephalin concentrations, reduce the blood alcohol concentration in different ways, or moderate hepatic steatosis. In this complex task, properly applied herbal preparations can help.

In the irreversible state, the above-mentioned agents are ineffective.

References

Abenavoli, L., Capasso, F., Addolorato, G., 2009. Phytotherapeutic approach to alcohol dependence: new old way? Phytomedicine 16, 638–644.

Annoni, G., Khlat, B., Lampertico, P., Dell'Oca, M., Dioguardi, F.S., 1988. Metadoxine (Metadoxil) in alcoholic liver diseases. Clin. Trials J. 25, 333–341.

Anstee, Q.M., Seth, D., Day, C.P., 2016. Genetic factors that affect risk of alcoholic and nonalcoholic fatty liver disease. Gastroenterology 150, 1728–1744.

Argawal, D.P., 1997. Molecular genetic aspects of alcohol metabolism and alcoholism. Pharmacopsychiatry 30, 79–84.

Azzi, A., Gysin, R., Kempná, P., Munteanu, A., Villacorta, L., Visarius, T., Zingg, J.M., 2004. Regulation of gene expression by alpha tocopherol. Biol. Chem. 385, 585–591.

Barnes, J., Anderson, L.A., Phillipson, J.D., 2001. St. John's wort (Hypericum perforatum L.): a review of its chemistry, pharmacology and clinical properties. J. Pharm. Pharmacol. 53, 583–600.

Baumert, T., Huber, M., Mayer, D., Kepper, D., 1989. Ethanol-induced inhibition of leucotriene degradation by omega-oxidation. Eur. J. Biochem. 182, 223–229.

Baylin, S.B., Ohm, J.E., 2006. Epigenetic gene silencing in cancer—a mechanism for early oncogenic pathway addiction? Nat. Rev. Cancer 6, 107–116.

Baylin, S.B., Herman, J.G., Graff, J.R., Vertino, P.M., Issa, J.P., 1998. Alterations in DNA methylation: a fundamental aspect of neoplasia. Adv. Cancer Res. 72, 141–196.

Becker, M.W., Lourençone, E.M.S., De Mello, A.F., Branco, A., Filho, E.M.R., Blatt, C.R., Mallmann, C.A., Schneider, M., Caregnato, R.C.A., Blatt, C.R., 2019. Liver transplantation and the use of kava: case report. Phytomedicine 15, 21–26.

Beilby, J., Olynyk, J., Ching, S., Prins, A., Swanson, N., Reed, W., Harley, H., Garcia-Webb, P., 1992. Transferrin index: an alternative method for calculating the iron saturation of transferring. Clin. Chem. 38, 2078–2081.

Bekő, G., Hagymási, K., Szentmihályi, K., Bányai, É.S., Osztovits, J., Fodor, J., Fehér, J., Blázovics, A., 2007. Sex-dependent alterations in erythrocyte trace element levels and antioxidant status after a month of moderate daily red wine consumption. Eur. J. Gastroenterol. Hepatol. 22, 185–191.

Bekő, G., Hagymási, K., Szentmihályi, K., Bíró, E., Osztovits, J., Szalay, F., Bárkovits, S., Blázovics, A., 2008. How can nutritional factor modify the cytokine pattern and redox parameters in alcoholic drink consuming women? Clin. Chem. Lab. Med. 46, S38.

Benlhabib, E., Baker, J.I., Keyler, D.E., Singh, A.K., 2004. Kudzu root extract suppresses voluntary alcohol intake and alcohol withdrawal symptoms in P rats receiving free access to water and alcohol. J. Med. Food 7, 168–179.

Bergmann, M.M., Hernandez, V., Hart, A., 2018. No controversial role of alcohol consumption in the development of inflammatory bowel diseases. Eur. J. Clin. Nutr. 72, 305–306.

Blázovics, A., 1999. Az alkoholos májkárosodás biokémiája (Biochemistry of alcoholic liver disease). Folia Hepatol. 4 (Suppl. 1), 9–18.

Blázovics, A., 2007. Redox homeostasis, bioactive agents and transduction therapy. Curr. Signal Transduct. Ther. Bentham Sci. 2, 226–239.

Blázovics, A., Fehér, J., 1996. Sikerek és kudarcok a retinoid terápiában (Successes and failures in retinoid therapy). Gyógyszereink 46, 124–129.

Blázovics, A., Sárdi, É., 2018. Methodological repertoire development to study the effect of dietary supplementation in cancer therapy. Microchem. J. 136, 121–127.

Blázovics, A., Vereckei, A., Cornides, A., Fehér, J., 1989. The effect of (+) cyanidanol-3 on the Na^+K^+ATP-ase and $Mg^{++}ATP$-ase activities of the rat brain in the presence and absence of ascorbic acid. Acta Physiol. Hung. 73, 9–14.

Blázovics, A., Szilvás, Á., Székely, G., Tordai, E., Székely, E., Czabai, G., Pallai, Z., Sárdi, É., 2008. Important bioactive molecules of erythrocytes in colorectal cancer patients after colectomy. Open Med. Chem. J. 2, 6–10.

Blázovics, A., Fébel, H., Bekő, G., Kleiner, D., Szentmihályi, K., Sárdi, É., 2019. Why do not red wine's polyphenols protect against the harmful effects of alcohol in alcoholism? Acta Aliment. 48, 358–361.

Bosron, W.F., Li, T.K., 1986. Genetic polymorphism of human liver alcohol and aldehyde dehydrogenases, and their relationship to alcohol metabolism and alcoholism. Hepatology 6, 502–510.

Bosron, W.F., Lumeng, L., Li, T.K., 1988. Genetic polymorphism of enzymes of alcohol metabolism and susceptibility to alcoholic liver disease. Mol. Aspects Med. 10, 147–158.

Brian, P., Lee, M.D., Vittinghoff, E., Dodge, J.L., Cullaro, G., Terrault, N.A., 2019. National trends and long-term outcomes of liver transplant for alcohol-associated liver disease in the United States. JAMA Intern. Med. 179, 340–348.

Broom, É., Worley, A., Gao, F., Hernandez, L.D., Ashton, C.E., Shih, L.C., Vander Horst, V.G., 2019. Translational methods to detect asymmetries in temporal and spatial walking metrics in parkinsonian mouse models and human subjects with Parkinson's disease. Sci. Rep. 9, 1–16.

Byun, H.J., Darvin, P., Kang, D.Y., Sp, N., Joung, Y.H., Park, J.H., Kim, S., Yang, Y.M., 2017. Silibinin downregulates MMP2 expression via Jak2/STAT3 pathway and inhibits the migration and invasive potential in MDA-MB-231 cells. Oncol. Rep. 37, 3270–3278.

Caballeria, J., Pares, A., Brú, C., Mercader, J., Garcia Plaza, A., Caballeria, L., 1998. Metadoxine accelerates fatty liver recovery in alcoholic patients: results of randomized double-blind, placebo-control trial. Spanish Group for the Study of Alcoholic Fatty Liver. J. Hepatol. 28, 54–60.

Calabrese, V., Renis, M., Calderone, A., Russo, A., Reale, S., Barcellona, M.L., Rizza, T., 1998. Stress proteins and SH-groups in oxidant-induced cellular injury after chronic ethanol administration in rat. Free Radic. Biol. Med. 24, 1159–1167.

Carai, M.A., Agabio, R., Bombardelli, E., Bourov, I., Gessa, G.L., Lobina, C., Morazzoni, P., Pani, M., Reali, R., Vacca, G., Colombo, G., 2000. Potential use of medicinal plants in the treatment of alcoholism. Fitoterapia 71 (Suppl. 1), S38–S42.

Cawte, J., 1986. Parameters of kava used as a challenge to alcohol. Aust. N. Z. J. Psychiatry 20, 70–76.

Chachay, V.S., Macdonald, G.A., Martin, J.H., Whitehead, J.P., O'Moore-Sullivan, T.M., Lee, P., Franklin, M., Klein, K., Taylor, P.J., Ferguson, M., Coombes, J.S., Thomas, G.P., Cowin, G.J., Kirkpatrick, C.M., Prins, J.B., Hickman, I.J., 2014. Resveratrol does not benefit patients with non-alcoholic fatty liver disease. Clin. Gastroenterol. Hepatol. 12, 2092–2103.

Chen, S.H., Zhong, G.S., Li, A.L., Li, S.H., Wu, L.K., 2006. Influence of *Hovenia dulcis* on alcohol concentration in blood and activity of alcohol dehydrogenase (ADH) of animals after drinking. Zhongguo Zhong Yao Za Zhi 31, 10941096.

Colombo, G., Serra, S., Vacca, G., Orrù, A., Maccioni, P., Morazzoni, P., Bombardelli, E., Riva, A., Gessa, G.L., Carai, M.A., 2006. Identification of miltirone as active ingredient of *Salvia miltiorrhiza* responsible for the reducing effect of root extracts on alcohol intake in rats. Alcohol. Clin. Exp. Res. 30, 754–762.

Corbin, K.D., Zeisel, S.H., 2012. Choline metabolism provides novel insights into nonalcoholic fatty liver disease and its progression. Curr. Opin. Gastroenterol. 28, 159–165.

Craig, S.A., 2004. Betaine in human nutrition. Am. J. Clin. Nutr. 80, 539–549.

Dan, L., Laposata, M., 1997. Ethyl palmitate and ethyl oleate are the predominant fatty acid ethyl esters in the blood after ethanol ingestion and their synthesis is differentially influenced by the extracellular concentrations of their corresponding fatty acids. Alcohol. Clin. Exp. Res. 21, 286–292.

Degrell, I., Molnar, G., Molnar, L., Kovacz, M., 1980. The effect of alcohol and alcohol withdrawal therapy on the concentration of carbohydrate products of metabolism and electrolytes (Na, K, Mg, Cl) in the blood and cerebrospinal fluid-changes in the oxidation-reduction in the brain. Psychiatr. Neurol. Med. Psychol. (Leipz) 32, 723–730.

Dupont, I., Lucas, D., Clot, P., Ménez, C., Albano, E., 1998. Cytochrome P4502E1 inducibility and hydroxyethyl radical formation among alcoholics. J. Hepatol. 28, 564–571.

Egresi, A., Lengyel, G., Somogyi, A., Blázovics, A., Hagymási, K., 2016. Az idült májbetegség progressziójához vezető folyamatok (Various pathways leading to the progression of chronic liver diseases). Orv. Hetil. 157, 290–297.

Egresi, A., Kovács, Á., Szilvás, Á., Blázovics, A., 2017. Bél-máj tengely vizsgálata colitis ulcerosaban—retrospektív tanulmány (Gut–liver axis in inflammatory bowel disease. A retrospective study). Orv. Hetil. 158, 1014–1021.

Elpek, G.Ö., 2014. Cellular and molecular mechanisms in the pathogenesis of liver fibrosis: an update. World J. Gastroenterol. 20, 7260–7276.

Esmaeil, N., Anaraki, S.B., Gharagozloo, M., Moayedi, B., 2017. Silymarin impacts on immune system as an immunomodulator: one key for many locks. Int. Immunopharmacol. 50, 194–201.

European Association for the Study of the Liver (EASL), 2018. Clinical Practice Guidelines: management of alcohol-related liver disease. J. Hepatol. 69, 154–181.

Ezhilarasan, D., Evraerts, J., Sid, B., Calderon, P.B., Karthikeyan, S., Sokal, E., Najimi, M., 2017. Silibinin induces hepatic stellate cell cycle arrest via enhancing p53/p27 and inhibiting Akt downstream signaling protein expression. Hepatobiliary Pancreat. Dis. Int. 16, 80–87.

Farooq, M.O., Bataller, R., 2016. Pathogenesis and management of alcoholic liver disease. Dig. Dis. 16, 347–355.

Fiebrich, F., Koch, H., 1979. Silymarin, an inhibitor of prostaglandin synthetase. Experienta 35, 1550–1552.

Finkelstein, J.D., Harris, B.J., Kyle, W.E., 1972. Methionine metabolism in mammals: kinetic study of betaine-homocysteine methyltransferase. Arch. Biochem. Biophys. 153, 320–324.

Fiorentino, D.E., Zlotnic, A., Masman, T.R., Howard, M., O'Garra, A., 1991. IL-10 inhibits cytochine production by activated macrophages. J. Immunol. 147, 3815–3822.

Frezza, M., DiPadova, C., Pozzato, G., Terpin, M., Baraona, E., Lieber, C.S., 1990. High blood alcohol levels in women. N. Engl. J. Med. 332, 95–99.

Fukunaga, T., Sillanaukee, P., Eriksson, C.J., 1993. Occurence of blood acetaldahyde in women during ethanol intoxication: pleriminary findings. Alcohol. Clin. Exp. Res. 17, 1198–2000.

Gao, Y., Wang, X., He, C., 2016. An isoflavonoid-enriched extract from *Pueraria lobata* (kudzu) root protects human umbilical vein endothelial cells against oxidative stress induced apoptosis. J. Ethnopharmacol. 4, 524–530.

Glick, S.D., Rossman, K., Steindorf, S., Maisonneuve, I.M., Carlson, J.N., 1991. Effects and after effects of ibogaine on morphine self-administration in rats. Eur. J. Pharmacol. 195, 341–345.

Grancini, V., Trombetta, M., Lunati, M.E., Zimbalatti, D., Boselli, M.L., Gatti, S., Donato, M.F., Resi, V., D'Ambrosio, R., Aghemo, A., Pugliese, G., Bonadonna, R.C., Orsi, E., 2015. Contribution of β-cell dysfunction and insulin resistance to cirrhosis-associated diabetes: role of severity of liver disease. J. Hepatol. 63, 1484–1490.

Gressner, O.A., Weiskirschen, R., Gressner, A.M., 2007. Biomarkers of liver fibrosis: clinical translation of molecular pathogenesis or based on liver-dependent malfunction tests. Clin. Chim. Acta 381, 107–113.

Groenbaeck, M., Deis, A., Sorensen, T.I.A., Becker, U., Schnohr, P., Jensen, G., 1995. Mortality associated with moderate intakes of wine, beer or spirits. Br. Med. J. 310, 1165–1169.

Grossman, C.J., Nienaber, M., Mendenhall, C.L., Hurtubise, P., Roselle, G.A., Rouster, S., Weber, N., Schmitt, G., Gartside, P.S., 1993. Sex differences and the effect of alcohol on immune response in male and female rats. Alcohol. Clin. Exp. Res. 17, 832–840.

Grove, J., Daly, A.K., Bassendine, M.F., Gilvarry, E., Day, C.P., 2000. Interleukin-10 promoter region polymorphisms and susceptibility to advanced alcoholic liver disease. Gut 46, 540–545.

Gyires, K., Fürst, Z., Ferdinándy, P., 2017. Farmakológia és klinikai farmakológia, [Pharcology and Clinical Pharmacology]. Medicina Könyvkiadó Zrt, Budapest.

Hagymási, K., Blázovics, A., 2004. Antioxidánsok a májvédelemben (Antioxidants in liver protection). Orv. Hetil. 145, 1421–1425.

Hagymási, K., Blázovics, A., Kocsis, I., Fehér, J., 2000. Effect of metadoxine-liver protecting agent on short-term extrahepatic cholestasis. Curr. Top. Biophys. 2, 69–73.

Hagymási, K., Blázovics, A., Lengyel, G., Kocsis, I., Fehér, J., 2001. Oxidative damage in alcoholic liver disese. Eur. J. Gastroenterol. Hepatol. 13, 49–53.

Hagymási, K., Lengyel, G., Tulassay, Z., 2013. A nem-alkoholos zsírmáj betegségről 2013-ban (Non alcoholic fatty liver in 2013). Magy. Belorv. Arch. 66, 185–191.

Hagymási, K., Bacsárdi, A., Egresi, A., Berta, E., Tulassay, Z., Lengyel, G., 2018. A bélflóra patofiziológai jelentősége és szerepe mint terápiás célpont májbetegégekben (The role of gut microbiota in chronic liver diseases, and treatment possibilities). Orv. Hetil. 159, 1465–1474.

Harada, S., 1990. Genetic polymorphism of aldehyde dehydrogenase and its physiological significance to alcohol metabolism. Prog. Clin. Biol. Res. 344, 289–294.

Harada, S., Tachiyashikim, K., Imaizumi, K., 1998. Effect of sex hormones on rat liver cytosolic alcohol dehydrogenase activity. J. Nutr. Sci. Vitaminol. (Tokyo) 44, 625–639.

Herbert, V., 1993. Viewpoint does mega C do more good than harm, or more harm than good? Nutr. Today 28, 126–133.

Horváth, T., Blázovics, A., 1992. Chemiluminescence in blood system of alcoholics and of patients with subliminal alcohol-drug use. Croat. J. Gastroenterol. Hepatol. 1, 159–163.

Horváth, T., Szabó, L., Nagy, Z., Blázovics, A., Gergely, K., Schwartz, T., 1992. Endogenous scavenger levels (vitamin E and A) of patients with chronic alcoholic liver disease under different environmental conditions. Acta Physiol. Hung. 80, 381–389.

Horváth, M.E., Gonzalez, C.R., Blázovics, A., Van der Looij, M., Barta, I., Müzes, G., Gergely, P., Fehér, J., 2001. Effect of silibinin and vitamin E on retardation of cellular immune response after partial. hepatectomy, J. Ethanopharmacol. 77, 227–232.

Hu, Y., Oscarson, M., Johansson, I., Yue, Q.Y., Dahl, M.l., Tabone, M., Arinco, S., Albano, E., Ingelman-Sundberg, M., 1997. Genetic polymorphism of human CYP 2EI: characterization of two variant alleles. Mol. Pharmacol. 51, 370–376.

Ioannides, C., 1996. Cytochromes p450 Metabolic and Toxicological Aspects. CRC Press, Boca Raton.

Jacob, R.A., Burri, B.J., 1996. Oxidative damage and defense. Am. J. Clin. Nutr. 63, 985S–990S.

Jahanafrooz, Z., Motamed, N., Rinner, B., Mokhtarzadeh, A., Baradaran, B., 2018. Silibinin to improve cancer therapeutic, as an apoptotic inducer, autophagy modulator, cell cycle inhibitor, and microRNAs regulator. Life Sci. 15, 236–247.

Jain, R., Balhara, Y.P., 2010. Indian impact of alcohol and substance abuse on adolescent brain: a preclinical perspective. J. Physiol. Pharmacol. 54, 213–234.

Keung, W.M., 2003. Anti-dipsotropic isoflavones: the potential therapeutic agents for alcohol dependence. Med. Res. Rev. 23, 669–696.

Keung, W.M., Vallee, B.L., 1993. Daidzin and daidzein suppress free-choice alcohol intake by Syrian golden hamsters. Proc. Natl. Acad. Sci. U. S. A. 90, 10008–10012.

Kim, Y.I., Miller, J.W., da Costa, K.A., Nadeau, M., Smith, D., Selhub, J., Zeisel, S.H., Mason, J.B., 1995. Folate deficiency causes secondary depletion of choline and phosphocholine in liver. J. Nutr. 124, 2197–2203.

Kim, H.J., Park, M.Y., Lee, Y.J., Kim, J.H., Kim, J.Y., Kwon, O., 2016. Effect of *Hovenia dulcis* fruit extract on alcohol-induced metabolism, inflammation and hangover following acute alcohol consumption: a randomized, double-blind, placebo-controlled study. In: Variability in Responses to Diet and Food. Published Online: 1 April 2016 (Abstract Number: lb209).

Kim, H., Kim, Y.J., Jeong, H.Y., Kim, J.Y., Choi, E.K., Chae, S.W., Kwon, O., 2017. A standardized extract of the fruit of *Hovenia dulcis* alleviated alcohol-induced hangover in healthy subjects with heterozygous ALDH2: a randomized, controlled, crossover trial. J. Ethnopharmacol. 14, 167–174.

Kmieć, Z., 2001. Cooperation of liver cells in health and disease. Adv. Anat. Embryol. Cell Biol. 161, 1–151.

Koivisto, T., Mishin, V.M., Mak, K.M., Cohen, P.A., Lieber, C.S., 1996. Induction of cytochrome P-450-2EI by ethanol in rat Kupffer cells. Alcohol. Clin. Exp. Res. 20, 207–212.

Kunitoh, S., Imaoka, S., Hiroi, T., Yabusaki, Y., Monna, T., Funae, Y., 1997. Acetaldehyde as well as ethanol is metabolized by human CYP2EI. J. Pharmacol. Exp. Ther. 280, 527–532.

Kwak, H.S., Joo, C.N., 1988. Effect of ginseng saponin fraction on ethanol metabolism in rat liver. Koryo Insam Hakhoechi 12, 76–86.

Kwo, P.Y., Ramchandani, V.A., O'Connor, S., Amann, D., Carr, L.G., Sandrasegaran, K., Kopecky, K.K., Li, T.K., 1998. Gender differences in alcohol metabolism: relationship to liver volume and effect of adjusting for body mass. Gastroenterology 115, 1552–1557.

Lee, F.C., Ko, J.H., Park, J.K., Lee, J.S., 1987. Effects of *Panax ginseng* on blood alcohol clearence in man. Clin. Exp. Pharmacol. Physiol. 14, 543–546.

Lee, C.M., Wong, H.N., Chui, K.Y., Choang, T.F., Hon, P.M., Chang, H.M., 1991. Miltirone, a central benzodiazepine receptor partial agonist from a Chinese medicinal herb *Salvia miltiorrhiza*. Neurosci. Lett. 24, 237–241.

Leo, M.A., Rosman, A.S., Lieber, C.S., 1993. Differential depletion of carotenoids and tocopherol in liver disease. Hepatology 17, 977–986.

Lewis, K.O., Paton, A., 1992. Could superoxide cause cirrhosis? Lancet ii, 188–189.

Li, D., Zhao, H., Gelernter, J., 2011. Strong association of the alcohol dehydrogenase 1B gene (ADH1B) with alcohol dependence and alcohol-induced medical diseases. Biol. Psychiatry 70, 504–512.

Li, D., Zhao, H., Gelernter, J., 2012. Strong protective effect of the aldehyde dehydrogenase gene (ALDH2) 504lys (*2) allele against alcoholism and alcohol induced medical diseases in Asians. Hum. Genet. 131, 725–737.

Li, Y.J., Li, Y.J., Yang, L.D., Zhang, K., Zheng, K.Y., Wei, X.M., Yang, Q., Niu, W.M., Zhao, M.G., Wu, Y.M., 2018. Silibinin exerts antidepressant effects by improving neurogenesis through BDNF/TrkB pathway. Behav. Brain Res. 1, 184–191.

Liao, C.S., Lin, J.S., Chang, C.P., Chao, T.J., Chao, Y.C., Cheng, T.C., Wu, C.W., Yin, S.J., 1991. Stomach and duodenal alcohol and aldehyde dehydrogenase isozymes in Chinese. Proc. Natl. Sci. Counc. Repub. China B 15, 92–96.

Lieber, C.S., 1990. Interaction of alcohol with other drugs and nutrients. Implication for the therapy of alcoholic liver disease. Drugs 40, 23–44.

Lieber, C.S., 1997a. Ethanol metabolism, cirrhosis, and alcoholism. Clin. Chim. Acta 257, 59–84.

Lieber, C.S., 1997b. Role of oxidative stress and antioxidant therapy in alcoholic and nonalcoholic liver diseases. Adv. Pharmacol. 38, 601–628.

Liu, X., Xu, Q., Long, X., Liu, W., Zhao, Y., Hayashi, T., Hattori, S., Fujisaki, H., Ogura, T., Tashiro, S.I., Onodera, S., Yamato, M., Ikejima, T., 2019. Silibinin-induced autophagy mediated by PPARα-sirt1-AMPK pathway participated in the regulation of type I collagen-enhanced migration in murine 3T3-L1 preadipocytes. Mol. Cell. Biochem. 450, 1–23.

Lu, Y., Cederbaum, A.I., 2018. Cytochrome P450s and alcoholic liver disease. Curr. Pharm. Des. 24, 1502–1517.

Lu, J., Cheng, Y., Wang, X., Woodson, K., Kemper, C., Disney, E., Wang, J., 2019. Alcohol intake enhances glutamatergic transmission from D2 receptor-expressing afferents onto D1 receptor-expressing medium spiny neurons in the dorsomedial striatum. Neuropsychopharmacology 44, 1123–1131.

Lunec, J., Holloway, K.A., Cooke, M.S., Faux, S., Griffits, H.R., Evans, M.D., 2002. Urinary 8-oxo-2'-deoxyguanosine: redox regulation of DNA repair in vivo. Free Radic. Biol. Med. 33, 875–885.

Ma, X., Baraona, E., Goozner, B.G., Lieber, C.S., 1999. Gender differences in medium-chain dicarboxylic aciduria in alcoholic men and women. Am. J. Med. 106, 70–75.

Marshall, A.W., Kingstone, D., Boss, M., Morgan, M.Y., 1983. Ethanol elimination in males and females: relationship to menstrual cycle and body composition. Hepatology 3, 701–706.

McGill, M.R., Du, K., Weemhoff, J.L., Jaeschke, H., 2015. Critical review of resveratrol in xenobiotic-induced hepatotoxicity. Food Chem. Toxicol. 86, 309–318.

Meyer, U.A., 1996. Overview of enzymes of drug metabolism. J. Pharmacokinet. Biopharm. 24, 449–459.

Mizoi, Y., Yamamoto, K., Ueno, Y., Fukunaga, T., Harada, S., 1994. Involvement of genetic polymorphysm of alcohol and aldehyde dehydrogenases in individual variation of alcohol metabolism. Alcohol Alcohol. 29, 707–710.

Molnár, V., Billes, F., Tyihák, E., Mikosch, H., 2008. Theoretical study on the vibrational spectra of methoxy- and formyl-dihydroxy-trans-stilbenes and their hydrolytic equilibria. Spectrochim. Acta A 69, 542–558.

Morales-Ibanez, O., Dominguez, M., Ki, S.H., Marcos, M., Chaves, J.F., Nguyen-Khac, E., Houchi, H., Affò, S., Sancho-Bru, P., Altamirano, J., Michelena, J., García-Pagán, J.C., Abraldes, J.G., Arroyo, V., Caballería, J., Laso, F.J., Gao, B., Bataller, R., 2013. Human and experimental evidence supporting a role for osteoportin in alcoholic hepatitis. Hepatology 58, 1742–1756.

Morgan, M.Y., Sherlock, S., 1977. Sex-related differences among 100 patients with alcoholic liver disease. BMJ 1, 939–941.

Neha Jaggi, A.S., Singh, N., 2016. Silymarin and its role in chronic diseases. Adv. Exp. Med. Biol. 929, 25–44.

Neuman, M.G., Maor, Y., Nanau, R.M., Melzer, E., Mell, H., Opris, M., Cohen, L., Malnick, S., 2015. Alcoholic liver disease: role of cytokines. Biomolecules 5, 2023–2034.

Niemelä, O., Parkkila, S., Pasanen, M., Viitala, K., Villanueva, J.A., Halsted, C.H., 1999. Induction of cytochrome P450 enzymes and generation of protein-aldehyde adducts are associated with sex-dependent sensitivity to alcohol-induced liver disease in micropigs. Hepatology 30, 1011–1017.

Nordmann, R., Rouach, H., 1996. Alcohol and free radicals: from basic research to clinical prospects. Ann. Gastroenterol. Hepatol. (Paris) 32, 128–133.

Nutrient Data Laboratory Agricultural Research Service U.S. Department of Agriculture, 2008. USDA Database for the Choline Content of Common Foods is Presented. http://ars.usda.gov/nutrientdata.

Oliva, F., Nibbio, G., Vizzuso, P., Jaretti Sodano, A., Ostacoli, L., Carletto, S., Picci, R.L., 2018. Gender differences in anxiety and depression before and after alcohol detoxification: anxiety and depression as gender-related predictors of relapse. Eur. Addict. Res. 24, 163–172.

Page, A., Mann, D.A., 2015. Epigenetic regulation of liver fibrosis. Clin. Res. Hepatol. Gastroenterol. 39, S64–S68.

Paolini, M., Antelli, A., Pozetti, L., Spetlova, D., Perocco, P., Valgimigli, L., Pedulli, G.F., Cantelli-Forti, G., 2001. Induction of cytochrome P450 enzymes and over-generation of oxygen radicals in beta-carotene-supplemented rats. Carcinogenesis 22, 483–1495.

Pár, A., 2000. A kezelés lehetősége alkoholos májbetegségekben. Absztinencia, táplálkozás, gyógyszerek, májtransplantáció (Treatment of alcoholic liver diseases. Abstinence, nutritional support, drug therapy, liver transplantation). Orv. Hetil. 141, 827–833.

Pár, A., Pár, G., 2019. Alkoholos májbetegség: a genetikai-epigenetikai tényezők szerepe és az absztinencia hatása, [Alcoholic liver disease: the roles of genetic-epigenetic factors and the effect of abstinence]. Orv. Hetil. 160, 524–532.

Park, S., Kim, D.S., Wu, X., Yi, Q.J., 2018. Mulberry and dandelion water extracts prevent alcohol-induced steatosis with alleviating gut microbiome dysbiosis. Exp. Biol. Med. (Maywood) 243, 882–894.

Rao, D.N., Yang, M.X., Lasker, J.M., Cederbaum, A.I., 1996. 1-Hydroxyethyl radical formation during NADPH- and NADH-dependent oxidation of ethanol by human liver microsomes. Mol. Pharmacol. 49, 814–821.

Rezvani, A.H., Overstreet, D.H., Lee, Y.W., 1995. Attenuation of alcohol intake by ibogaine in three strains of alcohol preferring rats. Pharmacol. Biochem. Behav. 52, 615–620.

Rezvani, A.H., Overstreet, D.H., Perfumi, M., Massi, M., 2003. Plant derivatives in the treatment of alcohol dependence. Pharmacol. Biochem. Behav. 75, 593–606.

Saito, H., Nagatome, Y., Bao, T., 1984. Effects of red ginseng, vitamins and their preparations. V. Effect on behaviours of alcohol-administerd mice. Yakuri Chiryo 12, 1482–1487.

Saxena, N.K., Anania, F.A., 2015. Adipocytokines and hepatic fibrosis. Trends Endocrinol. Metab. 26, 153–161.

Slater, T.F., Eakins, M.N., 1983. Interactions of (+)-cyanidanol-3 with free radical generating system. In: Bertelli, A. (Ed.), New Trends in the Therapy of Liver Diseases. Karger, Basel, Switzerland, pp. 84–89.

Smith, M., 1986. Genetics of human alcohol and aldehyde dehydrogenases. Adv. Hum. Genet. 15, 249–290.

Sonnenbichler, J., Zetl, I., 1984. Untersuchungen zum Wirkungsmechanismus von Silibinin: V. Einflub von Silibinin auf die Synthese ribosomaler RNA, mRNA und tRNA in Rattenlebern in vivo. Hoppe Seylers Z. Physiol. Chem. 365, 555–566.

Sonnenbichler, J., Goldberg, M., Hane, L., Madibunyi, I., Vogl, S., Zetl, I., 1986. Stimulatory effect of silibinin on the DNA synthesis in partially hepatectomized rat livers: non-response in hepatoma and other malign cell lines. Biochem. Pharmacol. 35, 538–541.

Stein, M.D., Cyr, M.G., 1997. Women and substance abuse. Med. Clin. North Am. 81, 979–998.

Steiner, G.G., 2001. Kava as an anticraving agent: preliminary data. Pac. Health Dialog 8, 335–339.

Stickel, F., Buch, S., Lau, K., et al., 2011. Genetic variation in the PNPLA3 gene is associated with alcoholic liver injury in Caucasians. Hepatology 53, 86–95.

Stickel, F., Datz, C., Hampe, J., Bataller, R., 2017. Pathophysiology and management of alcoholic liver disease: update 2016. Gut Liver 11, 173–188.

Süle, K., Szentmihályi, K., Szabó, G., Kleiner, D., Varga, I., Egresi, A., May, Z., Nyirády, P., Mohai Jr., M., Blázovics, A., 2018. Metal- and redox homeostasis in prostate cancer with vitamin D3 supplementation. Biomed. Pharmacother. 105, 558–565.

Sun, C., Fan, J.G., Qiao, L., 2015. Potential epigenetic mechanism in non-alcoholic fatty liver disease. Int. J. Mol. Sci. 16, 5161–5179.

Taga, K., Tosato, G., 1992. IL-10 inhibits human T-cell proliferation and IL-2 production. J. Immunol. 148, 1143–1148.

Tomczyk, M., Zovko-Koncić, M., Chrostek, L., 2012. Phytotherapy of alcoholism. Nat. Prod. Commun. 7, 273–280.

Trépo, E., Ouziel, R., Pradat, P., Momozawa, Y., Quertinmont, E., Gervy, C., Gustot, T., Degré, D., Vercruysse, V., Deltenre, P., Verset, L., Gulbis, B., Franchimont, D., Devière, J., Lemmers, A., Moreno, C., 2013. Marked 25-hydroxyvitamin D deficiency is associated with poor prognosis in patients with alcoholic liver disease. J. Hepatol. 59, 344–350.

Tsuritani, I., Ikai, E., Date, T., Suzuki, Y., Ishizaki, M., Yamada, Y., 1995. Polymorphism in ALDH2-genotype in Japanese men and the alcohol-blood pressure relationship. Am. J. Hypertens. 8, 1053–1059.

Tyihák, E., Albert, L., Németh, Z.I., Kátay, G., Király-Véghely, Z., Szende, B., 1998. Formaldehyde cycle and the natural formaldehyde generators and capturers. Acta Biol. Hung. 49, 225–238.

Umeno, M., Song, B.J., Kozak, C., Gelboin, H.V., Gonzalez, F.J., 1988. The rat P45011E1 gene-complete intron and exon sequence, chromosome mapping, and correlation of developmental expression with specific 5′ cytosine demethylation. J. Biol. Chem. 263, 4956–4962.

Verdura, S., Cuyàs, E., Llorach-Parés, L., Pérez-Sánchez, A., Micol, V., Nonell-Canals, A., Joven, J., Valiente, M., Sánchez-Martínez, M., Bosch-Barrera, J., Menendez, J.A., 2018. Silibinin is a direct inhibitor of STAT3. Food Chem. Toxicol. 116, 161–172.

Vidali, M., Stewart, S.F., Albano, E., 2008. Interplay between oxidative stress and immunity in the progression of alcohol-mediated liver injury. Trends Mol. Med. 14, 63–71.

Villanueva, A., Portela, A., Sayols, S., Battiston, C., Hoshida, Y., Méndez-González, J., Imbeaud, S., Letouzé, E., Hernandez-Gea, V., Cornella, H., Pinyol, R., Solé, M., Fuster, J., Zucman-Rossi, J., Mazzaferro, V., Esteller, M., Llovet, J.M., HEPTROMIC Consortium, 2015. DNA methylation-based prognosis and epidrivers in hepatocellular carcinoma. Hepatology 61, 1945–1956.

Wang, T.K., Weiner, H., Gorenstein, D.G., 1993. Import, processing, and two-dimensional NMR structure of a linker-deleted signal peptide of rat liver mitochondrial aldehyde dehydrogenase. J. Biol. Chem. 268, 19906–19914.

Wen, D.C., Hu, X.Y., Wang, Y.Y., Luo, J.X., Lin, W., Jia, L.Y., Gong, X.Y., 2016. Effects of aqueous extracts from *Panax ginseng* and *Hippophae rhamnoides* on acute alcohol intoxication: an experimental study using mouse model. J. Ethnopharmacol. 4, 67–73.

Whitfield, J.B., 1997. Meta-analysis of the effects of alcohol dehydrogenase genotype on alcohol dependence and alcoholic liver disease. Alcohol Alcohol. 32, 613–619.

WHO Library Cataloguing-in-Publication Data, 2014. World Health Organization. Global Status Report on Noncommunicable Diseases, Geneva.

Witting, L.A., 1980. Vitamin E and lipid antioxidants in free radical initiated reactions. In: Priyor, A. (Ed.), Free Radicals in Biology. New York Academi Press, New York, pp. 295–319.

Wong, N.A.C.S., Rae, F., Simpson, K.I., Murray, G.D., Harrison, D.I., 2000. Genetic polymorphisms of cytochrome p4502E1 and susceptibility to alcoholic liver disease and hepatocellular carcinoma in a white population: a study and literature review, including meta-analysis. Mol. Pharmacol. 53, 88–93.

Worral, S., Wilce, P.A., 1994. The effect of chronic ethanol feeding on cytokines in a rat model of alcoholic liver disease. Alcohol Alcohol. Suppl. 2, 447–451.

Worral, S., de Jersey, J., Shanley, B.C., 1991. Alcohol abusers exhibit a higher IgA response to acetaldehyde-modified proteins. Alcohol Alcohol. Suppl. 1, 261–264.

Worral, S., de Jersey, J., Nicholls, R., Wilce, P.A., 1993. Acetaldehyde/protein interactions: are they involved in the pathogenesis of alcoholic liver disease? Dig. Dis. 11, 265–277.

Wu, D., Wang, X., Zhou, R., Yang, L., Cederbaum, A.I., 2012. Alcohol steatosis and cytotoxicity: the role of cytochrome P4502E1 and autophagy. Free Radic. Biol. Med. 53, 1346–1357.

Yamada, S., Matsuoka, H., Harada, Y., Momosaka, Y., Izumi, H., Hohno, K., Yamaguchi, Y., Eto, S., 1999. Effect of long term ethanol consumption on ability to produce cytokine-induced neutrophil chemoatractant-1 in the rat liver and its gender difference. Alcohol. Clin. Exp. Res. 23 (Suppl. 4), 61S–66S.

Yang, X.Y., Wei, W.B., Zeng, L.R., He, J.H., Chen, P.F., 2018. Controversial role of alcohol consumption in the development of inflammatory bowel diseases. Eur. J. Clin. Nutr. 72, 304.

Yin, S.I., Chou, F.J., Chao, S.F., Tsai, S.F., Liao, C.S., Wang, S.L., Wu, C.W., 1993. Alcohol and aldehyde dehydrogenases in human esophagus: comparison with the stomach enzyme activities. Alcohol. Clin. Exp. Res. 17, 376–381.

Yin, S.I., Liao, C.S., Lee, Y.C., Wu, C.W., Jao, S.W., 1994. Genetic polymorphism and activities of age differences human colon alcohol and aldehyde dehydrogenases: no gender and alcohol. Clin. Exp. Res. 18, 1256–1260.

Yin, S.J., Liao, C.S., Wu, C.W., Li, T.T., Chen, L.L., Lai, C.L., Tsao, T.Y., 1997. Human stomach alcohol and aldehyde dehydrogenases: comparison of expression pattern and activities in alimentary tract. Gastroenterology 112, 766–775.

Yoshida, A., 1994. Genetic polymorphisms of alcohol metabolizing enzymes related to alcohol sensitivity and alcoholic diseases. Alcohol Alcohol. 29, 693–696.

Yoshida, A., Rzhetsky, A., Hsu, L.C., Chang, C., 1998. Human aldehyde dehydrogenase gene family. Eur. J. Biochem. 251, 549–557.

Zeisel, S.H., Blusztajn, J.K., 1994. Choline and human nutrition. Ann. Rev. Nutr. 14, 269–296.

Zeisel, S.H., da Costa, K.A., Franklin, P.D., Alexander, E.A., Lamont, J.T., Sheard, N.F., Beiser, A., 1991. Choline, an essential nutrient for humans. FASEB J. 5, 2093–2098.

Zeisel, S.H., Mar, M.H., Howe, J.C., Holden, J.M., 2003. Concentrations of choline-containing compounds and betaine in common foods. J. Nutr. 133, 1302–1307.

Hepatoprotective activity of natural compounds and plant extracts in nonalcoholic fatty liver disease

Antoni Sureda[a], Xavier Capó[a], and Silvia Tejada[b]
[a]Research Group on Community Nutrition and Oxidative Stress (NUCOX), Department of Fundamental Biology and Health Sciences, Health Research Institute of the Balearic Islands (IdISBa), and CIBEROBN (Physiopathology of Obesity and Nutrition CB12/03/30038), University of the Balearic Islands, Palma, Spain [b]Laboratory of Neurophysiology, Department of Biology, Health Research Institute of the Balearic Islands (IdISBa), and CIBEROBN (Physiopathology of Obesity and Nutrition CB12/03/30038), University of the Balearic Islands, Palma, Spain

5.1 Introduction

Nonalcoholic fatty liver disease (NAFLD) is the main cause of chronic liver disease (Fig. 5.1). The disorder is characterized by the presence of hepatic triglyceride accumulation in patients without alcohol consumption. NAFLD includes hepatic steatosis that consists of triglyceride liver infiltration, and inflammatory nonalcoholic steatohepatitis (NASH) based on the occurrence of fat with inflammation and different degrees of fibrosis even reaching hepatic cirrhosis. Simple hepatic steatosis is the benign form while NASH and hepatic cirrhosis can lead to liver failure or hepatocellular carcinoma (Angulo, 2002). Besides the liver triglyceride accumulation, NAFLD is characterized by macrovesicular steatosis, mild acute and chronic diffuse lobular inflammation, hepatocyte ballooning, perisinusoidal and perivenular deposition of collagen, defectively formed Mallory's hyaline, vacuolated nuclei in hepatocytes, lobular lipogranulomas, and diastase-resistant Kupffer cells (Brunt, 2001; Clark, 2006). In addition, NALFD is classified into two types, primary and secondary. Primary NAFLD is related to metabolic disorders including metabolic syndrome, whose risk factors include being overweight, type 2 diabetes, insulin resistance, altered triglycerides, and high-density lipoprotein (HDL) cholesterol. In addition, secondary NAFLD is associated with external factors such as jejuno-ileal bypass surgery, certain drugs, HIV infection, or certain hepatotoxins (Angulo, 2002; Clark, 2006). NAFLD prevalence has increased in the last 20 years (Perumpail et al., 2017). Some studies show that approximately 20%–30% of the general population suffers from NAFLD; this percentage is lower in Asiatic countries

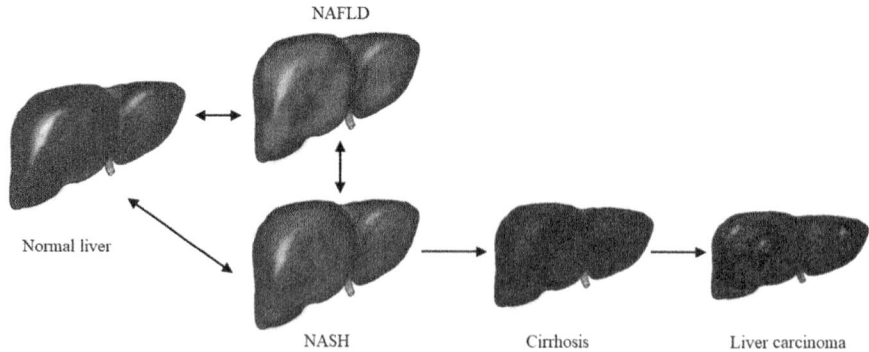

Fig. 5.1
Schematic representation of the progression of nonalcoholic fatty liver (NAFLD). *NASH,*
nonalcoholic steatohepatitis.

where the prevalence of this pathology is about 15% of the population. It has been observed that NAFLD affects all age ranges from children to old people. In children, the prevalence is lower than in adults. It is about 3% in children, and this percentage is higher (22.5%–52.8%) in obese children (Bellentani et al., 2010; Franzese et al., 1997). It has been observed that 30% of simple steatosis patients progress in NASH, about 20%–25% of these NASH patients develop cirrhosis, and 30–40% of patients with cirrhosis die from liver-related causes in 10 years (McCullough, 2004). Classically, the main risk factors for NAFLD are being female as well as age, type II diabetes, obesity, hyperlipidemia, and hypertransaminasemia (Clark, 2006; Mulhall et al., 2002). Other risk factors associated with NAFLD have been described (Table 5.1).

5.2 Nonalcoholic fatty liver disease pathogenesis and progression

As has been described previously, the main characteristic of NAFLD is the hepatic triglyceride accumulation. This increase may be due to several causes, including an increase in circulating free fatty acids from adipose tissue due to lipolysis, an increase in dietary fatty acids, an elevated hepatic lipogenesis, a reduction of very-low-density lipoprotein exports, and a decrease in β-oxidation (Pan et al., 2014). The fatty acid liver accumulation causes some changes in liver histology and in the hepatocytes, including lobular and portal inflammation, hepatocyte ballooning, apoptotic processes, increased aspartate aminotransferase (AST), collagen deposition, and hepatic fibrosis (Levene and Goldin, 2012). All these changes in the liver and hepatocytes cause hepatocyte lipotoxicity, increased oxidative stress associated with mitochondrial dysfunction, proinflammatory cytokine release, and the activation of immune and hepatic stellate cells (Pan et al., 2014). NAFLD progression has traditionally been considered from the point of view of the "two hits hypothesis," which proposes that a sedentary life style, hyperlipidic diets, obesity, and insulin resistance are

Table 5.1: Main NAFLD risk factors.

Insulin resistance	– Obesity
	– Sedentary lifestyle
	– Diabetes mellitus type 2
	– Hypertension
	– Dyslipidaemia
Drugs	– Tamoxifen
	– Corticosteroids
	– Amiodarone
	– Methotrexate
	– Estrogens
	– Valproic acid
	– Antiretroviral drugs
Other causes	– Excess carbohydrates
	– Rapid weight loss
Alterations of bowel anatomy	– Surgery for obesity
	– Pancreaticoduodenal resection
	– Short bowel
Metabolic diseases	– Hypobetalipoproteinemia
	– Abetalipoproteinemia
	– Wilson's disease
	– Lipodystrophies
	– Andersen's disease
	– Weber-Christian syndrome
Infections	– Chronic infection with the hepatitis C virus
	– Human immunodeficiency virus
	– Immunodeficiency syndrome acquired
Emerging associations	– Polycystic ovary syndrome
	– Hypothyroidism
	– Obstructive sleep apnea
	– Hypopituitarism
	– Hypogonadism

the first "hit" that causes an increase in liver lipid accumulation. This fact would suppose that hepatocytes are more predisposed to suffer a second "hit" from oxidative stress, mitochondrial disfunction, endoplasmic reticule stress, or proinflammatory adipokines. All of them could bring about the main characteristics of NAFLD, which are fibrosis, inflammation, and cellular death (Day and James, 1998). However, it has been observed that some steatosis subjects developed NASH without a second hit but other external injury. For this reason, nowadays it is proposed that NAFLD is caused by multiple factors that act synergistically with the advance and progression of NAFLD (Tilg and Moschen, 2010). This assumption is known as the "multiple parallel hits hypothesis." It supposes that several very diverse and parallel processes might often take place and could contribute to the development of liver inflammation. This theory has suggested that many elements such as genetic factors, extrahepatic tissues, high fat diets, diabetes, and/or obesity play significant roles in liver inflammation, fibrosis, and finally tumor development (Tilg and Moschen, 2010).

Insulin resistance has been described as playing a central role in NAFLD progression (Asrih and Jornayvaz, 2015). In a nonpathological situation, insulin regulates numerous cell functions in the liver, such as the stimulation of glucose uptake and storage, cell growth, and modulation of the energy balance and gene expression. In this sense, insulin modulates the lipid metabolism, inhibits fatty acid oxidation, promotes lipogenesis, and increases fatty acid uptake and very low-density lipoprotein (VLDL) secretion. When tissues become resistant to insulin action, the lipolysis of triglycerides increases and this triglyceride lipolysis causes an increase in plasma nonesterify fatty acids (NEFAs), raising liver fatty acid accumulation (Moller and Flier, 1991). In parallel, the accumulation of fatty acids in the liver increases insulin resistance (Pan et al., 2014). Hepatic triglyceride accumulation causes changes in hepatocyte function. Moreover, adipocytes release diverse proinflammatory cytokines. including tumor necrosis factor-α (TNF-α) or interleukin-6 (IL-6), which together with circulating NEFAs impair hepatic insulin signaling (Smith and Adams, 2011; Tarantino and Caputi, 2011) because inflammation is essential in NAFLD development. In fact, some studies have demonstrated that hepatocytes exposed to free fatty acids increase TNF-α and IL-1, both with proinflammatory effects. In this sense, it has been shown that high TNF-α levels can promote hepatocyte apoptosis (Schwabe et al., 2004). The TNF-α response involves the activation of the nuclear factor κβ (NFκβ), which is its major transcriptional regulator and is responsible for the many proinflammatory mediators such as cyclooxygenase-2 (COX-2) or the inducible oxide nitric synthase (iNOS) (Diehl, 2004; Pahl, 1999). At the same time, NFκβ activation reduces the activity of the peroxisome proliferator activated receptor (PPAR-γ). This is necessary for adipocyte differentiation and is a key transcriptional factor for adiponectin, which is a TNF-α antagonist (Diehl, 2004). However, not only is TNF-α responsible for liver inflammation, but also other proinflammatory mediators may participate in the development of steatosis because in diverse investigations, hepatic steatosis was not dependent on TNFα (Wieckowska et al., 2008; Yamaguchi et al., 2010). For instance, the role of IL-6 on NAFLD is still unclear. While some studies propose that IL-6 is hepatoprotective and promotes liver regeneration (Pan et al., 2014), other works suggest an important function on NAFLD because these patients presented high IL-6 plasma levels (Wieckowska et al., 2008) and the IL-6 receptor blocks elevated hepatic steatosis and improved hepatic injury in mice (Yamaguchi et al., 2010). A decrease in the adipokines adiponectin and leptin, with antiinflammatory properties, is also related to NAFLD (Tilg and Moschen, 2010). It has been observed that adiponectin was able to reduce liver fat accumulation and improve insulin resistance, and it is thought that sufficient production of adiponectin could prevent liver inflammation. Meanwhile, leptin is directly related to being overweight, being able to increase fatty acid oxidation, and reducing ectopic fat accumulation (Tilg and Moschen, 2010).

5.3 Oxidative stress and lipotoxicity

Oxygen is indispensable for life, but the respiratory chain is a source of radical oxygen species (ROS). ROS are oxygen-derived molecules with high reactivity that can react with biomolecules and consequently damage them. Organisms present various mechanisms to fight ROS; these mechanisms are antioxidant defenses that can be classified as enzymatic and nonenzymatic defenses. Among the antioxidant enzymes, various enzymes such as superoxide dismutase (SOD), catalase (CAT), glutathione peroxidase (GPx), glutathione reductase (GRd), or uncoupling proteins (UCPs) can be named (Capo et al., 2015). Nonenzymatic defenses are molecules with the capability to react with ROS and to reduce their damaging effects. The main nonenzymatic antioxidants are vitamins C and E, glutathione, and ubiquinone (Halliwell, 1995; Sureda et al., 2005). When ROS production is higher than ROS elimination, ROS could react with biomolecules such as lipids, proteins, or DNA, causing oxidative damage (Gutteridge and Halliwell, 1992). In NAFLD patients, liver fatty acid accumulation causes an increase in β-oxidation, which in turn provokes ROS overproduction in the respiratory chain (Ashraf and Sheikh, 2015; Videla et al., 2004). These ROS are able to activate proinflammatory cytokines in hepatocytes via NFκβ activation. One of the cytokines that increases as a consequence of ROS is TNF-α, the effects of which were already explained above. ROS also causes an increase of the transforming growth factor β (TGF-β), which activates collagen production by stellate cells, increasing hepatic fibrosis (Carter-Kent et al., 2008; Medina and Moreno-Otero, 2005). In addition, it has been observed that products of fat oxidation, especially malondialdehyde (MDA) and 4-hydroxinonenal (4-HNE), can exert cytotoxic effects in hepatocytes. For instance, it is known that products of lipid oxidation can increase collagen products or increase neutrophil chemiotactic activity, augmenting liver inflammation (Medina and Moreno-Otero, 2005; Singh et al., 2009).

Lipotoxicity is defined as cellular toxicity observed in the presence of abnormal fat accumulation (Unger, 2003). As has been described, NAFLD patients present elevated plasma triglycerides and abnormal hepatic triglyceride accumulation. However, this is not lipotoxic per se; nevertheless, free fatty acids and various lipid metabolites could be lipotoxic and can cause lipoapotosis in hepatocytes (Pan et al., 2014). The lipotoxic effect of free fatty acids may be due to several mechanisms such as lysosomal destabilization, mitochondrial pathways, death receptor signaling, and ER stress (Pan et al., 2014). Saturated fatty acids are able to induce hepatocyte apoptosis, activating JUN N-terminal kinase (JNK) and mitochondrial death pathways and increasing endoplasmic reticule stress (Schuster et al., 2018). Moreover, the high presence of fatty acids in the liver causes the synthesis of lipid derivates such as ceramides, diacylglycerols, lysophosphatidylcholine, and derivates from lipid oxidation that could have hepatotoxic effects and act as ROS (Han et al., 2008). Commonly, metabolic syndromes are associated with high plasma cholesterol levels. In this sense, it has been observed that cholesterol causes hepatotoxicity. Cholesterol can be accumulated in hepatic cells, where it can disrupt the integrity of membranes and alter mitochondrial function. This can cause an increase in ROS production and mitochondrial disfunction and a depletion in ATP production that together can cause apoptosis (Schuster et al., 2018).

5.4 Mediterranean diet and nonalcoholic fatty liver disease

NAFLD is a chronic liver disease that implies a possible development of cirrhosis, fibrosis, and hepatocellular carcinoma in developed countries. However, treatments are not totally effective or are being evaluated; in fact, there is no consensus on the adequate and specific pharmacological treatment (Jeznach-Steinhagen et al., 2019). Although 30% of the adult population (Kempinski et al., 2019) is diagnosed with NAFLD, few clinical assays have been performed up to now aimed at determining the effects of the Mediterranean diet on this chronic liver disease. In an Italian study, the relevance of lifestyle, including adherence to the Mediterranean diet and physical activity levels together with biochemical analyses, was investigated in 532 ultrasound-diagnosed NAFLD subjects and 667 non-NAFLD subjects (Trovato et al., 2016). The results showed a higher body mass index (BMI), insulin resistance, triglycerides, and alanine aminotransferase (ALT) levels in the NAFLD group while a higher adherence to the Mediterranean diet and a more active lifestyle were found in the control group. In a similar study (Baratta et al., 2017), 82.7% of patients ($n = 584$) presented steatosis (ultrasonography), although its prevalence diminished with the higher adherence to the Mediterranean diet. The authors also related the disease to higher ALT levels, hypertriglyceridemia, and waist circumference. NAFLD has been related to the patients' liver histology ($n = 82$) because adherence to the Mediterranean diet was associated with a smaller probability of developing steatohepatitis and steatosis, and also a positive relation existed between a high grade of NAFLD with weight, BMI, AST, and the homeostatic model assessment of insulin resistance (HOMA-IR) (Aller et al., 2015a). However, taking into account that NAFLD is initially diagnosed by the marker ALT, a first clinical assay included 259 obese type 2 diabetes patients because 70% of these patients also develop NAFLD (Fraser et al., 2008). The individuals were randomized in three groups with different diet recommendations but a similar total energy, plus 30 min of aerobic activity (3 times/week). The diets were the 2003 recommended American Diabetes Association diet (ADA), a low glycemic index (LGI) diet, and the Mediterranean diet. The authors reported lower ALT levels in the Mediterranean diet group at both 6 and 12 months after intervention with respect to the other diets; however, the NAFLD was not assessed. Other works have used ultrasound or magnetic resonance spectroscopy to assess the disease grade. In a nondietary intervention, 58 patients diagnosed with NAFLD by elastography for liver stiffness measurements and liver biopsies ($n = 34/58$) were compared with healthy controls (Kontogianni et al., 2014). A reduction in the severity of steatosis, ALT, insulin levels, and the insulin resistance index as well as increased serum adiponectin levels were observed in the adhered Mediterranean group. Fatty liver assessed by ultrasound was used to assess the steatosis grade of 90 patients with NAFLD following a Mediterranean diet during 6 months (Trovato et al., 2015). The authors reported an improvement in BMI, fatty liver content, HOMA-IR, and the performance of exercise, but no changes were observed in ALT levels. In fact, the clinical and Mediterranean diet intervention together with increased physical activity in 46 adults suffering from NAFLD during half a year (Gelli et al., 2017) induced reductions in the steatosis grade (e.g., 24 patients with grade 3 reduced to 4 patients), weight, hepatic enzymes levels (ALT, AST, and gamma glutamyl transferase (GGT)), or high-density lipoprotein (HDL) cholesterol. In addition, several indexes indicative of NAFLD were calculated, reporting significant improvements in the fatty liver index (FLI, which indicates the probability of significant steatosis), the Kotronen index (a predictor of liver fat percentage), the visceral adipose index (VAI, as visceral fat related to cardiometabolic risk), and the insulin resistance indices HOMA-IR and QUICKI. The authors concluded the benefits of a multidisciplinary intervention to improve the profile of these patients after a 6-month intervention, although the NAFLD diagnosis was not performed with MRS but with ultrasound and related indices. Ultrasound images were also used to measure the NAFLD score in 90 patients (Misciagna et al., 2017) who were asked to adhere to a control diet or a low glycemic index Mediterranean diet during half a year. The main outcome was a reduction on the NAFLD scores after the Mediterranean diet. In addition, FLI, serum glutamic-pyruvate transaminase, triglycerides, and glycemia levels were reduced after 6 months when compared to the baseline. Moreover, the GGT and HDL cholesterol levels were only reduced in the Mediterranean group. In a cross-over study (Ryan et al., 2013), 12 nondiabetic patients but with a positive biopsy of NAFLD were asked to participate in a randomized diet intervention undertaking a control diet (low fat-high carbohydrate diet) or a Mediterranean diet during 6 weeks each. Even though no significant changes were detected in weight, the subjects displayed a hepatic steatosis (evaluated by MRS), circulating insulin reduction, and better insulin sensitivity after the Mediterranean diet. Despite the positive results, the limitations of this study were the low number of patients enrolled and the short time follow-up. In addition to the diet, an antioxidant supplement containing silybin, chlorogenic acid, and vitamin E was also studied in overweight NAFLD patients (Abenavoli et al., 2015a, 2017), who were randomized in control, the Mediterranean diet, and the same diet plus a daily antioxidant supplement for half a year. An improvement in body weight and anthropometric parameters as well as lipid profile was reported after following the Mediterranean diet. Moreover, when antioxidant supplementation was given, the indices related to insulin resistance in these NAFLD patients were reduced in addition to the hepatic fat accumulation and liver stiffness. In that line, the effects of the Mediterranean diet supplemented with olive oil or nuts have been described for patients ($n = 276$, 57% NAFLD) of the PREDIMED-Malaga trial, observing that nut supplementation had lower increases in FLI (Cueto-Galan et al., 2017). In another work (Properzi et al., 2018), MRS was applied to discern the hepatic steatosis in 48 patients ad libitum who adhered to a Mediterranean diet or a low-fat diet for 12 weeks. After intervention, the reduction in weight was similar between both groups when compared with the baseline. Also, a reduction of the hepatic steatosis was observed in both groups, with slightly better results in the Mediterranean group although it was not statistically significant with respect to the low-fat group. Also, the lipid profile (total cholesterol and triglycerides) improved after the Mediterranean intervention in addition to ALT, glycated hemoglobin

(HbA1c) levels, and the Framingham Risk Score (FRS, to assess the 10-year risk of coronary heart disease). GGT levels were only statistically reduced in the Mediterranean group as was previously reported by other research groups (Gelli et al., 2017; Ryan et al., 2013). The differences in results could be related to the shorter follow-up of patients. In a recent cross-over study, the same diets were used to assess the intestinal permeability in 20 NAFLD patients diagnosed by biopsy (Biolato et al., 2019). Every diet intervention was followed during 16 weeks with the same period of wash-out between both low-fat and Mediterranean diets. Even though no changes were observed in the primary outcome, reduced mean body weight, waist circumference, and ALT and AST levels were observed after the Mediterranean diet intervention. These positive results were maintained after the wash-out period and after the low-fat diet.

5.5 Natural compound effects on nonalcoholic fatty liver disease

NAFLD is a multisystem disease whose progression leads to hepatic complications. To date, there is no effective pharmacological treatment available for the disorder, with modifications in lifestyle, including a healthy diet, regular physical activity, and moderate weight loss as the first line of defense for managing NAFLD. This lack of treatment has increased interest in finding new therapeutic agents that contribute to prevent or slow the progression of NAFLD. Supplementation with natural compounds, in their native form, as extracts or as isolated compounds is emerging as a coadjuvant treatment for NAFLD, considering the beneficial effects on inflammatory markers, metabolic risk factors, and histological markers in the liver observed in animal models (Pan et al., 2014).

Resveratrol (3,5,4'-trihydroxy-trans-stilbene) is a nonflavonoid phenolic compound present in significant amounts in plants and spices, with grapes and red wine, apples, peanuts, and berries the main sources in the human diet (Harikumar and Aggarwal, 2008) (Fig. 5.2). The effectiveness of resveratrol against NAFLD was initially examined in a randomized, double-blind, controlled clinical trial (Faghihzadeh et al., 2014). In this study, 50 NAFLD subjects with significant steatosis were supplemented with resveratrol (a daily capsule of 500 mg) or an equivalent placebo for 12 weeks and all of them were instructed to follow a healthy diet and get regular exercise. Resveratrol supplementation significantly diminished the hepatic steatosis grade and the hepatic tissue echogenicity evaluated by ultrasound as well as diminished the serum levels of ALT, proinflammatory cytokines, cytokeratin-18 M30 (CK-18), and peripheral blood mononuclear cell NF-κB activity with respect to the control group. In the same procedure, the authors did not see additional effects of resveratrol in the anthropometric data, lipid profile, insulin resistance, and blood pressure (Faghihzadeh et al., 2015). In another double-blind, randomized, placebo-controlled trial comprising 60 subjects with NAFLD, resveratrol (150 mg twice daily) or a placebo was taken during 3 months (Chen et al., 2015). Although no significant differences were shown between the groups in

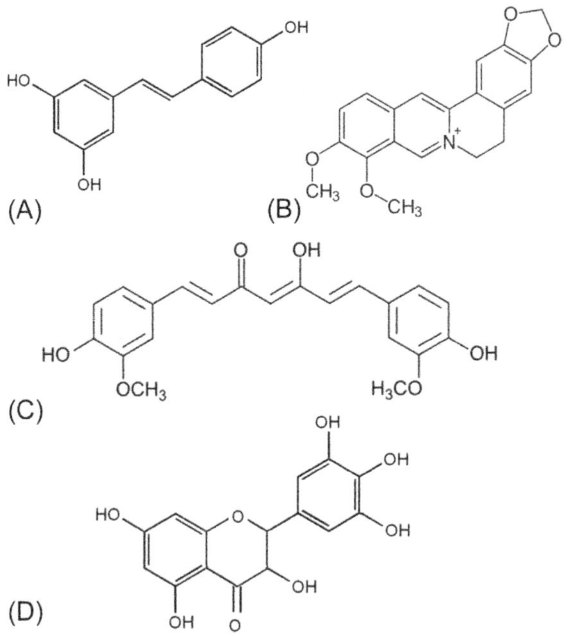

Fig. 5.2
General chemical structure of some polyphenols with potential hepatoprotective effects.
(A) Resveratrol; (B) berberine; (C) curcurmin; (D) dihydromyricetin.

the severity of hepatic fatty accumulation determined by ultrasound, resveratrol significantly reduced the circulating levels of AST and ALT, improved insulin resistance, glucose, and the lipid metabolism. In addition, after the intervention period, resveratrol supplementation reduced serum concentrations of tumor necrosis factor alpha (TNF-α), CK-18, and fibroblast growth factor 21 (FGF21) and elevated adiponectin. The effects of 1.5 g of resveratrol daily were monitored for 6 months in a randomized clinical trial with 28 overweight patients with histological NAFLD confirmed by ultrasound (Heeboll et al., 2016). The results reported that although resveratrol treatment slightly alleviated liver function markers and liver fat accumulation, the intervention had no reliable therapeutic effects in ameliorating the clinical or histological markers of NAFLD with respect to the control group. The authors concluded that larger and longer clinical trials were needed because their findings presented a limited effect-size only. Similarly, another randomized, placebo-controlled clinical trial including 112 NAFLD patients with a 12-week intervention with resveratrol 150 mg/day in two oral doses did not show significant effects on liver fat content and markers of cardiometabolic risk (Kantartzis et al., 2018). The great variability in baseline liver fat content can be a limiting factor to show effects by intervention because resveratrol was related to a reduction of liver fat content in patients with very high levels of liver fat. Finally, 16 obese patients with NAFLD diagnosed with magnetic resonance spectroscopy were randomized to intake resveratrol (500 mg, 3 times daily) or a placebo during 6 months (Poulsen et al., 2018).

The intervention did not improve very low-density lipoprotein triglyceride (VLDL-TG) kinetics, insulin resistance or body composition, and liver fat depots.

Berberine is an isoquinoline quaternary alkaloid present in many natural plants, including *Berberis vulgaris* L. and *B. aristata* DC. (family Berberidaceae), *Hydrastis Canadensis* L. (family Ranunculaceae), and members of the genus *Coptis* (family Ranunculaceae) (Imenshahidi and Hosseinzadeh, 2019; Tillhon et al., 2012). Several studies written in Chinese have investigated the effects of berberine in dosages of 500 mg/day during a period of 3–4 months in patients with fatty liver. In these studies, an improvement in insulin resistance, the lipid profile, and the fatty liver condition and a decrease of the liver enzymes AST, ALT, and GGT were observed (Bai et al., 2011; Cao et al., 2012; Li, 2015; Ning et al., 2013; Xie et al., 2011). The berberine efficacy in the NAFLD treatment was also investigated by Yan and Collaborators (2015) in a randomized, parallel-controlled, open-label clinical trial. 184 Subjects with NAFLD underwent a lifestyle intervention (dietary adjustments and physical activity promotion) alone or with the addition of pioglitazone (15 mg/day) or berberine (500 mg, 3 times/day) during 16 weeks. The treatment of berberine together with lifestyle intervention exerted better effects on hepatic fat content and body weight, serum lipid profile, and HOMA-IR with respect to the lifestyle intervention alone. Although berberine-modulated genes related to energy metabolism in a rat model, these effects on human need to be further studied. The same group of researchers applied lipidomic analyses to characterize the changes in lipid metabolism in a subsample of the previous study (Chang et al., 2016). Berberine significantly modified the serum lipid profile compared to the lifestyle intervention alone. The alteration of the sphingolipid metabolism by the compound, especially a reduction in serum ceramides, was the most significant change. Additional studies are essential to confirm the use of these variations in lipids as early markers of NAFLD.

Silybin is the major flavonolignan isolated from the medicinal plant milk thistle (*Silybum marianum* L. Gaernt., family Asteraceae) (Bijak, 2017). In a preliminary study, the beneficial effects of the silybin-phosphatidylcholine complex, formulated to increase the bioavailability of silybin, together with vitamin E (silybin 94 mg, phosphatidylcholine 194 mg, vitamin E 90 mg, 4 pieces/day) were assayed in a randomized clinical trial with NAFLD overweight patients (Federico et al., 2006). The treatment with the silybin complex significantly improved the transaminase levels and insulin resistance. The same researchers also investigated the effects of the silybin complex twice daily for 12 months in a randomized, double-blind clinical trial (Loguercio et al., 2012). The subjects included in the intervention group showed significant improvement in plasma liver enzymes (AST, ALT, and GGT), insulin resistance, and liver histology with a reduction in the mean severity score for liver steatosis and liver fibrosis, but without increases in body weight. Finally, in a randomized clinical trial with 30 overweight NAFLD patients, the same group also investigated the effects of a personalized Mediterranean diet together with the silybin complex (Abenavoli et al., 2015b). A personalized Mediterranean diet was designed for two groups of 10 patients during

6 months, whereas a third group was refused any treatment. One group, in addition to the diet, was supplemented with the silybin complex. The obtained results were similar to the previous data with significant improvements in the silybin group in insulin sensitivity, HOMA-IR, and fasting glucose. Also, the hepatic fat accumulation grade (according to the Hamaguchi score), anthropometric parameters, and lipid profile were significantly reduced in both intervention groups.

Silymarin, the extract of milk thistle, is characterized by the presence of several flavonolignans, mainly silybin, and the flavonoid taxifolin (Kim et al., 2003). A group of 36 patients with NALFD confirmed by percutaneous liver biopsy was randomized to two groups: an intervention group treated with two silymarin tablets of 540 mg plus vitamin E of 36 mg/day, a hypocaloric diet, and a lifestyle modification program; and a second placebo group only with the hypocaloric diet (Aller et al., 2015b). After the intervention, both groups evidenced a decrease in body weight, BMI, waist circumference, GGT, FLI, and the NAFLD-fibrosis score. The improvement in liver parameters was also found in patients without a loss of 5% of weight in the silymarin group. In another assay, subjects with metabolic syndrome and liver steatosis confirmed with ultrasound participated in an open, controlled study (Sorrentino et al., 2015). The intervention group received a supplement of silymarin formulation (two tablets of 210 mg daily containing 125 mg of silibinin and 30 IU of vitamin E) during 3 months and both intervention and placebo groups were subjected to hypocaloric diet and exercise. Improvements in the reduction of abdominal circumference, BMI, and the ultrasound determination of the right liver lobe were greater in the supplemented group, whereas the hepatic steatosis index and lipid accumulation product index response were similar in both groups. The efficacy of silymarin in patients with NASH was investigated in a randomized, double-blind, placebo-controlled trial (Wah Kheong et al., 2017). Patients were randomly allocated to receive silymarin (700 mg, 3 times/day) or placebo during 48 weeks. Silymarin treatment significantly reduced hepatic fibrosis, serum HbA1c, TG, ALT, AST, and GGT levels, and elevated HDL-C levels with respect to the placebo group. However, silymarin did not reduce the NAFLD Activity Score (NAS) during the intervention by 30% or more in a significantly better amount of silymarin patients than the placebo.

Anthocyanins comprise a diverse group of water-soluble bioactive compounds belonging to the flavonoid polyphenols responsible for the red, blue, and purple coloration in flowers, fruits, and vegetables (Castañeda-Ovando et al., 2009; Wallace et al., 2016). In a clinical trial, healthy humans with borderline hepatitis were supplemented with purple sweet potato beverage containing acylated anthocyanins (200 mg twice daily) for 8 weeks (Suda et al., 2008). The consumption of the beverage significantly reduced the serum levels of hepatic enzymes with respect to the placebo group. In a randomized controlled trial, 74 subjects with NAFLD received purified anthocyanins (4 capsules of 80 mg daily) from black currant and bilberry or a placebo during a 12-week period (Zhang et al., 2015). Patients from the intervention group showed a decrease in serum ALT, CK-18, and myeloperoxidase concentrations as well as improved insulin resistance. Although the supplemented group showed a mild improvement in the fibrosis score, no significant differences were found in the clinical evolution of NAFLD between the supplemented and placebo groups.

Dihydromyricetin is a flavonoid isolated from *Ampelopsis grossedentata* (Hand.-Mazz.) W.T. Wang (family Vitaceae), an edible plant used in traditional Chinese medicine (Li et al., 2017). One double-blind clinical trial comprising 60 NALFD patients confirmed by ultrasound investigated the effects of the intake of 2 capsules of dihydromyricetin (150 mg twice daily) or a placebo for 3 months (Chen et al., 2015). The supplementation did not modify the severity of fatty infiltration; nevertheless, a significant reduction in serum liver enzymes, low-density cholesterol (LDL-C), TNF-α, CK-18, FGF21, and HOMA-IR and increased adiponectin were found.

The curcuminoid curcumin (difeurloylmethane) is a yellow pigment and the primary active ingredient of turmeric (*Curcuma longa* L., family Zingiberaceae), widely used as a spice and flavoring agent (Martin et al., 2012). Randomized NAFLD patients, confirmed by liver sonography, were allocated to receive curcumin (1000 mg/day twice daily) ($n = 50$) or control ($n = 52$) during 8 weeks (Panahi et al., 2016, 2017). Curcumin intake significantly improved the serum lipid profile, uric acid, and AST and ALT, whereas no differences were reported in glucose control parameters. In another placebo-controlled trial, NAFLD patients diagnosed with ultrasonography were randomly allocated to intake an amorphous dispersion curcumin preparation (500 mg/day equivalent to 70 mg curcumin) or placebo during 8 weeks (Rahmani et al., 2016). Curcumin intake was related to a significant decrease in liver fat content. They also showed a significant reduction in BMI and serum levels of total cholesterol, LDL-C, triglycerides, AST, ALT, glucose, and glycated hemoglobin with respect to the placebo group. The protective effects of 250 mg phospholipid curcumin (equivalent to 50 mg/day pure curcumin) or placebo during 8 weeks were investigated on the serum metabolomic profile in NAFLD patients (Chashmniam et al., 2019). Metabolomic analysis showed that some targets of curcumin, including amino acids, tricarboxylic acid (TCA) cycle, bile acids, and gut microbiota-derived metabolites, presented significant differences between both groups. In another recent placebo-controlled study, NAFLD patients who were overweight and had impaired fasting glucose received phytosomal curcumin containing 200 mg curcumin, 480 mg phosphatidylcholine, 120 mg phosphatidylserine, and 8 mg piperine from *Piper nigrum* L. during 8 weeks (Cicero et al., 2020). Improvements in fasting plasma insulin and tryglycerides, hepatic function (liver transaminases and FLI), blood pressure, and serum cortisol levels were shown after the phytosomal curcumin supplementation compared with the placebo group. Mirhafez et al. (2019) administered curcumin with piperine (500 mg/day curcumin and 5 mg/day piperine) or a placebo during 8 weeks to NAFLD patients in a randomized, double-blind, placebo-controlled trial. Oxidative stress assessed by measuring serum prooxidant and antioxidant balance did not show differences between the groups, suggesting that the curcumin dose was low to find beneficial effects.

The green cardamom seed (*Elettaria cardamomom* (L.) Maton, family Zingiberaceae) is a spice mainly used in India and the Middle East that contains multiple polyphenols such as luteolin, quercetin, kaempferol, and pelargonidin (Bhaswant et al., 2015). Green cardamom (2 capsules of 500 mg 3 times/day) was provided to overweight/obese NAFLD patients in a double-blind, randomized, placebo-controlled clinical trial for 3 months (Daneshi-Maskooni et al., 2018). Green cardamom intake significantly increased serum histone deacetylase Sirtuin-1 (Sirt1) and reduced inflammatory mediators (high-sensitivity C-reactive protein (hs-CRP), TNF-α, IL-6), ALT, and the degree of liver accumulation of fat. It also improved the grade of fatty liver determined by ultrasonography, serum lipid profile (increased high-density lipoprotein (HDL-C) and reduced LDL-C and TG), glucose indices, and increased irisin levels (Daneshi-Maskooni et al., 2019).

Cinnamon is a spice that has been used for thousands of years to provide flavor to different dishes, especially curries. This spice derives from the brown bark of the cinnamon tree (*Cinnamomum verum* L., family Lauraceae) and contains diverse bioactive compounds including cinnamaldehyde, cinnamic acid, eugenol, coumarin, and procyanidin oligomers (Broadhurst et al., 2000). In a randomized clinical trial, patients diagnosed with NAFLD by ultrasonography were randomized to receive capsules of cinnamon (750 mg each capsule twice daily) or a placebo for 12 weeks (Askari et al., 2014). After the intervention period, the fasting blood glucose, HOMA-IR, triglycerides, total cholesterol, hepatic enzymes (AST, ALT, and GGT) and hs-CRP were reduced with respect to the placebo group.

Green tea is one of the most widely consumed beverages worldwide. Tea leaves from *Camellia sinensis* (L.) Kuntze (family Theaceae) contain a variety of bioactive components, such as flavonoids, caffeine, tannins, and essential oils (Fang et al., 2019). Sakata and Collaborators (2013) examined the effect of supplementation with green tea rich in high-density catechins in NAFLD subjects in a double-blind, placebo-controlled study for 12 weeks. Participants consumed 700 mL green tea containing high levels of catechins (1080 mg), low levels (200 mg catechins), or a placebo. The supplementation with high levels induced better improvements in body fat, serum ALT, and urine 8-isoprostane with respect to the other groups. A greater increase in the liver-to-spleen computed tomography attenuation ratio was also found in the high catechin group. The activity of green tea extract consumption on live enzymes was analyzed in a double-blind, placebo-controlled, randomized clinical trial (Pezeshki et al., 2016). NALFD patients diagnosed with ultrasonography were allocated to receive green tea extract supplement (500 mg/day) or a placebo during 90 days. The BMI and serum alkaline phosphatase (ALP) were significantly diminished in both groups after the intervention period, although the decrease was higher in the green tea extract group. Serum transaminases were reduced only in the supplemented group. In a similar procedure, overweight NAFLD patients were randomized for treatment with green tea extract (500 mg twice/day) or a placebo during 12 weeks (Hussain et al., 2017). Green tea supplementation improved the lipid profile and anthropometric parameters; reduced HOMA-IR, aminotransferases, and hs-CRP; and increased the serum levels of adiponectin. Moreover, green tea extract ameliorated fatty liver changes measured with ultrasound. Another double-blind clinical trial investigated the efficacy of 550 mg of green tea tablets daily for 3 months together with nutritional education in NAFLD patients (Tabatabaee et al., 2017). BMI, AST, and fasting blood sugar significantly decreased in the green tea group after the intervention with respect to the placebo group.

Garlic (*Allium sativum* L., family Amaryllidaceae) can be considered a functional food with diverse bioactive compounds such as organosulfur compounds, mainly allicin, and flavonoids that has been extensively utilized as herbal therapy in traditional medicine (Martins et al., 2016). Garlic powder consumption was tested on body composition in NAFLD patients in a randomized, double-blind, placebo-controlled design (Soleimani et al., 2016). Subjects ($n = 110$) were randomly allocated to the intervention group (two tablets containing 400 mg garlic powder daily) or placebo for 15 weeks. Weight and body fat content were significantly reduced in the supplemented group with respect to the placebo after the intervention period. One limitation was the fact that the clinical and biochemical parameters were not determined. In another study, the beneficial effects of fermented garlic extract, designed to reduce its pungent smell and taste, in hepatic function in adults with elevated serum GGT levels were analyzed (Kim et al., 2017). The supplementation with fermented garlic extract (one sachet of 20 g, twice daily) during 12 weeks significantly improved the serum ALT and GGT levels with respect to the control group.

Olive oil, a characteristic constituent of the Mediterranean diet derived from the fruits—olives—of *Olea europaea* L. (family Oleaceae) trees, presents elevated levels of monounsaturated fatty acids and phenolic compounds such as hydroxytyrosol and oleuropein (Cicerale et al., 2010; Serreli and Deiana, 2018). In a 6-month intervention, 93 NAFLD ultrasound diagnosed males were divided into three groups receiving either olive oil, canola oil, or soybean/safflower oil as the control group as a cooking medium (not exceeding 20 g/day) (Nigam et al., 2014). After the intervention, the fasting insulin, HOMA-IR, and severity of the fatty liver were significantly decreased in both the olive and canola oil groups with respect to the control group, whereas BMI decreased significantly only in the olive oil group. Another clinical trial evaluated the effects of virgin olive oil on aminotransferases and the severity of steatosis in the NAFLD patients subjected to a hypocaloric diet to lose weight (Shidfar et al., 2018). Participants were randomly allocated to the olive oil group (consuming about 20% of their total daily energy requirements from olive oil) or the control group (with normal consumption of oil) during 12 weeks. Serum levels of ALT and AST significantly diminished in the intervention group with respect to the control one, and although the severity of liver steatosis improved in both groups, no significant differences were observed between both groups. In a recent clinical trial, NAFLD patients were divided to intake either olive or sunflower oil (20 g/day) for 12 weeks together with a hypocaloric diet (Rezaei et al., 2019). Olive oil consumption improved the degree of fatty liver and reduced the percentage of body fat in patients with NAFLD, but did not affect liver enzymes or cardiometabolic risk factors. The reductions in weight, waist circumference, blood pressure, and serum aminotransferases were similar in both groups and could be attributed to the hypocaloric diet.

Licorice (*Glycyrrhiza glabra* L., family Leguminosae) is a plant used since antiquity in traditional medicine (Isbrucker and Burdock, 2006). Licorice root extracts contain as the main bioactive component glycyrrhizin, a saponin with notable pharmacological but also potential toxic effects (Nazari et al., 2017). The effects of licorice were evaluated in NAFLD patients with elevated liver enzymes confirmed by sonography in a double-blind randomized clinical trial (Hajiaghamohammadi et al., 2012). 66 Patients were assigned to aqueous licorice root extract (2 g) or placebo intake for 2 months. Following the intervention period, the ALT and AST were reduced in both groups, although the decrease was only significant in the licorice group. However, liver function or liver histology was not evaluated.

Bayberry comprises about 35–50 species of the genus *Myrica* (family Myricaceae) native to China and Southeast Asia with many different bioactive compounds, including anthocyanins and phenolic acids (Ge et al., 2018; Kang et al., 2012). The hepatoprotective effects of bayberry juice were evaluated in young individuals diagnosed with NAFLD (abdominal ultrasonographic examination) (Guo et al., 2014). Bayberry juice (250 mL) or a placebo was given to the participants twice daily for 4 weeks. Bayberry juice decreased the plasma levels of protein carbonyl groups, inflammatory markers (TNFα and IL-18), polypeptide-specific antigen, and CK-18.

5.6 Conclusions

It is clear that a relation between NAFLD and the Mediterranean diet exists. However, clinical trials are scarce and different limitations of the published works related to the methodology should be taken into account, such as a low sample size or a short time follow-up. Moreover, ultrasound imaging, ALT levels as the initial diagnosis marker, or different indices have been used to assess the NAFLD presence, and only a few works have used magnetic resonance spectroscopy as the main tool to establish the disease diagnosis. The Mediterranean diet is rich in polyphenols; in fact, much evidence seems to support the fact that some natural compounds can improve the indicators of liver damage and reduce the accumulation of fat. However, other studies do not observe clear effects with respect to a hypocaloric diet and exercise regime. Although it should not be ruled out that some of these compounds may have some beneficial effects on NAFLD, these cannot replace a balanced and hypocaloric diet and regular physical exercise as the main mechanism to revert the disease. The use of bioactive natural compounds such as resveratrol or berberine, spices, and plant extracts with the ability to improve or reverse liver steatosis complementary to a dietary intervention and healthy lifestyle may contribute to the treatment and/or prevention of NAFLD progression.

Acknowledgments

This work was supported by the Spanish Ministry of Economy and Competitiveness, Instituto de Salud Carlos III (CIBEROBN-CB12/03/30038) and Fundación la "Marató de TV3" (549/U/2016). X Capó was funded by a FOLIUM program of the Health Research Institute of the Balearic Islands (IdISBa). The authors thank Xavier Canyelles for the design of Fig. 5.1.

References

Abenavoli, L., Di Renzo, L., Guzzi, P.H., Pellicano, R., Milic, N., Lorenzo, A.D.E., 2015a. Non-alcoholic fatty liver disease severity, central fat mass and adinopectin: a close relationship. Clujul Med. 88, 489–493.

Abenavoli, L., Greco, M., Nazionale, I., Peta, V., Milic, N., Accattato, F., Foti, D., Gulletta, E., Luzza, F., 2015b. Effects of Mediterranean diet supplemented with silybin-vitamin E-phospholipid complex in overweight patients with non-alcoholic fatty liver disease. Expert Rev. Gastroenterol. Hepatol. 9, 519–527.

Abenavoli, L., Greco, M., Milic, N., Accattato, F., Foti, D., Gulletta, E., Luzza, F., 2017. Effect of Mediterranean diet and antioxidant formulation in non-alcoholic fatty liver disease: a randomized study. Nutrients 9.

Aller, R., Izaola, O., de la Fuente, B., De Luis Roman, D.A., 2015a. Mediterranean diet is associated with liver histology in patients with non alcoholic fatty liver disease. Nutr. Hosp. 32, 2518–2524.

Aller, R., Izaola, O., Gomez, S., Tafur, C., Gonzalez, G., Berroa, E., Mora, N., Gonzalez, J.M., de Luis, D.A., 2015b. Effect of silymarin plus vitamin E in patients with non-alcoholic fatty liver disease. A randomized clinical pilot study. Eur. Rev. Med. Pharmacol. Sci. 19, 3118–3124.

Angulo, P., 2002. Nonalcoholic fatty liver disease. N. Engl. J. Med. 346, 1221–1231.

Ashraf, N.U., Sheikh, T.A., 2015. Endoplasmic reticulum stress and oxidative stress in the pathogenesis of non-alcoholic fatty liver disease. Free Radic. Res. 49, 1405–1418.

Askari, F., Rashidkhani, B., Hekmatdoost, A., 2014. Cinnamon may have therapeutic benefits on lipid profile, liver enzymes, insulin resistance, and high-sensitivity C-reactive protein in nonalcoholic fatty liver disease patients. Nutr. Res. 34, 143–148.

Asrih, M., Jornayvaz, F.R., 2015. Metabolic syndrome and nonalcoholic fatty liver disease: is insulin resistance the link? Mol. Cell. Endocrinol. 418 (Pt 1), 55–65.

Bai, R.M., Zheng, B.B., Zhang, R.D., Wei, J., 2011. Effects of berberine on insulin resistance and serumadiponectin of nonalcoholic fatty liver patients. Pract. Geriatr. 25, 423–426.

Baratta, F., Pastori, D., Polimeni, L., Bucci, T., Ceci, F., Calabrese, C., Ernesti, I., Pannitteri, G., Violi, F., Angelico, F., Del Ben, M., 2017. Adherence to Mediterranean diet and non-alcoholic fatty liver disease: effect on insulin resistance. Am. J. Gastroenterol. 112, 1832–1839.

Bellentani, S., Scaglioni, F., Marino, M., Bedogni, G., 2010. Epidemiology of non-alcoholic fatty liver disease. Dig. Dis. 28, 155–161.

Bhaswant, M., Poudyal, H., Mathai, M.L., Ward, L.C., Mouatt, P., Brown, L., 2015. Green and black cardamom in a diet-induced rat model of metabolic syndrome. Nutrients 7, 7691–7707.

Bijak, M., 2017. Silybin, a major bioactive component of milk thistle (*Silybum marianum* L. Gaernt.)—chemistry, bioavailability, and metabolism. Molecules 22.

Biolato, M., Manca, F., Marrone, G., Cefalo, C., Racco, S., Miggiano, G.A., Valenza, V., Gasbarrini, A., Miele, L., Grieco, A., 2019. Intestinal permeability after Mediterranean diet and low-fat diet in non-alcoholic fatty liver disease. World J. Gastroenterol. 25, 509–520.

Broadhurst, C.L., Polansky, M.M., Anderson, R.A., 2000. Insulin-like biological activity of culinary and medicinal plant aqueous extracts in vitro. J. Agric. Food Chem. 48, 849–852.

Brunt, E.M., 2001. Nonalcoholic steatohepatitis: definition and pathology. Semin. Liver Dis. 21, 3–16.

Cao, Y.F., Cai Wei, W., Zhang, L.L., Fang, Y., 2012. Clinical observation on the Berberine plus metformin in treatment of type 2 diabetes complicated by nonalcoholic fatty liver disease. Mod. Prevent. Med. 39, 4885–4887.

Capo, X., Martorell, M., Sureda, A., Llompart, I., Tur, J.A., Pons, A., 2015. Diet supplementation with DHA-enriched food in football players during training season enhances the mitochondrial antioxidant capabilities in blood mononuclear cells. Eur. J. Nutr. 54, 35–49.

Carter-Kent, C., Zein, N.N., Feldstein, A.E., 2008. Cytokines in the pathogenesis of fatty liver and disease progression to steatohepatitis: implications for treatment. Am. J. Gastroenterol. 103, 1036–1042.

Castañeda-Ovando, A., Pacheco-Hernández, M.L., Páez-Hernández, M.E., Rodríguez, J.A., Galán-Vidal, C.A., 2009. Chemical studies of anthocyanins: a review. Food Chem. 113, 589–871.

Chang, X., Wang, Z., Zhang, J., Yan, H., Bian, H., Xia, M., Lin, H., Jiang, J., Gao, X., 2016. Lipid profiling of the therapeutic effects of berberine in patients with nonalcoholic fatty liver disease. J. Transl. Med. 14, 266.

Chashmniam, S., Mirhafez, S.R., Dehabeh, M., Hariri, M., Azimi Nezhad, M., Nobakht, M.G.B.F., 2019. A pilot study of the effect of phospholipid curcumin on serum metabolomic profile in patients with non-alcoholic fatty liver disease: a randomized, double-blind, placebo-controlled trial. Eur. J. Clin. Nutr. 73, 1224–1235.

Chen, S., Zhao, X., Ran, L., Wan, J., Wang, X., Qin, Y., Shu, F., Gao, Y., Yuan, L., Zhang, Q., Mi, M., 2015. Resveratrol improves insulin resistance, glucose and lipid metabolism in patients with non-alcoholic fatty liver disease: a randomized controlled trial. Dig. Liver Dis. 47, 226–232.

Cicerale, S., Lucas, L., Keast, R., 2010. Biological activities of phenolic compounds present in virgin olive oil. Int. J. Mol. Sci. 11, 458–479.

Cicero, A.F.G., Sahebkar, A., Fogacci, F., Bove, M., Giovannini, M., Borghi, C., 2020. Effects of phytosomal curcumin on anthropometric parameters, insulin resistance, cortisolemia and non-alcoholic fatty liver disease indices: a double-blind, placebo-controlled clinical trial. Eur. J. Nutr. 59, 477–483.

Clark, J.M., 2006. The epidemiology of nonalcoholic fatty liver disease in adults. J. Clin. Gastroenterol. 40 (Suppl. 1), S5–10.

Cueto-Galan, R., Baron, F.J., Valdivielso, P., Pinto, X., Corbella, E., Gomez-Gracia, E., Warnberg, J., 2017. Changes in fatty liver index after consuming a Mediterranean diet: 6-year follow-up of the PREDIMED-Malaga trial. Med. Clin. (Barc.) 148, 435–443.

Daneshi-Maskooni, M., Keshavarz, S.A., Qorbani, M., Mansouri, S., Alavian, S.M., Badri-Fariman, M., Jazayeri-Tehrani, S.A., Sotoudeh, G., 2018. Green cardamom increases Sirtuin-1 and reduces inflammation in overweight or obese patients with non-alcoholic fatty liver disease: a double-blind randomized placebo-controlled clinical trial. Nutr. Metab. (Lond.) 15, 63.

Daneshi-Maskooni, M., Keshavarz, S.A., Qorbani, M., Mansouri, S., Alavian, S.M., Badri-Fariman, M., Jazayeri-Tehrani, S.A., Sotoudeh, G., 2019. Green cardamom supplementation improves serum irisin, glucose indices, and lipid profiles in overweight or obese non-alcoholic fatty liver disease patients: a double-blind randomized placebo-controlled clinical trial. BMC Complement. Altern. Med. 19, 59.

Day, C.P., James, O.F., 1998. Steatohepatitis: a tale of two "hits". Gastroenterology 114, 842–845.

Diehl, A.M., 2004. Tumor necrosis factor and its potential role in insulin resistance and nonalcoholic fatty liver disease. Clin. Liver Dis. 8, 619–638. x.

Faghihzadeh, F., Adibi, P., Rafiei, R., Hekmatdoost, A., 2014. Resveratrol supplementation improves inflammatory biomarkers in patients with nonalcoholic fatty liver disease. Nutr. Res. 34, 837–843.

Faghihzadeh, F., Adibi, P., Hekmatdoost, A., 2015. The effects of resveratrol supplementation on cardiovascular risk factors in patients with non-alcoholic fatty liver disease: a randomised, double-blind, placebo-controlled study. Br. J. Nutr. 114, 796–803.

Fang, J., Sureda, A., Silva, A.S., Khan, F., Xu, S., Nabavi, S.M., 2019. Trends of tea in cardiovascular health and disease: a critical review. Trends Food Sci. Technol. 88, 385–396.

Federico, A., Trappoliere, M., Tuccillo, C., de Sio, I., Di Leva, A., Del Vecchio Blanco, C., Loguercio, C., 2006. A new silybin-vitamin E-phospholipid complex improves insulin resistance and liver damage in patients with non-alcoholic fatty liver disease: preliminary observations. Gut 55, 901–902.

Franzese, A., Vajro, P., Argenziano, A., Puzziello, A., Iannucci, M.P., Saviano, M.C., Brunetti, F., Rubino, A., 1997. Liver involvement in obese children. Ultrasonography and liver enzyme levels at diagnosis and during follow-up in an Italian population. Dig. Dis. Sci. 42, 1428–1432.

Fraser, A., Abel, R., Lawlor, D.A., Fraser, D., Elhayany, A., 2008. A modified Mediterranean diet is associated with the greatest reduction in alanine aminotransferase levels in obese type 2 diabetes patients: results of a quasi-randomised controlled trial. Diabetologia 51, 1616–1622.

Ge, S., Wang, L., Ma, J., Jiang, S., Peng, W., 2018. Biological analysis on extractives of bayberry fresh flesh by GC-MS. Saudi J. Biol. Sci. 25, 816–818.

Gelli, C., Tarocchi, M., Abenavoli, L., Di Renzo, L., Galli, A., De Lorenzo, A., 2017. Effect of a counseling-supported treatment with the Mediterranean diet and physical activity on the severity of the non-alcoholic fatty liver disease. World J. Gastroenterol. 23, 3150–3162.

Guo, H., Zhong, R., Liu, Y., Jiang, X., Tang, X., Li, Z., Xia, M., Ling, W., 2014. Effects of bayberry juice on inflammatory and apoptotic markers in young adults with features of non-alcoholic fatty liver disease. Nutrition 30, 198–203.

Gutteridge, J.M., Halliwell, B., 1992. Comments on review of Free Radicals in Biology and Medicine, second edition, by Barry Halliwell and John M. C. Gutteridge. Free Radic. Biol. Med. 12, 93–95.

Hajiaghamohammadi, A.A., Ziaee, A., Samimi, R., 2012. The efficacy of licorice root extract in decreasing transaminase activities in non-alcoholic fatty liver disease: a randomized controlled clinical trial. Phytother. Res. 26, 1381–1384.

Halliwell, B., 1995. How to characterize an antioxidant: an update. Biochem. Soc. Symp. 61, 73–101.

Han, M.S., Park, S.Y., Shinzawa, K., Kim, S., Chung, K.W., Lee, J.H., Kwon, C.H., Lee, K.W., Park, C.K., Chung, W.J., Hwang, J.S., Yan, J.J., Song, D.K., Tsujimoto, Y., Lee, M.S., 2008. Lysophosphatidylcholine as a death effector in the lipoapoptosis of hepatocytes. J. Lipid Res. 49, 84–97.

Harikumar, K.B., Aggarwal, B.B., 2008. Resveratrol: a multitargeted agent for age-associated chronic diseases. Cell Cycle 7, 1020–1035.

Heeboll, S., Kreuzfeldt, M., Hamilton-Dutoit, S., Kjaer Poulsen, M., Stodkilde-Jorgensen, H., Moller, H.J., Jessen, N., Thorsen, K., Kristina Hellberg, Y., Bonlokke Pedersen, S., Gronbaek, H., 2016. Placebo-controlled, randomised clinical trial: high-dose resveratrol treatment for non-alcoholic fatty liver disease. Scand. J. Gastroenterol. 51, 456–464.

Hussain, M., Habib Ur, R., Akhtar, L., 2017. Therapeutic benefits of green tea extract on various parameters in non-alcoholic fatty liver disease patients. Pak. J. Med. Sci. 33, 931–936.

Imenshahidi, M., Hosseinzadeh, H., 2019. Berberine and barberry (*Berberis vulgaris*): a clinical review. Phytother. Res. 33, 504–523.

Isbrucker, R.A., Burdock, G.A., 2006. Risk and safety assessment on the consumption of Licorice root (*Glycyrrhiza* sp.), its extract and powder as a food ingredient, with emphasis on the pharmacology and toxicology of glycyrrhizin. Regul. Toxicol. Pharmacol. 46, 167–192.

Jeznach-Steinhagen, A., Ostrowska, J., Czerwonogrodzka-Senczyna, A., Boniecka, I., Shahnazaryan, U., Kurylowicz, A., 2019. Dietary and pharmacological treatment of nonalcoholic fatty liver disease. Medicina (Kaunas) 55.

Kang, W., Li, Y., Xu, Y., Jiang, W., Tao, Y., 2012. Characterization of aroma compounds in Chinese bayberry (*Myrica rubra* Sieb. et Zucc.) by gas chromatography mass spectrometry (GC-MS) and olfactometry (GC-O). J. Food Sci. 77, C1030–C1035.

Kantartzis, K., Fritsche, L., Bombrich, M., Machann, J., Schick, F., Staiger, H., Kunz, I., Schoop, R., Lehn-Stefan, A., Heni, M., Peter, A., Fritsche, A., Haring, H.U., Stefan, N., 2018. Effects of resveratrol supplementation on liver fat content in overweight and insulin-resistant subjects: a randomized, double-blind, placebo-controlled clinical trial. Diabetes Obes. Metab. 20, 1793–1797.

Kempinski, R., Lukawska, A., Krzyzanowski, F., Slosarz, D., Poniewierka, E., 2019. Clinical outcomes of non-alcoholic fatty liver disease: Polish-case control study. Adv. Clin. Exp. Med. 28, 1615–1620.

Kim, N.C., Graf, T.N., Sparacino, C.M., Wani, M.C., Wall, M.E., 2003. Complete isolation and characterization of silybins and isosilybins from milk thistle (*Silybum marianum*). Org. Biomol. Chem. 1, 1684–1689.

Kim, H.N., Kang, S.G., Roh, Y.K., Choi, M.K., Song, S.W., 2017. Efficacy and safety of fermented garlic extract on hepatic function in adults with elevated serum gamma-glutamyl transpeptidase levels: a double-blind, randomized, placebo-controlled trial. Eur. J. Nutr. 56, 1993–2002.

Kontogianni, M.D., Tileli, N., Margariti, A., Georgoulis, M., Deutsch, M., Tiniakos, D., Fragopoulou, E., Zafiropoulou, R., Manios, Y., Papatheodoridis, G., 2014. Adherence to the Mediterranean diet is associated with the severity of non-alcoholic fatty liver disease. Clin. Nutr. 33, 678–683.

Levene, A.P., Goldin, R.D., 2012. The epidemiology, pathogenesis and histopathology of fatty liver disease. Histopathology 61, 141–152.

Li, H.L., 2015. Observation of the clinical effects of Berberine combined with Yi-gan-Ling in the treatment of metabolize syndrome with nonalcoholic steatohepatitis. Anhui Med. Pharm. J. 19, 363–366.

Li, H., Li, Q., Liu, Z., Yang, K., Chen, Z., Cheng, Q., Wu, L., 2017. The versatile effects of dihydromyricetin in health. Evid. Based Complement. Alternat. Med. 2017, 1053617.

Loguercio, C., Andreone, P., Brisc, C., Brisc, M.C., Bugianesi, E., Chiaramonte, M., Cursaro, C., Danila, M., de Sio, I., Floreani, A., Freni, M.A., Grieco, A., Groppo, M., Lazzari, R., Lobello, S., Lorefice, E., Margotti, M., Miele, L., Milani, S., Okolicsanyi, L., Palasciano, G., Portincasa, P., Saltarelli, P., Smedile, A., Somalvico, F., Spadaro, A., Sporea, I., Sorrentino, P., Vecchione, R., Tuccillo, C., Del Vecchio Blanco, C., Federico, A., 2012. Silybin combined with phosphatidylcholine and vitamin E in patients with nonalcoholic fatty liver disease: a randomized controlled trial. Free Radic. Biol. Med. 52, 1658–1665.

Martin, R.C., Aiyer, H.S., Malik, D., Li, Y., 2012. Effect on pro-inflammatory and antioxidant genes and bioavailable distribution of whole turmeric vs curcumin: similar root but different effects. Food Chem. Toxicol. 50, 227–231.

Martins, N., Petropoulos, S., Ferreira, I.C., 2016. Chemical composition and bioactive compounds of garlic (*Allium sativum* L.) as affected by pre- and post-harvest conditions: a review. Food Chem. 211, 41–50.

McCullough, A.J., 2004. The clinical features, diagnosis and natural history of nonalcoholic fatty liver disease. Clin. Liver Dis. 8, 521–533. viii.

Medina, J., Moreno-Otero, R., 2005. Pathophysiological basis for antioxidant therapy in chronic liver disease. Drugs 65, 2445–2461.

Mirhafez, S.R., Farimani, A.R., Gholami, A., Hooshmand, E., Tavallaie, S., Nobakht, M.G.B.F., 2019. The effect of curcumin with piperine supplementation on pro-oxidant and antioxidant balance in patients with non-alcoholic fatty liver disease: a randomized, double-blind, placebo-controlled trial. Drug Metab. Pers. Ther. 34. https://doi.org/10.1515/dmpt-2018-0040.

Misciagna, G., Del Pilar Diaz, M., Caramia, D.V., Bonfiglio, C., Franco, I., Noviello, M.R., Chiloiro, M., Abbrescia, D.I., Mirizzi, A., Tanzi, M., Caruso, M.G., Correale, M., Reddavide, R., Inguaggiato, R., Cisternino, A.M., Osella, A.R., 2017. Effect of a low glycemic index Mediterranean diet on non-alcoholic fatty liver disease. A randomized controlled clinical trial. J. Nutr. Health Aging 21, 404–412.

Moller, D.E., Flier, J.S., 1991. Insulin resistance—mechanisms, syndromes, and implications. N. Engl. J. Med. 325, 938–948.

Mulhall, B.P., Ong, J.P., Younossi, Z.M., 2002. Non-alcoholic fatty liver disease: an overview. J. Gastroenterol. Hepatol. 17, 1136–1143.

Nazari, S., Rameshrad, M., Hosseinzadeh, H., 2017. Toxicological effects of *Glycyrrhiza glabra* (Licorice): a review. Phytother. Res. 31, 1635–1650.

Nigam, P., Bhatt, S., Misra, A., Chadha, D.S., Vaidya, M., Dasgupta, J., Pasha, Q.M., 2014. Effect of a 6-month intervention with cooking oils containing a high concentration of monounsaturated fatty acids (olive and canola oils) compared with control oil in male Asian Indians with nonalcoholic fatty liver disease. Diabetes Technol. Ther. 16, 255–261.

Ning, J., Zhang, H.T., Liu, D.D., Wang, X.Q., 2013. The efficiency of Berberine combined with metformin in the treatment of type 2 diabetes mellitus with nonalcoholic fatty liver disease. Chin. J. Mod. Drug. Appl. 7, 155–157.

Pahl, H.L., 1999. Activators and target genes of Rel/NF-kappaB transcription factors. Oncogene 18, 6853–6866.

Pan, M.H., Lai, C.S., Tsai, M.L., Ho, C.T., 2014. Chemoprevention of nonalcoholic fatty liver disease by dietary natural compounds. Mol. Nutr. Food Res. 58, 147–171.

Panahi, Y., Kianpour, P., Mohtashami, R., Jafari, R., Simental-Mendia, L.E., Sahebkar, A., 2016. Curcumin lowers serum lipids and uric acid in subjects with nonalcoholic fatty liver disease: a randomized controlled trial. J. Cardiovasc. Pharmacol. 68, 223–229.

Panahi, Y., Kianpour, P., Mohtashami, R., Jafari, R., Simental-Mendia, L.E., Sahebkar, A., 2017. Efficacy and safety of phytosomal curcumin in non-alcoholic fatty liver disease: a randomized controlled trial. Drug Res. (Stuttg.) 67, 244–251.

Perumpail, B.J., Khan, M.A., Yoo, E.R., Cholankeril, G., Kim, D., Ahmed, A., 2017. Clinical epidemiology and disease burden of nonalcoholic fatty liver disease. World J. Gastroenterol. 23, 8263–8276.

Pezeshki, A., Safi, S., Feizi, A., Askari, G., Karami, F., 2016. The effect of green tea extract supplementation on liver enzymes in patients with nonalcoholic fatty liver disease. Int. J. Prev. Med. 7, 28.

Poulsen, M.K., Nellemann, B., Bibby, B.M., Stodkilde-Jorgensen, H., Pedersen, S.B., Gronbaek, H., Nielsen, S., 2018. No effect of resveratrol on VLDL-TG kinetics and insulin sensitivity in obese men with nonalcoholic fatty liver disease. Diabetes Obes. Metab. 20, 2504–2509.

Properzi, C., O'Sullivan, T.A., Sherriff, J.L., Ching, H.L., Jeffrey, G.P., Buckley, R.F., Tibballs, J., MacQuillan, G.C., Garas, G., Adams, L.A., 2018. *Ad libitum* Mediterranean and low-fat diets both significantly reduce hepatic steatosis: a randomized controlled trial. Hepatology 68, 1741–1754.

Rahmani, S., Asgary, S., Askari, G., Keshvari, M., Hatamipour, M., Feizi, A., Sahebkar, A., 2016. Treatment of non-alcoholic fatty liver disease with curcumin: a randomized placebo-controlled trial. Phytother. Res. 30, 1540–1548.

Rezaei, S., Akhlaghi, M., Sasani, M.R., Barati Boldaji, R., 2019. Olive oil lessened fatty liver severity independent of cardiometabolic correction in patients with non-alcoholic fatty liver disease: a randomized clinical trial. Nutrition 57, 154–161.

Ryan, M.C., Itsiopoulos, C., Thodis, T., Ward, G., Trost, N., Hofferberth, S., O'Dea, K., Desmond, P.V., Johnson, N.A., Wilson, A.M., 2013. The Mediterranean diet improves hepatic steatosis and insulin sensitivity in individuals with non-alcoholic fatty liver disease. J. Hepatol. 59, 138–143.

Sakata, R., Nakamura, T., Torimura, T., Ueno, T., Sata, M., 2013. Green tea with high-density catechins improves liver function and fat infiltration in non-alcoholic fatty liver disease (NAFLD) patients: a double-blind placebo-controlled study. Int. J. Mol. Med. 32, 989–994.

Schuster, S., Cabrera, D., Arrese, M., Feldstein, A.E., 2018. Triggering and resolution of inflammation in NASH. Nat. Rev. Gastroenterol. Hepatol. 15, 349–364.

Schwabe, R.F., Uchinami, H., Qian, T., Bennett, B.L., Lemasters, J.J., Brenner, D.A., 2004. Differential requirement for c-Jun NH_2-terminal kinase in TNFalpha- and Fas-mediated apoptosis in hepatocytes. FASEB J. 18, 720–722.

Serreli, G., Deiana, M., 2018. Biological relevance of extra virgin olive oil polyphenols metabolites. Antioxidants (Basel) 7.

Shidfar, F., Bahrololumi, S.S., Doaei, S., Mohammadzadeh, A., Gholamalizadeh, M., Mohammadimanesh, A., 2018. The effects of extra virgin olive oil on alanine aminotransferase, aspartate aminotransferase, and ultrasonographic indices of hepatic steatosis in nonalcoholic fatty liver disease patients undergoing low calorie diet. Can. J. Gastroenterol. Hepatol. 2018, 1053710.

Singh, R., Wang, Y., Schattenberg, J.M., Xiang, Y., Czaja, M.J., 2009. Chronic oxidative stress sensitizes hepatocytes to death from 4-hydroxynonenal by JNK/c-Jun overactivation. Am. J. Physiol. Gastrointest. Liver Physiol. 297, G907–G917.

Smith, B.W., Adams, L.A., 2011. Nonalcoholic fatty liver disease and diabetes mellitus: pathogenesis and treatment. Nat. Rev. Endocrinol. 7, 456–465.

Soleimani, D., Paknahad, Z., Askari, G., Iraj, B., Feizi, A., 2016. Effect of garlic powder consumption on body composition in patients with nonalcoholic fatty liver disease: a randomized, double-blind, placebo-controlled trial. Adv. Biomed. Res. 5, 2.

Sorrentino, G., Crispino, P., Coppola, D., De Stefano, G., 2015. Efficacy of lifestyle changes in subjects with non-alcoholic liver steatosis and metabolic syndrome may be improved with an antioxidant nutraceutical: a controlled clinical study. Drugs R D 15, 21–25.

Suda, I., Ishikawa, F., Hatakeyama, M., Miyawaki, M., Kudo, T., Hirano, K., Ito, A., Yamakawa, O., Horiuchi, S., 2008. Intake of purple sweet potato beverage affects on serum hepatic biomarker levels of healthy adult men with borderline hepatitis. Eur. J. Clin. Nutr. 62, 60–67.

Sureda, A., Tauler, P., Aguilo, A., Cases, N., Fuentespina, E., Cordova, A., Tur, J.A., Pons, A., 2005. Relation between oxidative stress markers and antioxidant endogenous defences during exhaustive exercise. Free Radic. Res. 39, 1317–1324.

Tabatabaee, S.M., Alavian, S.M., Ghalichi, L., Miryounesi, S.M., Mousavizadeh, K., Jazayeri, S., Vafa, M.R., 2017. Green tea in non-alcoholic fatty liver disease: a double blind randomized clinical trial. Hepat. Mon. 17, e14993.

Tarantino, G., Caputi, A., 2011. JNKs, insulin resistance and inflammation: a possible link between NAFLD and coronary artery disease. World J. Gastroenterol. 17, 3785–3794.

Tilg, H., Moschen, A.R., 2010. Evolution of inflammation in nonalcoholic fatty liver disease: the multiple parallel hits hypothesis. Hepatology 52, 1836–1846.

Tillhon, M., Guaman Ortiz, L.M., Lombardi, P., Scovassi, A.I., 2012. Berberine: new perspectives for old remedies. Biochem. Pharmacol. 84, 1260–1267.

Trovato, F.M., Catalano, D., Martines, G.F., Pace, P., Trovato, G.M., 2015. Mediterranean diet and non-alcoholic fatty liver disease: the need of extended and comprehensive interventions. Clin. Nutr. 34, 86–88.

Trovato, F.M., Martines, G.F., Brischetto, D., Trovato, G., Catalano, D., 2016. Neglected features of lifestyle: their relevance in non-alcoholic fatty liver disease. World J. Hepatol. 8, 1459–1465.

Unger, R.H., 2003. Minireview: weapons of lean body mass destruction: the role of ectopic lipids in the metabolic syndrome. Endocrinology 144, 5159–5165.

Videla, L.A., Rodrigo, R., Araya, J., Poniachik, J., 2004. Oxidative stress and depletion of hepatic long-chain polyunsaturated fatty acids may contribute to nonalcoholic fatty liver disease. Free Radic. Biol. Med. 37, 1499–1507.

Wah Kheong, C., Nik Mustapha, N.R., Mahadeva, S., 2017. A randomized trial of silymarin for the treatment of nonalcoholic steatohepatitis. Clin. Gastroenterol. Hepatol. 15, 1940–1949 e1948.

Wallace, T.C., Slavin, M., Frankenfeld, C.L., 2016. Systematic review of anthocyanins and markers of cardiovascular disease. Nutrients 8.

Wieckowska, A., Papouchado, B.G., Li, Z., Lopez, R., Zein, N.N., Feldstein, A.E., 2008. Increased hepatic and circulating interleukin-6 levels in human nonalcoholic steatohepatitis. Am. J. Gastroenterol. 103, 1372–1379.

Xie, X.M., Meng, X.J., Zhou, X.J., Shu, X.C., Kong, H.J., 2011. The effency of Berberine in newly diagnosed type 2 diabetes mellitus with nonalcoholic fatty liver disease patients and the influence of blood rheology. China J. Chin. Mater. Med. 36, 3032–3035.

Yamaguchi, K., Itoh, Y., Yokomizo, C., Nishimura, T., Niimi, T., Fujii, H., Okanoue, T., Yoshikawa, T., 2010. Blockade of interleukin-6 signaling enhances hepatic steatosis but improves liver injury in methionine choline-deficient diet-fed mice. Lab. Invest. 90, 1169–1178.

Yan, H.M., Xia, M.F., Wang, Y., Chang, X.X., Yao, X.Z., Rao, S.X., Zeng, M.S., Tu, Y.F., Feng, R., Jia, W.P., Liu, J., Deng, W., Jiang, J.D., Gao, X., 2015. Efficacy of berberine in patients with non-alcoholic fatty liver disease. PLoS One 10, e0134172.

Zhang, P.W., Chen, F.X., Li, D., Ling, W.H., Guo, H.H., 2015. A CONSORT-compliant, randomized, double-blind, placebo-controlled pilot trial of purified anthocyanin in patients with nonalcoholic fatty liver disease. Medicine (Baltimore) 94, e758.

CHAPTER 6

Liver cancer

Ismail Shah[a], Sajjad Ali Khan[a], Sadiq Hussain[a], Fazlullah Khan[b], and Kamal Niaz[c]

[a]Department of Pharmacy, Abdul Wali Khan University, Garden Campus, Mardan, Pakistan
[b]Department of Allied Health Sciences, Bashir Institute of Health Sciences, Bhara Kahu, Islamabad, Pakistan [c]Department of Pharmacology and Toxicology, Faculty of Bio-Sciences, Cholistan University of Veterinary and Animal Sciences (CUVAS), Bahawalpur, Pakistan

6.1 Introduction

The liver is an accessory digestive gland present in vertebrates that helps in the detoxification of different metabolites, the synthesis of proteins, and the production of essential biochemicals for digestion (Abdel-Misih and Bloomston, 2010). Moreover, it regulates glycogen storage, red blood cell breakdown, hormones (Mustafa et al., 2015), and bile production (Tortora and Derrickson, 2008). It is a highly specialized tissue mainly made up of cells called hepatocytes and other cells that line the liver's small tubes (Bile ducts) and cells that line its blood vessels. The bile ducts come out of the liver carrying bile to the gallbladder or directly to the intestines. These different types of liver cells can form various types of benign (noncancerous) and malignant (cancerous) tumors. These tumors differ widely in causes, treatment, and prognosis.

Liver (hepatic) cancer appears to be the second principal reason for cancer-related mortalities in developing countries and sixth in developed countries (Choo et al., 2016). Approximately, 782,500 and 745,500 hepatic carcinoma and fatalities occurred throughout the world, respectively, in which 50% just in China (Tang et al., 2016). It is a serious disease that has turned into a serious medical and social problem (Li and Wang, 2016).

Patients with hepatic carcinoma when diagnosed in the beginning usually undergo surgical resection or hepatic transplantation based on their hepatic preserve. Although hepatic carcinoma is frequently hard to treat surgically, even at an early diagnosis, numerous cases are diagnosed at an advanced stage that are difficult to treat surgically. Even after surgical treatment, hepatic cancer often persists and metastasizes. Although chemotherapy along with molecular targeting therapy is a substitute cure for extremely developed hepatic carcinoma, its curative properties are narrow, leading to pitiful overall survival. The recurrence of cancer, metastasis, and resistance to chemo- and radiotherapy of the solid tumor is attributed to the existence of cancer stem cells (Nio et al., 2017).

Influence of Nutrients, Bioactive Compounds, and Plant Extracts in Liver Diseases. https://doi.org/10.1016/B978-0-12-816488-4.00004-8

6.2 Classification of hepatic cancers

The majority of primary liver cancers (PLC) originate from epithelial cells, either from cells of the intrahepatic bile duct or hepatocytes (Srivatanakul et al., 2004). Nonepithelial hepatic cancers are rare. Among hepatocyte line cancers, hepatocellular carcinoma (HCC) is the most widespread, occurring throughout the world (Shin et al., 2010). On the basis of spreading capacity (metastasis), liver cancer is broadly classified into benign tumors and malignant tumors as follows:

6.2.1 Benign tumors

Hepatic hemangioma: This is the most common benign hepatic tumor with a high frequency rate in females. Levels of estrogen and pregnancy may affect the size of the tumor. It is generally asymptomatic and hardly ever grows or bleeds. Surgical excision is necessary in several symptomatic cases. Several cases are incidentally discovered.

Focal nodular hyperplasia (FNH): It is the second most frequent benign hepatic tumor with an 80%–90% prevalence frequency in women. All the normal hepatic constituents are present in a hyperplastic lesion, but in a peculiarly structured pattern. Oral contraceptives, a basic congenital arteriovenous abnormality, and several medicines including azathioprine are thought to play a role in the disease. Several imaging procedures in combination may be needed for exact diagnosis.

Hepatocellular adenoma: Adenomas arise frequently in younger females. Several studies have showed this to be due to oral contraceptives. Most of the cases are asymptomatic and found by chance while scanning for any other disease. They may be complicated occasionally by bleeding after trauma or even spontaneously.

Angiomyolipoma: It is a comparatively rare tumor and possesses blood vessels, fatty cells, and smooth muscle cells in changeable proportions. Thick-walled blood vessels are generally arranged in the shape of an island.

Bile duct cystadenoma: It is a rare multilocular cystic tumor possibly because of congenital bile duct defects. It generally arises from ducts close to the hepatic hilum and is more prevalent in women. Because of its malignant degeneration capability, surgical excision may be suggested.

6.2.2 Malignant tumors

Hepatocellular carcinoma (HCC): This is the most common type among hepatocyte line cancers, occurring worldwide. It is more prevalent in men. HBV or HCV and chronic liver disease/cirrhosis are its frequent underlying cause.

Intrahepatic cholangiocarcinoma (CCA): It is the second most occurring intrahepatic primary cancer, arising from the epithelium of the intrahepatic bile duct. Primarily, it occurs in middle-aged and elders of any gender. Its frequency varies with geography and it presents the highest prevalence in Southeast Asia. Hepatolithiasis, liver fluke infection, primary sclerosing cholangitis, and carcinogenic nitroso-compounds are its predisposing factors (Alvarez et al., 1999).

Combined hepatocellular and cholangiocarcinoma: It is a rare type with violent malignancy that has unambiguous elements of both cholangio and hepatocellular carcinoma that are closely admixed with a low prognosis. Its frequency varies broadly, but patients having primary hepatic cancer possess a 1.0%–6.5% prevalence rate. Usually these tumors arise mostly in men in their 60s. In Asia, it is greatly linked with HBV/HCV and cirrhosis (Hermanek et al., 1999).

Hepatoblastoma: It is the most frequent juvenile hepatic tumor with twice the prevalence rate in boys; it arises in the hepatic endodermal epithelium (Karlsson et al., 1999).

Bile duct cystadenocarcinoma: It is a rare epithelium-lined cystic tumor with papillary infoldings secreting either mucus or, less commonly, serous. Lesions develop from ducts proximal to the hepatic hilum. It arises from congenital liver cysts (Iemoto et al., 1983), bile ducts (Cruickshank and Sparshott, 1971), fibropolycystic disease (Theise et al., 1993), biliary cystadenoma (Wee et al., 1993), and a hepatoduodenal ligament (Inoue et al., 1995). After surgical removal, there is good prognosis (Hermanek et al., 1999). Different types of liver cancers and their causative agents are shown in Table 6.1.

6.3 Causes of liver cancer

Viral hepatitis: Viral hepatitis is a major infectious disease and currently is a challenge to health worldwide. In developing countries, the hepatitis A virus (HAV) and the hepatitis E virus (HEV) are widespread diseases. Usually, they cause self-limiting hepatitis and then sporadically lead to liver failure, chronic HEV infection, and unusual immune suppression (Stanaway et al., 2016). Several studies have demonstrated that HBV and HCV play a key role in the development of HCC. The infection of the hepatitis virus is linked with cellular inflammation, DNA damage, and oxidative stress and consequentially causes major hepatic injuries such as cirrhosis, fibrosis, chronic hepatitis, and ultimately HCC. The genotypic characteristics and the presence of viral proteins are mostly responsible for their direct oncogenic properties, due to which it interacts easily with host proteins, changing the balance of cell molecular pathways. Recently, different studies stated that viral hepatitis can trigger hepatic cancer stem cells (Sukowati et al., 2016).

Cirrhosis (scarring): Cirrhosis is the major cause of hepatic diseases leading to disrupted changes in liver units. This commonly occurs through the continuous loss

Table 6.1: Various types of hepatic cancer and their causative agents.

S. no.	Types	Causative agents
1	Hepatic hemangioma	Unknown (genetic factor plays role)
2	Focal nodular hyperplasia	Oral contraceptives, basic congenital arteriovenous abnormality, medicines (azathioprine)
3	Hepatocellular adenoma	Oral contraceptives
4	Angiomyolipoma	Unknown (genetic factor plays role)
5	Bile duct cystadenoma	Congenital bile duct defects
6	Hepatocellular carcinoma	HBV/HCV/chronic liver disease/cirrhosis
7	Intrahepatic cholangiocarcinoma	Hepatolithiasis, liver fluke infection, primary sclerosing cholangitis, carcinogenic nitroso-compounds
8	Combined hepatocellular and cholangiocarcinoma	HBV/HCV/cirrhosis
9	Hepatoblastoma	Wilson disease, Beckwith-Wiedemann syndrome, familial adenomatous polyposis, *Porphyria cutanea* tarda, inborn metabolic disorders such as glycogen storage diseases, tyrosinemia, and alpha1-antitrypsin deficiency
10	Bile duct cystadenocarcinoma	Congenital liver cysts, bile ducts, fibro polycystic disease, biliary cystadenoma, and hepatoduodenal ligament

of organ function via the use of antivirals, immunosuppressants, or antiinflammatory agents. Liver cirrhosis is a fundamental precancerogenic abrasion ultimately resulting in HCC (Mueller, 2016). Cirrhosis is the end stage in most chronic hepatic diseases that are mainly composed of fatal, harsh resource impediments such as hepato-cellular carcinoma, gastrointestinal hemorrhage, hepatic encephalopathy, renal failure, and many other infections, among others. The major cause of cirrhosis, the hepatitis C virus, was abolished by the advanced and feasible effective antiviral therapy that tends to be continued. Researchers estimated that there will be triple the deaths due to cirrhosis up to 2030. Due to high epidemics and the development of alcoholic liver diseases and nonalcoholic fatty liver diseases, cirrhosis has received more attention (Tapper and Parikh, 2018).

Aflatoxins (AF): Aflatoxins (AF) are composed of very toxic metabolites produced by the fungi *Aspergillus flavus, Aspergillus clavatus,* and *Aspergillus parasiticus.* In various foods such as grains, maize, and groundnuts, large amounts of AF (B1, B2, G1, and G2) are present, with B1 being the highly toxic form. AFM1 is known to be the principal metabolite of AFB1, excreted in milk and mammal urine along with addicted food or AF contaminated feed. AF B1-8,9-epoxide is formed from AFB1 through cytochrome p450, which can bind with RNA, DNA, and proteins leading to toxicity and cancer.

AF toxicity is mainly related to food safety and is a public health issue. It causes acute or chronic aflatoxicosis. Acute aflatoxicosis consists of conditions in which binding of the AFB1-epoxide to diverse cellular macromolecules takes place. This results in acute hepatotoxicity and leads to hepatocellular injury with acute liver damage, edema of the limbs, rapid progressive jaundice, abdominal pain, high fever, fulminant hepatic failure, vomiting, and eventually death (mortality rate 39%). Chronic aflatoxicosis is characterized by liver carcinoma. Epidemiological and animal studies reveal that an improvement in HCC is due to the synergistical working of HBV and AF (Afum et al., 2016). AF exposure causes conditions such as liver cancer and immune suppression. These both conditions further lead to increased susceptibility toward different diseases such as HIV, malaria and also in potential conciliation to vaccine efficacy as well. Acute aflatoxicosis prompts death while prolonged pathological conditions such as cancer and immunosuppression are usually caused by chronic aflatoxicosis. AFB1 primarily targets the liver and causes liver damage mostly in poultry and rodents, among others (Ogodo and Ugbogu, 2016).

Alcohol: Hepatic injury caused by alcohol is a primary cause of liver cirrhosis and HCC in the West (Morgan et al., 2004) and in Japanese men (Makimoto and Higuchi, 1999). It is also a major threat for hepatocarcinogenesis in areas with low hepatitis virus prevalence (Hellerbrand et al., 2001).

Hemochromatosis: It is an iron disorder in which the body absorbs too much iron with no proper way of getting rid of it. This is genetic and a mutated transporter of iron (HEF protein) is involved in it. If the condition is not treated, the excess iron can damage organs and joints, ultimately becoming fatal.

Heterozygotes for HFE mutations preexposed to viral hepatitis or alcohol abusers have a high risk of cirrhosis and later hepatic cancer than those with no mutations exposed to the same risks. The excess of iron is more associated with HCC with an increased death risk of 45% (Lauret et al., 2002).

Tyrosinemia: This autosomal recessive defect is caused by fumarylacetoacetate; an enzyme for the phenylalanine and tyrosine degradation. The deposition of upstream products results in serious hepatic disease and juvenile HCC. HCC affects 37% of patients who live to an age of 2 years, and liver transplants may occur in patients (Schagdarsurengin et al., 2003).

Alpha-1-antitrypsin deficiency: This autosomal-recessive defect results in elevated trypsin activity, and may cause cirrhosis and HCC development (Teckman and Lindblad, 2006).

Oral contraceptives: There is an increased risk of HCC among users of oral contraceptives. There is a dose-response relationship with an exposure period in women with HCC (Maheshwari et al., 2007).

Cigarette smoking: Several studies have shown a significant association between tobacco smoking and liver cancer and stomach cancer. However, basic evidence should be recorded carefully due to deficient information on known risk factors (Park et al., 2008).

Liver flukes: An association of liver flukes with chronic infection and cholangiocarcinoma (malignant neoplasm of the biliary duct system) risk has been demonstrated. *Opisthorchis viverrini* was considered to be carcinogenic (Srivatanakul et al., 2004). Several research studies have shown that liver flukes, *O. viverrini*, and *Clonorchis sinensis* play key roles as risk factors of CCA in Asia, particularly in Thailand (Sithithaworn et al., 2014).

Infection-induced chronic inflammation leads to the sustained production of molecules in the body that fight infection and act as carcinogens. Such chronic inflammations have key roles in several cancers, especially hepatic and stomach cancer (Srivatanakul, 2001). During inflammation, reactive oxygen and nitrogen species are produced that destroy the infectious agent. However, they can damage normal tissues as well by damaging DNA, leading to mutations and chromosomal aberrations accompanied by a raised cell division rate with decreased DNA repair efficiency. Chronic exposure to these agents can lead to damaging mutations.

Nitrosamines: Certain research studies have shown that nitrosamine compounds are a risk for the development of cholangiocarcinoma and hepatocellular carcinoma. These compounds are present in high levels in preserved protein products such as sausages, dried fish, fermented fish products, cured pork, dried shrimps, salty meat, common salts, and ground water (Rundlöf et al., 2000).

Hepatolithiasis: Several studies have shown a link between hepatolithiasis (recurrent pyogenic cholongitis) with CCA (Sugihara and Kojiro, 1987).

Inflammatory bowel disease and primary sclerosing cholangitis: According to several scientific studies, these are also predisposing factors to develop not only colorectal neoplasia but also carcinoma of the bile duct, including CCA (Harrison, 1999).

Arsenic compounds: The medicinal or environmental exposure to arsenic compounds is frequently related to hepato-cellular and hepatic angio-sarcomas. Hepatoportal sclerosis, hepatomegaly, fibrosis, and cirrhosis frequently occur following prolonged exposure to arsenic. Several mechanisms for hepatocarcinogenesis induced by arsenic include DNA damage through oxidation, damaged DNA repair impairment, altered methylation of DNA, acquired tolerance to apoptosis, hyperproliferation, and abnormal signaling of estrogen. Several of these mechanisms are liver selective. Overall, evidence indicates that the liver is a central target of arsenic carcinogenesis (Liu and Waalkes, 2008).

Thorotrast accumulation: Several studies have experimentally shown that thorium has a role in the development of bile duct epithelial cell and sinusoidal lining cell cancers (Srivatanakul et al., 2004).

Several other causes of hepatic cancer include diabetes (Campbell et al., 2016), obesity, chronic exposure to organic solvents such as xylene and toluene (Ferrand et al., 2008), family history, and polycyclic aromatic hydrocarbons (Johnson et al., 2010).

6.4 Diagnosis

Ultrasonography: Abdominal ultrasonography/abdominal ultrasound imaging/abdominal sonography is a type of medical ultrasonography. The main purpose of this technology is to visualize the internal organs through sound wave transmission. Abdominal ultrasound examination is performed by gastroenterologists or other trained professionals. It is used to diagnose abnormalities in internal organs such as the kidney, liver, pancreas, spleen, etc.

In hepatic imaging examination, abdominal ultrasonography is mainly used because it is easy to operate, clearer, pliable, noninvasive, and more satisfactory. Regular ultrasonography assessment can help to identify an intrahepatic space-occupying lesion at the initial stage as well as very precisely distinguish and detect cystic or space-occupying and metastatic lesions in the abdomen or liver. All HCC imaging techniques have improved considerably over the past decades. A high-resolution ultrasound scan can detect liver lesions smaller than 1 cm, and it is a useful screening tool. A fast multislice computed and magnetic resonance (MR) scanner provides multiphasic contrast enhanced imaging, which is required for lesion characterization and to assess the loco regional extent, number, and size of the lesion (Dittrich et al., 2016). Color Doppler sonography is a significant diagnostic noninvasive procedure for hepatic vasculature and portal venous system abnormality detection (Raman et al., 2013). Color Doppler flow recognizes the proximity correlation between the lesion and the main vessels rather than visualizing the supply of blood within the lesion. Contrast ultrasonography creates a clear picture of hemodynamic variability within hepatic carcinoma and enables the differences and diagnoses of changed types of hepatic cancer. This procedure has led us to the assessment of microvascular perfusion and intercessional measures for hepatic tumors due to its real-time multisectional imaging.

Computed tomography (CT): The multislice, multiphasic (improved, arterial, portal, and delayed phase) CT scan is the mostly applied standard imaging technique for determining the extent of hepatocellular carcinoma (DiSaia et al., 2017). It gives a three-dimensional (3D) size of the liver and the volume of the tumor as well as a metastasis assessment.

For clearer and superior scanning, contrast iodinated agents are applied. Their competency is to sense and diagnose minute tumors.

Magnetic resonance imaging (MRI): An MRI is an excellent procedure to detect intrahepatic lesions, especially T2-weighted spin-echo sequences that are the most efficient for tumor detection. Plain and improved scans are frequently used to observe and diagnose the response of hepatic carcinoma in clinical practice because of the absence of irradiation, high tissue resolution, multiparameter and multidirectional imaging, a structure combining topographies (comprising diffusion-weighted imaging, perfusion-weighted imaging, and spectrum analysis), and extensive imaging technique competency. When the hepatocyte specific contrast agents (Gd-EOB_DTPAs) are used in combination, the discovery rates for < 1.0 cm liver cancer, diagnostic precession, and the differential diagnosis of hepatic carcinoma are enhanced.

Largely in the late arterial phase of CT or MRI, liver cancer exhibits a clear heterogeneous augmentation or intermittently shows homogeneous promulgation. Specifically, liver cancer with ≤ 5.0 cm shows less improvement in the portal venous phase and/or parenchyma balance phase scan. This enhanced manner of "rapid wash in and out" is distinctive of hepatic carcinoma. The diagnosis of hepatic carcinoma by CT and MRI needs the assimilation of other specifically related signs shown in sequences of MRI in order to have a detailed judgment and improved diagnosis.

Digital subtraction angiography (DSA): This is a fluoroscopy procedure applied in interventional radiology to picture blood vessels clearly in a dense soft or bony tissue area. DSA is an invasive technique and is suggested to be executed via the selective or ultraselective hepatic artery. Mostly, this procedure is used for hepatic cancer local treatment or for acute bleeding from a hepatic cancer rupture. A hepatic carcinoma chiefly shows staining of tumors and blood vessels in the tumor on DSA. It helps in identifying the size, number, and blood supply of hepatic carcinoma and gives correct results about the anatomic disparity of vessels and significant vascular anatomic interaction along with tumor invasion to the portal vein.

6.4.1 Nuclear medical imaging

Positron emission tomography (PETCT): 18F-fluorodeoxyglucose-positron emission tomography/CT (18F-FDG PET/CT) has been recently introduced to detect extrahepatic metastases and predict the posttransplant prognosis in hepatic transplantation. Through this procedure, the PET/CT of the whole body is carried out using 18F-FDG for the detection of several cancerous lesions, including HCC (Beyer et al., 2000). Hepatic tissues, however, showed an elevated glucose-6-phosphatase level and discharged FDG-6-phosphate. This procedure verified the decreased discrimination between the usual liver and HCC. Thus, 18F-FDG PET/CT showed an average false-negative rate of 40%–50% for HCC detection (Lee and Kim, 2016).

6.4.2 Single photon emission computed tomography (SPECT)

Current improvements in nuclear imaging techniques using SPECT provide superior 3D spatial resolution. These techniques are able to differentiate the biochemistry and functional metabolism of neoplastic and normal tissue (Gritters and Wahl, 1993). Through SPECT, a tiny HCC of 1.9 cm in diameter can be detected (Yumoto et al., 1984).

6.4.3 Liver puncture biopsy

In this procedure, a needle is inserted into the liver for tissue sample collection. This is typically not essential in patients with space-occupying lesions. This should be carried out under CT or ultrasonography guidelines. A histological diagnosis for liver biopsy or cytological diagnosis can be achieved using an 18- or 16-gauge core needle or a fine needle for puncture. The platelet count and blood clotting should be done prior to the procedure because the key risk of a liver puncture biopsy is bleeding or needle tract implementation. A liver puncture biopsy should not be done in those patients who have serious hemorrhagic tendencies or serious diseases that affect the brain, heart, lungs, and kidneys or with systemic failure. To avoid rupturing tumor nodules and needle tract implementation, normal liver tissues should pass through using the puncture tract to avoid the direct puncture of nodules found on the surface of the liver. It is recommended that one piece of tissue each in the tumor and in the para-tumor liver tissue should be punctured for improved diagnostic accuracy based on objective comparison. Some false-negative results accompany the pathological diagnosis of a liver puncture. Approximately 33% of false negativity is counted in a biopsy. Negative results cannot completely eradicate the possibility of liver cancer. This test delivers a pathological diagnosis and is very significant to diagnose liver cancer, treatment management, and prognosis.

6.4.4 Serological molecular markers for liver cancer

Alpha fetoprotein (AFP) level determination in the blood gives some information regarding HCC. About 50% of HCCs secrete AFP (Song et al., 2016) and a plasma AFP concentration > 400 ng/mL is generally considered reliable to support the diagnosis of HCC with the omission of embryonal tumors of the ovary or testis, liver cirrhosis, active or chronic hepatitis, and pregnancy. Because the precision of the AFP level is challenged, it has been removed from the updated international guidelines for HCC surveillance (Bai et al., 2017).

6.4.5 Pathological diagnosis of liver cancer

This is generally combined with clinical signs and symptoms as well as knowing the history of the patient, HBV/HCV infection, tumor serum markers, and imaging examination. The pathological diagnosis is comprised of the uncultured illustration of specimens, microscopic examination, immune histochemical observation, and typical pathological photos (Zhou et al., 2018).

6.4.6 Prevention

During the last two decades, it was expected that more than half of hepatic cancers could be prohibited by counseling and sharing knowledge among individuals. It is not always possible to control hepatic cancer. However, several steps can help in controlling hepatic cancer, including vaccination against infection from HBV and HCV; reduced alcohol intake; cessation of tobacco smoking (Liu et al., 2018); careful needle use (source of HBV, HCV, and HIV) (Yang et al., 2018); use of clean water with no carcinogens such as arsenic, etc.; avoiding chronic exposure to organic solvents and chemicals including benzopyrene, acrylamide, vinyl chloride, and trichloroethylene; weight reduction; nonalcoholic fatty disease (linked with obesity); and controlling type 2 diabetes (Mantovani and Targher, 2017).

6.4.7 Treatment

Regardless of the advancement in treatment strategies, hepatic cancer is still one of the most difficult cancers to treat because of its reappearance, which is a main problem after treatment with a frequency greater than 70% after 5 years (Llovet et al., 2005). Therefore, several treatment regimens are applied, including:

Treatment for advanced disease: Hepatic cancers in the advanced stage are treated with standard frontline therapy (Liu et al., 2006), cytotoxic chemotherapy (Burroughs et al., 2004), immunotherapy (Hanahan and Weinberg, 2011), and oncolytic virus therapy (Russell et al., 2012).

Treatment for intermediate stage: Transarterial embolization (TAE) (embolic particles without chemotherapy) or TACE (chemotherapeutic drugs and embolic particles) (Llovet et al., 2002) therapy is applied for treating hepatic cancer in the intermediate stage.

Treatment for early stage: The early stage of hepatic cancer is treated with surgical resection (partial hepatectomy) (Kamiyama et al., 2014), liver transplantation (Mazzaferro et al., 1996), and locoregional therapy (Liu et al., 2015).

In spite of the abovementioned treatment options, many types of hepatic cancers remain untreatable and the emergence of drug resistance is constant (Gao et al., 2010). Consequently, new approaches for treatment are necessary. Almost half of the drugs used today in liver therapy are either natural products or their derivatives (Paterson and Anderson, 2005). The use of natural products to prevent/treat liver diseases dates back several thousand years. Natural products have gained attention globally for improving healthcare, disease prevention, and as conventional or complementary medicines for curable and incurable diseases (López et al., 2009). Several drugs prescribed nowadays are either directly isolated from natural products or are their artificially modified forms (Bringmann et al., 2008). These include compounds such as:

6.4.7.1 Glycyrrhizin

It is the main biological active agent of the root of *Glycyrrhiza glabra* L. It is a triterpene with antiviral potential applied for the protection of liver functions and the treatment of chronic hepatitis and tumors. It has nonspecific strong antiinflammatory potential and decreases the risk of water and sodium retention (Wan et al., 2009) (Fig. 6.1).

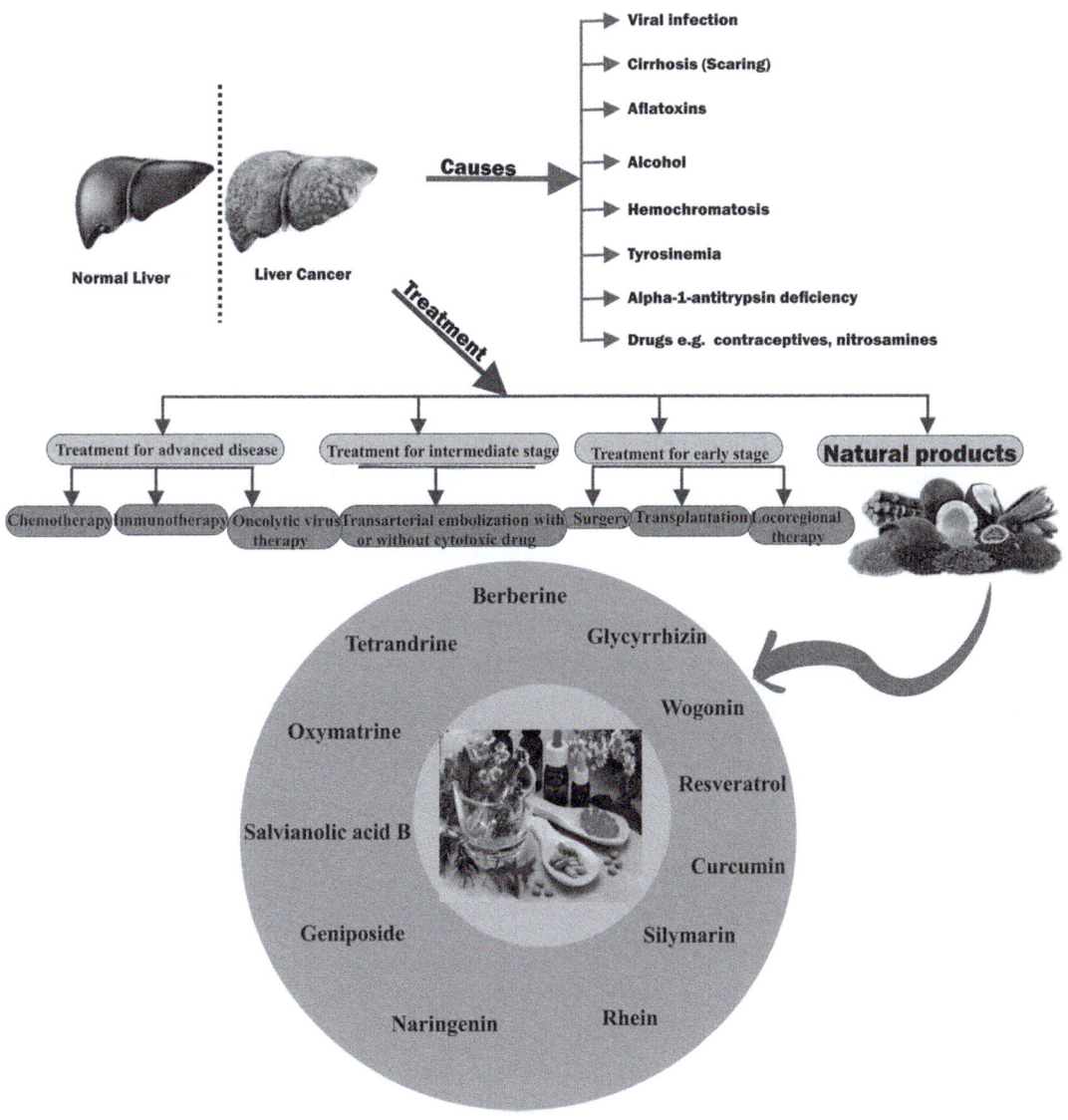

Fig. 6.1
Liver cancer, causes, and remedies based on natural products.

In a proper animal model, glycyrrhizin demonstrated the inhibition of acute liver injury, which may be due to the downregulation of MMP-9 (Abe et al., 2008). It also considerably inhibited hepatocyte apoptosis by decreasing caspase-3 expression and inhibiting cytochrome C release into the cytoplasm (Tang et al., 2007). It has the potential to augment proliferating cell nuclear antigen expression, aiding in enhancing the regeneration of livers injured by lipopolysaccharide. It prevents liver injury during hepato-biliary surgery as well (Ogiku et al., 2011).

6.4.7.2 Wogonin

It is a monoflavonoid obtained from *Scutellaria radix*. It has been applied for inflammatory diseases and hepatitis for thousands of years (Guo et al., 2007). It suppresses the secretion of hepatitis B surface antigen (HBsAg) in cell culture. It has cytotoxic properties via the induction of apoptosis in hepatocellular carcinoma cells SK-HEP-1; caspase-3 cascade activation; initiation of the p53 protein; and alternative expression of the p21 protein (Chen et al., 2002).

6.4.7.3 Resveratrol

It is a polyphenolic compound found in wine, grapes, and berries having considerable potential in the treatment of hepatic diseases. Several studies have shown its hepatoprotective, antiinflammatory, antiaging, antioxidant, and anticarcinogenic potential (Smoliga et al., 2011) as well as beneficial effects in cholestatic liver injury. It potentially decreases IL-6, TNF-α, and mRNA and reduces the Kupffer cell number recruited in the damaged liver. In a proper animal model, it has shown enhanced regeneration of the hepatocyte, decreased fibrosis (Chan et al., 2011), significant inhibition of the growth of liver tumors and angiogenesis, and a protective capability of hepatic injury caused by methotrexate (Tunalı-Akbay et al., 2010). Its oral administration in a dose of 20 mg/kg/day for 4 weeks significantly prevented the dimethyl nitrosamine-induced loss in liver and body weight, and inhibited serum elevation aspartate transaminase, alanine transaminase, bilirubin, and alkaline phosphatase levels in a proper animal model (Lee et al., 2010). It also had a decreased mRNA expression of genes related to fibrosis such as transforming growth factor beta1, collagen type I, alpha-smooth muscle actin, and hydroxyproline (Hong et al., 2010).

6.4.7.4 Curcumin

It is present in the plant *Curcuma longa* L., and it was isolated for the first time two centuries ago. It was applied for many diseases of the skin as well as diarrhea, rheumatism, intestinal worms, body aches, intermittent fevers, biliousness, hepatic disorders, dyspepsia, urinary discharges, constipation, inflammations, colic, amenorrhea, and leukoderma. It performs its action through the modulation of numerous molecular targets (Pari et al., 2008). It inhibits nuclear factor-kappa B that adjusts many profibrotic and proinflammatory cytokines. It has antioxidant potential that provides a molecular rationale for its application in hepatic disorders. It attenuates hepatic damage induced by iron overdose, ethanol, cholestasis, thioacetamide, and carbon tetrachloride (CCl_4) intoxication along with a reversal potential of CCl_4 cirrhosis to some extent (Rivera-Espinoza and Muriel, 2009).

6.4.7.5 Silymarin

It is a flavonolignan obtained from *Silybum marianum* (L.) Gaertn. that has been well known as a liver tonic for centuries that is applied to prevent or reverse the hepatotoxicity of naturally occurring toxins or reactive drug metabolites (Rašković et al., 2011). It reduces the production of free radicals and the peroxidation of lipids while having antifibrotic properties. It is a toxin-blocking agent that inhibits toxin binding to the receptors of the hepatocyte cell membrane (Muthumani and Prabu, 2012). In a proper animal model, it decreased hepatic damage induced by radiation, acetaminophen, iron overload, carbon tetrachloride, phenyl hydrazine, cold ischemia by *Amanita phalloides*, and alcohol (Chen et al., 2012). It has antioxidant and membrane-stabilizing properties and enhances the regeneration of the hepatocyte. Moreover, it decreases the inflammatory reaction and inhibits hepatic fibrogenesis (Feher and Lengyel, 2012) with a significant reduction in the proliferation and angiogenesis of tumor cells and insulin resistance. A significant increased survival rate has been observed in patients with liver cirrhosis induced by alcohol.

6.4.7.6 Rhein

It is an anthraquinone derivative obtained from *Rheum rhabarbarum* L. with the potential to inhibit the proliferation of various cancer cells. It arrests the cell cycle by decreasing oncogene c-Myc and apoptosis via a caspase-dependent pathway (Shi et al., 2008). In a proper animal model, it improves fatty liver disease via the negative balance of energy, the regulation of hepatic lipogen, and immune modulation (Sheng et al., 2011). It has antioxidant and antiinflammatory properties and inhibits TGF-beta-1 expression and suppresses hepatic stellate cell activation (Guo et al., 2002). It shows a protective effect against hepatic injury and can inhibit ethanol/CCl_4-induced hepatic fibrosis in a proper animal model (Wang et al., 2011). The mechanisms most probably contribute to its antiinflammatory and antioxidant properties, its inhibition of TGF-beta1, and its suppression of hepatic stellate cell activation.

6.4.7.7 Naringenin

It is a citrus flavanone present in tomatoes and grapefruit with diverse pharmacological properties. Citrus flavonoids exhibit anticancer activity via inducing cell apoptosis and inhibiting proliferation. According to the nitrosodiethylamine induction hepatocarcinogenesis in a rat model, the naringenin ability was due to the reduction in cell proliferation and apoptosis induction. Also, it involved various decreasing factors such as NF-jB downregulation, vascular endothelial growth factor (VEGF), MMPs, and mitochondrial pathway modulation. In the molecular mechanism of naringenin-induced cell proliferation and apoptosis, in which Phytochem Rev 123 expression of Bcl-2 played a key role and improved expression of Bax and caspase-3, among others. By regulating the expression of these apoptosis-related proteins, it has been demonstrated via in vitro and in vivo results that nobiletin possesses good anticancer hepatic activities, as it holds the induction of apoptosis and the cell cycle. Its oral administration between 20 and 50 mg/kg/day amazingly prohibited DMN-induced liver and body weight loss and prohibited serum aspartate transaminase, alanine transaminase, alkaline phosphatase, and bilirubin level elevation (Lee et al., 2004), along with offering hepatoprotective and antifibrogenic properties. It also has antioxidant potential, decreasing the peroxidation of lipids against oxytetracycline-induced liver oxidative stress (Pari and Gnanasoundari, 2006). In a proper animal model, it showed hepatoprotective potential against cadmium-induced oxidative injury (Renugadevi and Prabu, 2010). It also significantly decreased levels of alanine transaminases and serum aspartate, tissue thiobarbituric acid reactive substances, gamma-glutamyl transpeptidase, conjugate dienes, protein carbonyl content, and lipid hydroperoxides. It significantly increased catalase, glutathione peroxidase, superoxide dismutase, glutathione-*S*-transferase, and glutathione reductase activities in ethanol-induced liver damage (Jayaraman et al., 2009).

6.4.7.8 Geniposide

It is an iridoid glycoside found in the *Gardenia jasminoides* Ellis fruit, used against fatty liver and hyperlipidemia (Kojima et al., 2011) and to restrain liver fibrosis (Ma et al., 2011) along with the expression of CYP2E1 suppression and enhanced expression of peroxisome proliferator-activated receptor-a (PPARa), which are linked with enhanced superoxide dismutase and decreased malondialdehyde in the liver. In a proper animal model, it demonstrated hepatoprotective potential against hepatic steatosis with the suggested mechanism based on its antioxidant properties or adipocytokine release regulation and PPARa expression. It also has antiangiogenic and antiinflammatory potential with the induction of apoptotic cell death in rat hepatoma cells and human hepatocarcinoma Hep3B cells (Kim et al., 2005).

6.4.7.9 Salvianolic acid B (or magnesium lithospermate B, SAB)

It is a water-soluble polyphenolic acid found in *Salviae miltiorrhizae* Bunge (Sm), a common herbal medicine used in China for thousands of years as an accelerator of blood circulation and/or an antioxidant agent along with applications in hepatitis B, early-stage cirrhosis (Yu et al., 1994), late-stage schistosomial cirrhosis, fibrosis, and splenomegaly (Wu et al., 1958). Its mechanism of action may be the inhibition of activated HSCs that propagate and provide collagen materials to the hepatic extracellular matrix (ECM), leading to a fibrotic mass and the apoptosis induction of activated stellate cells.

6.4.7.10 Oxymatrine (or kwoninone, OM)

It is an alkaloid present in the Chinese herb *Sophora alopecuraides* L., with antiviral, antibacterial, antitumor, immunosuppression, and antiinflammatory potential. In a proper animal model, it suppressed the RNA of intracellular HCV, showing its role in the prevention of fibrosis in chronic hepatitis (Chen et al., 2001). In a multicenter randomized double-blind controlled clinical study, it significantly improved hepatic fibrosis and inflammation, improved HA and type III procollagen peptide (Mao et al., 2004), enhanced IFN-g and IL-2 expression, and decreased TNF-a and IL-10 expression in liver tissues (Yu et al., 2004).

6.4.7.11 Tetrandrine

It is an isoquinoline alkaloid found in *Stephania tetrandra* S. Moore, a Chinese herbal medicine (Li et al., 2001) applied to treat lung and liver fibrosis in China. In a proper animal model, it has demonstrated prominent attenuation of DNA and collagen synthesis via the suppression of HSC activation (Chen et al., 2005b), inhibiting signaling of PDGF (Tian et al., 1997), apoptosis induction (Zhao et al., 2004), decreasing of the autocrine of the TGF-b1-PDGF-PDGF-Rb1 loop (Liu et al., 1998), enhancement of Smad 7 protein to stop TGF-mediated matrix synthesis (Chen et al., 2005a), improvement of the fluidity of the mitochondria membrane, and lowering the Ca21 level lipid peroxidation inhibition (Chen et al., 1996).

6.4.7.12 Berberine

It is present in *Coptis chinensis Franch*. It prevents liver damage via lowering glutathione *S*-transferase and g-glutamyl transpeptidase (Anis et al., 2001) and repressing *tert*-butyl hydroperoxide (*t*-BHP)-induced cytotoxicity and lipid peroxidation in a proper animal model (Hwang et al., 2002). It presents free radical scavenging ability and is also cytotoxic to several HCC cell lines, inducing apoptosis through the caspase-mitochondria pathway, stopping the proliferation of tumor cells (Lin et al., 2004), and restricting the cell cycle S phase (Liu et al., 1994) along with the inhibition of AP-1 (Fukuda et al., 1999) and cyclo-oxygenase-2 (COX-2) activity (Fukuda et al., 1999). These are important regulators in cellular proliferation, carcinogenesis, and angiogenesis (Sawaoka et al., 1999). Various active plant constituents, sources, and their potential use in the treatment of liver cancer are shown in Table 6.2.

6.4.7.13 Others

The traditional medicine system is a complex combination with hundreds or thousands of several constituents hat have prime roles in the treatment and prevention of diseases, particularly liver diseases. Different studies reported that *Cyphomandra betacea* (Cav.) Sendtn. possessed advanced antioxidant and antiproliferative potential. The species has been reported to be valuable for breast and liver cancer cells. It possesses a 7.63 mg gallic acid equivalent/g of total phenolic content, which may be responsible for the antiproliferative and antioxidant activity of *C. betacea* fruits (Mutalib et al., 2016).

It has been stated that novel cereal-derived proteins and peptides also hold a significant level of preventive assets against diverse stages of cancer such as initiation, promotion, and

Table 6.2: Plant constituents, sources, and their use in hepatoprotection.

S. no.	Constituent	Source	Use
1	Glycyrrhizin	*Glycyrrhiza glabra*	Hepatoprotective/chronic hepatitis and tumors.
2	Wogonin	*Scutellaria radix*	Inflammatory diseases and hepatitis, As cytotoxic, HBsAg suppression.
3	Resveratrol	*Vitis vinifera, Rubusfruticosus,* and *Rubusidaeus*	Hepatoprotective, antiinflammatory, antiaging, antioxidant, anticarcinogenic, used in cholestatic liver injury, decrease IL-6, TNF-a, mRNA, and reduces Kupffer cell number recruited in the damaged liver.
4	Curcumin	*Curcuma longa*	Skin disorders, diarrhea, rheumatism, intestinal worms, body ache, intermittent fevers, biliousness, hepatic disorders, dyspepsia, urinary discharges, constipation, inflammations, colic, amenorrhea, and leukoderma. Inhibits nuclear factor-kappa B.
5	Silymarin	*Silybum marianum*	Liver tonic, antioxidant, reduces free radicals, lipid peroxidation, as toxin blocking agent, membrane-stabilizing property, enhances hepatocyte regeneration, decreases inflammatory reaction, and inhibits hepatic fibrogenesis.
6	Rhein	*Rheum rhabarbarum*	Inhibit cancer cell proliferation, arrest cell cycle by decreasing oncogene c-Myc and apoptosis via caspase-dependent pathway.
7	Naringenin	*Solanum lycopersicum* and *Vitis vinifera*	Inhibit DMN-induced liver weight loss, serum aspartate transaminase, alanine transaminase, alkaline phosphatase and bilirubin level elevation, along with hepatoprotective, antifibrogenic, antioxidant, decrease lipid peroxidation.
8	Geniposide	*Gardenia jasminoides* Ellis fruit	Used in fatty liver, hyperlipidemia, restrain liver fibrosis, expression of CYP2E1 suppression, enhanced expression of peroxisome proliferator-activated receptor-a (PPARa).
9	Salvianolic acid B	*Salviae miltiorrhizae*	Blood-circulation accelerator, antioxidant used in hepatitis B, early-stage cirrhosis, late-stage schistosomial cirrhosis, fibrosis, and splenomegaly.
10	Oxymatrine	*Sophora alopecuraides*	Immunosuppression, antiinflammatory, antibacterial, antiviral, and antitumor.
11	Tetrandrine	*Stephania tetrandra*	Attenuation of DNA and collagen synthesis, used in lung and liver fibrosis.
12	Berberine	*Coptis chinensis*	Prevents liver damage via lowering glutathione S-transferase and g-glutamyl transpeptidase, and repressing *tert*-butyl hydroperoxide (*t*-BHP)-induced cytotoxicity and lipid peroxidation.

progression. It has now become an area of interest for researchers over the past few years. Chemotherapy is an effective urgent treatment for cancers and hence chemoprevention becomes a viable anticancer approach. The natural chemopreventive agents are expected to be safe, inexpensive, and plentiful compared to synthetic compounds. Therefore, peptides, which have a wide range of availability and acceptability, are deemed fit to use. As dietary proteins, peptides and amino acids are naturally produced or they can also be formed by fermentation, gastrointestinal digestion, or enzymatic hydrolysis. Studies reveal that these molecules have good anticancer potential in the regulation of apoptosis and angiogenesis, which is an important step in controlling tumor metastasis (de Mejia and Dia, 2010).

The antitumor activities of bioactive peptides consist of different central mechanisms such as (a) Apoptosis induction, which is composed of an energy-dependent cascade arbitrating through specific proteases or caspases, the activation of proapoptotic receptors to overcome tumor resistance in apoptotic pathways, caspase modulation, p53 activity restoration, and proteasome inhibition, among others; (b) Intermediate tumor generation blocking via regulating the cellular mechanisms connected with cell proliferation and the survival or cell growth controlling biosynthetic pathways, and (c) An immune system function regulation via enhancing the tumor-linked antigen (antigenicity) expression in cancer cells by triggering tumor cells to release danger signals that activate immune responses (immunogenicity) or by increasing the identification of tumor cell predisposition, which are then eliminated by the immune system (susceptibility).

Many anticancer-associated peptides have proapoptotic potential and these processes are promoted through several mechanisms in different cancer cells involving autophagy and apoptosis. In vitro models have been used for maize peptides to evaluate the anticancer properties. HepG2 cells, obtained from the enzymatic hydrolysis of proteins that were extracted from corn gluten meal, showed more activity than maize peptides. Also, for H22-tumor bearing mice, the maize peptides were tested and the results revealed that at a dose of 400 mg/kg, the maize peptides showed significant inhibition of hepatic tumor cells and also increased the immune system activity as compared to the control group.

Neohesperidin, hesperidin, and naringin are the active citrus flavonoids present in citrus seeds that showed a greater cytotoxic effect on human HepG2 cells. Among these, hesperidin is the most active flavonoid and its activity has mainly been associated with the mitochondrial and death receptor pathways. Naringin has a lower potential of inhibition but also has been used to induce human hepatocellular carcinoma in HepG2 cell apoptosis through caspase-9 mitochondrial-mediated activation and caspase-8-mediated proteolysis of Bid. Hesperetin (the aglycone of hesperidin) activity is related with the inhibition of proliferation and the apoptosis induction of hepatocellular carcinoma via activating the mitochondrial pathway by increasing the intracellular Ca^{2+}, ROS, and ATP level.

Paraptosis, a wide topic of interest in recent years, is morphologically and biochemically different from apoptosis and is usually associated with the nonapoptotic programmed cell death. It has been characterized by cytoplasmic vacuolation with swelling of the mitochondria or endoplasmic reticulum, and many apoptotic characteristics are absent such as DNA fragmentation, pyknosis, etc. It has been reported that ERK1/2 activation causes hesperidin-induced paraptosis (cell death in HepG2 cells) and involved more production of ROS and loss of membrane potential (Yumnam et al., 2014). Various research studies have shown that in the invasion and metastasis of various tumor cells, the matrix metalloproteinases (MMPs) and a family of zinc-dependent endopeptidases are normally involved. The potential ability of hesperidin to prevent invasion or metastasis of human hepatocellular carcinoma cells is due to the suppression of nicotine-activated MMPs. The expression of MMP-9 is suppressed by hesperidin via inhibiting both activator protein-1 (AP-1) and NF-κB through the NF-κB (IκB), JNK, and p38 signaling pathway inhibition. Furthermore, various other agents have been reported to play an important role in the control of tumor growth and invasion such as the hepatocyte growth factor (HGF), the motility and morphogenic factor, and the paracrine cellular growth factor. Nobiletin executed inhibition via ERK2 or Akt signaling pathways and comparatively showed better activity than the other three flavones (Yi et al., 2017).

6.5 Conclusion

The liver is an accessory digestive gland found in vertebrates that perform various vital functions. This gland sometimes develops tumors that are either malignant or nonmalignant because of several causal factors. Several approaches are applied for its treatment, among which the natural product-based treatment is widespread and is thought to be the one with the least toxic effects so far.

According to knowledge on herbal medicine and clinical experience accumulated for centuries, several herbal species can provide new avenues for alternative treatments of liver disease. These have the ability to protect hepatic cells from the detrimental effects of various chemical agents, suppress cancerous cell proliferation, and display a cytotoxic effect on hepatic cells.

Natural products have been applied for thousands of years to treat liver disorders and have now become a promising therapy in this regard. There are numerous herbal species that have hepatoprotective properties. They serve as a main treasury of new and potential therapeutic drugs, presenting a wide number of bioactive molecules with roles in hepatic disease management. The active phytochemicals demonstrating hepatoprotective potential have been isolated from several species. These phytochemicals can be purified and developed into drugs with the standards and quality of modern developed medicine. Several serious challenges are faced by the pharmaceutical industry because the drug discovery procedure is becoming costly, riskier, and seriously ineffective. These products have served for centuries as a basis of drugs with about half the drugs in use nowadays of natural origin. The 21st century has seen a great move toward the therapeutic valuation of natural products in hepatic ailments by vigilantly synergizing the strengths of conventional medicine systems with the current evidence-based concept of medicinal evaluation, herbal product standardization, and placebo-controlled randomized clinical trials to support medical efficiency. Natural products possess a prime role in our life and presently are used globally as a promising therapy for several hepatic ailments.

Conflict of interest

The authors declare that they have no conflict of interest.

References

Abdel-Misih, S.R., Bloomston, M., 2010. Liver anatomy. Surg. Clin. North Am. 90, 643–653.

Abe, K., Ikeda, T., Wake, K., Sato, T., Sato, T., Inoue, H., 2008. Glycyrrhizin prevents of lipopolysaccharide/D-galactosamine-induced liver injury through down-regulation of matrix metalloproteinase-9 in mice. J. Pharm. Pharmacol. 60, 91–97.

Afum, C., Cudjoe, L., Hills, J., Hunt, R., Padilla, L., Elmore, S., Afriyie, A., Opare-Sem, O., Phillips, T., Jolly, P., 2016. Association between aflatoxin M1 and liver disease in HBV/HCV infected persons in Ghana. Int. J. Environ. Res. Public Health 13, 377.

Alvarez, F., Berg, P., Bianchi, F., Bianchi, L., Burroughs, A., Cancado, E., Chapman, R., Cooksley, W., Czaja, A., Desmet, V., 1999. International Autoimmune Hepatitis Group Report: review of criteria for diagnosis of autoimmune hepatitis. J. Hepatol. 31, 929–938.

Anis, K., Rajeshkumar, N., Kuttan, R., 2001. Inhibition of chemical carcinogenesis by berberine in rats and mice. J. Pharm. Pharmacol. 53, 763–768.

Bai, D.-S., Zhang, C., Chen, P., Jin, S.-J., Jiang, G.-Q., 2017. The prognostic correlation of AFP level at diagnosis with pathological grade, progression, and survival of patients with hepatocellular carcinoma. Sci. Rep. 7, 12870.

Beyer, T., Townsend, D.W., Brun, T., Kinahan, P.E., Charron, M., Roddy, R., Jerin, J., Young, J., Byars, L., Nutt, R., 2000. A combined PET/CT scanner for clinical oncology. J. Nucl. Med. 41, 1369–1379.

Bringmann, G., Brun, R., Kaiser, M., Neumann, S., 2008. Synthesis and antiprotozoal activities of simplified analogs of naphthylisoquinoline alkaloids. Eur. J. Med. Chem. 43, 32–42.

Burroughs, A., Hochhauser, D., Meyer, T., 2004. Systemic treatment and liver transplantation for hepatocellular carcinoma: two ends of the therapeutic spectrum. Lancet Oncol. 5, 409–418.

Campbell, P.T., Newton, C.C., Freedman, N.D., Koshiol, J., Alavanja, M.C., Freeman, L.E.B., Buring, J.E., Chan, A.T., Chong, D.Q., Datta, M., 2016. Body mass index, waist circumference, diabetes, and risk of liver cancer for US adults. Cancer Res. 76, 6076–6083.

Chan, C.C., Cheng, L.Y., Lin, C.L., Huang, Y.H., Lin, H.C., Lee, F.Y., 2011. The protective role of natural phytoalexin resveratrol on inflammation, fibrosis and regeneration in cholestatic liver injury. Mol. Nutr. Food Res. 55, 1841–1849.

Chen, X.-H., Hu, Y.-M., Liao, Y.-Q., 1996. Protective effects of tetrandrine on CCl$_4$-injured hepatocytes. Zhongguo Yao Li Xue Bao 17, 348–350.

Chen, Y., Li, J., Zeng, M., Lu, L., Qu, D., Mao, Y., Fan, Z., Hua, J., 2001. The inhibitory effect of oxymatrine on hepatitis C virus in vitro. Zhonghua Gan Zang Bing Za Zhi 9, 12–14.

Chen, Y.-C., Shen, S.-C., Lee, W.-R., Lin, H.-Y., Ko, C.-H., Shih, C.-M., Yang, L.-L., 2002. Wogonin and fisetin induction of apoptosis through activation of caspase 3 cascade and alternative expression of p21 protein in hepatocellular carcinoma cells SK-HEP-1. Arch. Toxicol. 76, 351–359.

Chen, Y.-w., LI, D.-g., WU, J.-x., Chen, Y.-w., LU, H.-m., 2005a. Effects of tetrandrine on transmembrane signaling in rat hepatic stellate cells. Chin. J. Hepatol. 13, 609–610.

Chen, Y.-W., Wu, J.-X., Chen, Y.-W., Li, D.-G., Lu, H.-M., 2005b. Tetrandrine inhibits activation of rat hepatic stellate cells in vitro via transforming growth factor-β signaling. World J. Gastroenterol. 11, 2922.

Chen, I.S., Chen, Y.C., Chou, C.H., Chuang, R.F., Sheen, L.Y., Chiu, C.H., 2012. Hepatoprotection of silymarin against thioacetamide-induced chronic liver fibrosis. J. Sci. Food Agric. 92, 1441–1447.

Choo, S.P., Tan, W.L., et al., 2016. Comparison of hepatocellular carcinoma in Eastern versus Western populations. Cancer 122 (22), 3430–3446.

Cruickshank, A., Sparshott, S.M., 1971. Malignancy in natural and experimental hepatic cysts: experiments with aflatoxin in rats and the malignant transformation of cysts in human livers. J. Pathol. 104, 185–190.

de Mejia, E.G., Dia, V.P., 2010. The role of nutraceutical proteins and peptides in apoptosis, angiogenesis, and metastasis of cancer cells. Cancer Metastasis Rev. 29 (3), 511–528.

DiSaia, P.J., Creasman, W.T., Mannel, R.S., McMeekin, D.S., Mutch, D.G., 2017. SPEC—Clinical Gynecologic Oncology. Elsevier Health Sciences.

Dittrich, C., Kosty, M., Jezdic, S., Pyle, D., Berardi, R., Bergh, J., El-Saghir, N., Lotz, J.-P., Österlund, P., Pavlidis, N., 2016. ESMO/ASCO recommendations for a global curriculum in medical oncology edition 2016. ESMO Open 1, e000097.

Feher, J., Lengyel, G., 2012. Silymarin in the prevention and treatment of liver diseases and primary liver cancer. Curr. Pharm. Biotechnol. 13, 210–217.

Ferrand, J.-F., Cénée, S., Laurent-Puig, P., Loriot, M.-A., Trinchet, J.C., Degos, F., Bronovicky, J.-P., Pelletier, G., Stücker, I., 2008. Hepatocellular carcinoma and occupation in men: a case-control study. J. Occup. Environ. Med. 50, 212–220.

Fukuda, K., Hibiya, Y., Mutoh, M., Koshiji, M., Akao, S., Fujiwara, H., 1999. Inhibition of activator protein 1 activity by berberine in human hepatoma cells. Planta Med. 65, 381–383.

Gao, M., Nettles, R.E., Belema, M., Snyder, L.B., Nguyen, V.N., Fridell, R.A., Serrano-Wu, M.H., Langley, D.R., Sun, J.-H., O'Boyle II, D.R., 2010. Chemical genetics strategy identifies an HCV NS5A inhibitor with a potent clinical effect. Nature 465, 96.

Gritters, L., Wahl, R., 1993. Single photon emission computed tomography in cancer imaging. Oncology (Williston Park) 7, 59–63. 66 discussion 66, 69–70.

Guo, M.-Z., Li, X.-S., Xu, H.-R., Mei, Z.-C., Shen, W., Ye, X.-F., 2002. Rhein inhibits liver fibrosis induced by carbon tetrachloride in rats. Acta Pharmacol. Sin. 23, 739–744.

Guo, Q., Zhao, L., You, Q., Yang, Y., Gu, H., Song, G., Lu, N., Xin, J., 2007. Anti-hepatitis B virus activity of wogonin in vitro and in vivo. Antiviral Res. 74, 16–24.

Hanahan, D., Weinberg, R.A., 2011. Hallmarks of cancer: the next generation. Cell 144, 646–674.

Harrison, P., 1999. Diagnosis of primary sclerosing cholangitis. J. Hepatobiliary Pancreat. Surg. 6, 356–360.

Hellerbrand, K., Papadimitriou, A., Winter, G., 2001. Process for Stabilizing Proteins. Google Patents.

Hermanek, P., Hutter, R.V., Sobin, L.H., Wittekind, C., 1999. Classification of isolated tumor cells and micrometastasis. Cancer 86, 2668–2673.

Hong, S.-W., Jung, K.H., Zheng, H.-M., Lee, H.-S., Suh, J.-K., Park, I.-S., Lee, D.-H., Hong, S.-S., 2010. The protective effect of resveratrol on dimethylnitrosamine-induced liver fibrosis in rats. Arch. Pharm. Res. 33, 601–609.

Hwang, J.-M., Wang, C.-J., Chou, F.-P., Tseng, T.-H., Hsieh, Y.-S., Lin, W.-L., Chu, C.-Y., 2002. Inhibitory effect of berberine on tert-butyl hydroperoxide-induced oxidative damage in rat liver. Arch. Toxicol. 76, 664–670.

Iemoto, Y., Kondo, Y., Nakano, T., Tsuchiya, K., Ohto, M., 1983. Biliary cystadenocarcinoma diagnosed by liver biopsy performed under ultrasonographic guidance. Gastroenterology 84, 399–403.

Inoue, S., Harada, A., Nakao, A., Itoh, T., Torii, A., Nonami, T., Takagi, H., 1995. A case of extrahepatic biliary cystadenocarcinoma arising in the hepatoduodenal ligament. Am. J. Gastroenterol. 90, 156.

Jayaraman, J., Veerappan, M., Namasivayam, N., 2009. Potential beneficial effect of naringenin on lipid peroxidation and antioxidant status in rats with ethanol-induced hepatotoxicity. J. Pharm. Pharmacol. 61, 1383–1390.

Johnson, N.M., Qian, G., Xu, L., Tietze, D., Marroquin-Cardona, A., Robinson, A., Rodriguez, M., Kaufman, L., Cunningham, K., Wittmer, J., 2010. Aflatoxin and PAH exposure biomarkers in a US population with a high incidence of hepatocellular carcinoma. Sci. Total Environ. 408, 6027–6031.

Kamiyama, T., Tahara, M., Nakanishi, K., Yokoo, H., Kamachi, H., Kakisaka, T., Tsuruga, Y., Matsushita, M., Todo, S., 2014. Long-term outcome of laparoscopic hepatectomy in patients with hepatocellular carcinoma. Hepatogastroenterology 61, 405–409.

Karlsson, A., Stöcker, M., Schmidt, R., 1999. Composites of micro-and mesoporous materials: simultaneous syntheses of MFI/MCM-41 like phases by a mixed template approach. Microporous Mesoporous Mater. 27, 181–192.

Kim, B.-C., Kim, H.-G., Lee, S.-A., Lim, S., Park, E.-H., Kim, S.-J., Lim, C.-J., 2005. Genipin-induced apoptosis in hepatoma cells is mediated by reactive oxygen species/c-Jun NH_2-terminal kinase-dependent activation of mitochondrial pathway. Biochem. Pharmacol. 70, 1398–1407.

Kojima, K., Shimada, T., Nagareda, Y., Watanabe, M., Ishizaki, J., Sai, Y., Miyamoto, K.-i., Aburada, M., 2011. Preventive effect of geniposide on metabolic disease status in spontaneously obese type 2 diabetic mice and free fatty acid-treated HepG2 cells. Biol. Pharm. Bull. 34, 1613–1618.

Lauret, E., Rodríguez, M., González, S., Linares, A., López-Vázquez, A., Martínez-Borra, J., Rodrigo, L., López-Larrea, C., 2002. HFE gene mutations in alcoholic and virus-related cirrhotic patients with hepatocellular carcinoma. Am. J. Gastroenterol. 97, 1016.

Lee, S.D., Kim, S.H., 2016. Role of positron emission tomography/computed tomography in living donor liver transplantation for hepatocellular carcinoma. Hepatobiliary Surg. Nutr. 5, 408.

Lee, M.-H., Yoon, S., Moon, J.-O., 2004. The flavonoid naringenin inhibits dimethylnitrosamine-induced liver damage in rats. Biol. Pharm. Bull. 27, 72–76.

Lee, E.-S., Shin, M.-O., Yoon, S., Moon, J.-O., 2010. Resveratrol inhibits dimethylnitrosamine-induced hepatic fibrosis in rats. Arch. Pharm. Res. 33, 925–932.

Li, L., Wang, H., 2016. Heterogeneity of liver cancer and personalized therapy. Cancer Lett. 379, 191–197.

Li, D.-G., Wang, Z.-R., Lu, H.-M., 2001. Pharmacology of tetrandrine and its therapeutic use in digestive diseases. World J. Gastroenterol. 7, 627.

Lin, C.C., Ng, L.T., Hsu, F.F., Shieh, D.E., Chiang, L.C., 2004. Cytotoxic effects of *Coptis chinensis* and *Epimedium sagittatum* extracts and their major constituents (berberine, coptisine and icariin) on hepatoma and leukaemia cell growth. Clin. Exp. Pharmacol. Physiol. 31, 65–69.

Liu, J., Waalkes, M.P., 2008. Liver is a target of arsenic carcinogenesis. Toxicol. Sci. 105, 24–32.

Liu, P., Kawada, N., Mizoguchi, Y., Morisawa, S., 1994. Effects of magnesium lithospermate B on cyclooxygenase activity in rat liver, adherent cells and enzyme's product. Zhongguo Zhong Yao Za Zhi 19, 110–113. 128.

Liu, D., Li, G., Cao, Y., 1998. Blocking action of tetrandrine on the scar-collagen matrix contraction stimulated by transforming growth factor beta. Zhongguo Zhong Xi Yi Jie He Za Zhi 18, 429–430.

Liu, L., Cao, Y., Chen, C., Zhang, X., McNabola, A., Wilkie, D., Wilhelm, S., Lynch, M., Carter, C., 2006. Sorafenib blocks the RAF/MEK/ERK pathway, inhibits tumor angiogenesis, and induces tumor cell apoptosis in hepatocellular carcinoma model PLC/PRF/5. Cancer Res. 66, 11851–11858.

Liu, C.-Y., Chen, K.-F., Chen, P.-J., 2015. Treatment of liver cancer. Cold Spring Harb. Perspect. Med. 5, a021535.

Liu, X., Baecker, A., Wu, M., Zhou, J.Y., Yang, J., Han, R.Q., Wang, P.H., Jin, Z.Y., Liu, A.M., Gu, X., 2018. Interaction between tobacco smoking and hepatitis B virus infection on the risk of liver cancer in a Chinese population. Int. J. Cancer 142, 1560–1567.

Llovet, J.M., Real, M.I., Montaña, X., Planas, R., Coll, S., Aponte, J., Ayuso, C., Sala, M., Muchart, J., Solà, R., 2002. Arterial embolisation or chemoembolisation versus symptomatic treatment in patients with unresectable hepatocellular carcinoma: a randomised controlled trial. Lancet 359, 1734–1739.

Llovet, J.M., Schwartz, M., Mazzaferro, V., 2005. Resection and liver transplantation for hepatocellular carcinoma. In: Seminars in Liver Disease. Copyright© 2005 by Thieme Medical Publishers, Inc., New York, pp. 181–200.

López, D., Fischbach, M.A., Chu, F., Losick, R., Kolter, R., 2009. Structurally diverse natural products that cause potassium leakage trigger multicellularity in Bacillus subtilis. Proc. Natl. Acad. Sci. U. S. A. 106, 280–285.

Ma, T., Huang, C., Zong, G., Zha, D., Meng, X., Li, J., Tang, W., 2011. Hepatoprotective effects of geniposide in a rat model of nonalcoholic steatohepatitis. J. Pharm. Pharmacol. 63, 587–593.

Maheshwari, S., Sarraj, A., Kramer, J., El-Serag, H.B., 2007. Oral contraception and the risk of hepatocellular carcinoma. J. Hepatol. 47, 506–513.

Makimoto, K., Higuchi, S., 1999. Alcohol consumption as a major risk factor for the rise in liver cancer mortality rates in Japanese men. Int. J. Epidemiol. 28, 30–34.

Mantovani, A., Targher, G., 2017. Type 2 diabetes mellitus and risk of hepatocellular carcinoma: spotlight on nonalcoholic fatty liver disease. Ann. Transl. Med. 5.

Mao, Y.-M., Zeng, M.-D., Lu, L.-G., Wan, M.-B., Li, C.-Z., Chen, C.-W., Fu, Q.-C., Wang, J.-Y., She, W.-M., Cai, X., 2004. Capsule oxymatrine in treatment of hepatic fibrosis due to chronic viral hepatitis: a randomized, double blind, placebo-controlled, multicenter clinical study. World J. Gastroenterol. 10, 3269.

Mazzaferro, V., Regalia, E., Doci, R., Andreola, S., Pulvirenti, A., Bozzetti, F., Montalto, F., Ammatuna, M., Morabito, A., Gennari, L., 1996. Liver transplantation for the treatment of small hepatocellular carcinomas in patients with cirrhosis. N. Engl. J. Med. 334, 693–700.

Morgan, T.R., Mandayam, S., Jamal, M.M., 2004. Alcohol and hepatocellular carcinoma. Gastroenterology 127, S87–S96.

Mueller, S., 2016. Does pressure cause liver cirrhosis? The sinusoidal pressure hypothesis. World J. Gastroenterol. 22, 10482.

Mustafa, M.E., Mansoor, M.M., Mohammed, A., Babker, A.A.A., 2015. Evaluation of platelets count and coagulation parameters among patients with liver disease. World J. Pharm. Res. 4, 360–368.

Mutalib, M.A., Ali, F., Othman, F., Ramasamy, R., Rahmat, A., 2016. Phenolics profile and anti-proliferative activity of *Cyphomandra betacea* fruit in breast and liver cancer cells. SpringerPlus 5, 2105.

Muthumani, M., Prabu, S.M., 2012. Silibinin potentially protects arsenic-induced oxidative hepatic dysfunction in rats. Toxicol. Mech. Methods 22, 277–288.

Nio, K., Yamashita, T., Kaneko, S., 2017. The evolving concept of liver cancer stem cells. Mol. Cancer 16, 4.

Ogiku, M., Kono, H., Hara, M., Tsuchiya, M., Fujii, H., 2011. Glycyrrhizin prevents liver injury by inhibition of high-mobility group box 1 production by Kupffer cells after ischemia-reperfusion in rats. J. Pharmacol. Exp. Ther. 339, 93–98.

Ogodo, A.C., Ugbogu, O.C., 2016. Public health significance of aflatoxin in food industry—a review. Eur. J. Clin. Biomed. Sci. 2, 51–58.

Pari, L., Gnanasoundari, M., 2006. Influence of naringenin on oxytetracycline mediated oxidative damage in rat liver. Basic Clin. Pharmacol. Toxicol. 98, 456–461.

Pari, L., Tewas, D., Eckel, J., 2008. Role of curcumin in health and disease. Arch. Physiol. Biochem. 114, 127–149.

Park, S., Bae, J., Nam, B.-H., Yoo, K.-Y., 2008. Aetiology of cancer in Asia. Asian Pac. J. Cancer Prev. 9, 371–380.

Paterson, I., Anderson, E.A., 2005. The renaissance of natural products as drug candidates. Science 310, 451–453.

Raman, S., Salaria, S., Hruban, R., Fishman, E., 2013. Groove pancreatitis: spectrum of imaging findings and radiology—pathology correlation. http://www.ajronline.org/doi/abs/10.2214.AJR.

Rašković, A., Stilinović, N., Kolarović, J., Vasović, V., Vukmirović, S., Mikov, M., 2011. The protective effects of silymarin against doxorubicin-induced cardiotoxicity and hepatotoxicity in rats. Molecules 16, 8601–8613.

Renugadevi, J., Prabu, S.M., 2010. Cadmium-induced hepatotoxicity in rats and the protective effect of naringenin. Exp. Toxicol. Pathol. 62, 171–181.

Rivera-Espinoza, Y., Muriel, P., 2009. Pharmacological actions of curcumin in liver diseases or damage. Liver Int. 29, 1457–1466.

Rundlöf, T., Olsson, E., Wiernik, A., Back, S., Aune, M., Johansson, L., Wahlberg, I., 2000. Potential nitrite scavengers as inhibitors of the formation of N-nitrosamines in solution and tobacco matrix systems. J. Agric. Food Chem. 48, 4381–4388.

Russell, S.J., Peng, K.-W., Bell, J.C., 2012. Oncolytic virotherapy. Nat. Biotechnol. 30, 658.

Sawaoka, H., Tsuji, S., Tsujii, M., Gunawan, E.S., Sasaki, Y., Kawano, S., Hori, M., 1999. Cyclooxygenase inhibitors suppress angiogenesis and reduce tumor growth in vivo. Lab. Invest. 79, 1469–1477.

Schagdarsurengin, U., Wilkens, L., Steinemann, D., Flemming, P., Kreipe, H.H., Pfeifer, G.P., Schlegelberger, B., Dammann, R., 2003. Frequent epigenetic inactivation of the RASSF1A gene in hepatocellular carcinoma. Oncogene 22, 1866.

Sheng, X., Wang, M., Lu, M., Xi, B., Sheng, H., Zang, Y.Q., 2011. Rhein ameliorates fatty liver disease through negative energy balance, hepatic lipogenic regulation, and immunomodulation in diet-induced obese mice. Am. J. Physiol. Endocrinol. Metab. 300, E886–E893.

Shi, P., Huang, Z., Chen, G., 2008. Rhein induces apoptosis and cell cycle arrest in human hepatocellular carcinoma BEL-7402 cells. Am. J. Chin. Med. 36, 805–813.

Shin, H.-R., Oh, J.-K., Masuyer, E., Curado, M.-P., Bouvard, V., Fang, Y., Wiangnon, S., Sripa, B., Hong, S.-T., 2010. Comparison of incidence of intrahepatic and extrahepatic cholangiocarcinoma—focus on East and South-Eastern Asia. Asian Pac. J. Cancer Prev. 11, 1159–1166.

Sithithaworn, P., Yongvanit, P., et al., 2014. Roles of liver fluke infection as risk factor for cholangiocarcinoma. J. Hepatobiliary Pancreat. Sci. 21 (5), 301–308.

Smoliga, J.M., Baur, J.A., Hausenblas, H.A., 2011. Resveratrol and health—a comprehensive review of human clinical trials. Mol. Nutr. Food Res. 55, 1129–1141.

Song, P.-P., Xia, J.-F., Inagaki, Y., Hasegawa, K., Sakamoto, Y., Kokudo, N., Tang, W., 2016. Controversies regarding and perspectives on clinical utility of biomarkers in hepatocellular carcinoma. World J. Gastroenterol. 22, 262.

Srivatanakul, P., 2001. Epidemiology of liver cancer in Thailand. Asian Pac. J. Cancer Prev. 2, 117–121.

Srivatanakul, P., Sriplung, H., Deerasamee, S., 2004. Epidemiology of liver cancer: an overview. Asian Pac. J. Cancer Prev. 5, 118–125.

Stanaway, J.D., Flaxman, A.D., Naghavi, M., Fitzmaurice, C., Vos, T., Abubakar, I., Abu-Raddad, L.J., Assadi, R., Bhala, N., Cowie, B., 2016. The global burden of viral hepatitis from 1990 to 2013: findings from the Global Burden of Disease Study 2013. Lancet 388, 1081–1088.

Sugihara, S., Kojiro, M., 1987. Pathology of cholangiocarcinoma. In: Neoplasms of the Liver. Springer, pp. 143–158.

Sukowati, C.H., El-Khobar, K.E., Ie, S.I., Anfuso, B., Muljono, D.H., Tiribelli, C., 2016. Significance of hepatitis virus infection in the oncogenic initiation of hepatocellular carcinoma. World J. Gastroenterol. 22, 1497.

Tang, B., Qiao, H., Meng, F., Sun, X., 2007. Glycyrrhizin attenuates endotoxin-induced acute liver injury after partial hepatectomy in rats. Braz. J. Med. Biol. Res. 40, 1637–1646.

Tang, J.-C., Feng, Y.-L., et al., 2016. Circulating tumor DNA in hepatocellular carcinoma: trends and challenges. Cell Biosci. 6 (1), 32.

Tapper, E.B., Parikh, N.D., 2018. Mortality due to cirrhosis and liver cancer in the United States, 1999-2016: observational study. BMJ 362, k2817.

Teckman, J.H., Lindblad, D., 2006. Alpha-1-antitrypsin deficiency: diagnosis, pathophysiology, and management. Curr. Gastroenterol. Rep. 8, 14–20.

Theise, N., Miller, F., Worman, H., Morris, P., Schwartz, M., Miller, C., Thung, S., 1993. Biliary cystadenocarcinoma arising in a liver with fibropolycystic disease. Arch. Pathol. Lab. Med. 117, 163–165.

Tian, Z., Liu, S., Li, D., 1997. Blocking action of tetrandrine on the cell proliferation induced by PDGF in human lung fibroblasts and liver Ito cell of rats. Zhonghua Yi Xue Za Zhi 77, 50–53.

Tortora, G.J., Derrickson, B.H., 2008. Principles of Anatomy and Physiology. John Wiley & Sons.

Tunalı-Akbay, T., Sehirli, O., Ercan, F., Sener, G., 2010. Resveratrol protects against methotrexate-induced hepatic injury in rats. J. Pharm. Pharm. Sci. 13, 303–310.

Wan, X.-y., Luo, M., Li, X.-d., He, P., 2009. Hepatoprotective and anti-hepatocarcinogenic effects of glycyrrhizin and matrine. Chem. Biol. Interact. 181, 15–19.

Wang, X., Sun, H., Zhang, A., Jiao, G., Sun, W., Yuan, Y., 2011. Pharmacokinetics screening for multi-components absorbed in the rat plasma after oral administration traditional Chinese medicine formula Yin-Chen-Hao-Tang by ultra performance liquid chromatography-electrospray ionization/quadrupole-time-of-flight mass spectrometry combined with pattern recognition methods. Analyst 136, 5068–5076.

Wee, A., Nilsson, B., Kang, J., Tan, L., Rauff, A., 1993. Biliary cystadenocarcinoma arising in a cystadenoma. Report of a case diagnosed by fine needle aspiration cytology. Acta Cytol. 37, 966–970.

Wu, Y., Yang, C., Jiang, J., 1958. Primary report of radix salviae miltorrhizae in treatment of late-stage schistosomial cirrhosis and splenomegaly. Zhonghua Yixue Zazhi, 542–545.

Yang, J., Zhang, Y., Luo, L., Meng, R., Yu, C., 2018. Global mortality burden of cirrhosis and liver cancer attributable to injection drug use, 1990–2016: an age-period-cohort and spatial autocorrelation analysis. Int. J. Environ. Res. Public Health 15, 170.

Yi, L., Ma, S., Ren, D., 2017. Phytochemistry and bioactivity of citrus flavonoids: a focus on antioxidant, anti-inflammatory, anticancer and cardiovascular protection activities. Phytochem. Rev. 16, 479–511.

Yu, Y., Yang, H., Zhu, L., Cao, L., Liu, Z., Zhu, L., Zhang, E., Tian, Y., Shen, H., Teng, S., 1994. Clinical trial of large-dose radix salviae miltorrhizae in treatment of liver fibrosis. Shanghai Zhongyiyao Zazhi 1, 8–10.

Yu, X.-H., Zhu, J.-S., Yu, H.-F., Zhu, L., 2004. Immunomodulatory effect of oxymatrine on induced CCl_4-hepatic fibrosis in rats. Chin. Med. J. 117, 1856.

Yumnam, S., Park, H.S., et al., 2014. Hesperidin induces paraptosis like cell death in hepatoblatoma, HepG2 cells: Involvement of ERK1/2 MAPK. PLoS One 9 (6).

Yumoto, Y., Jinno, K., Tokuyama, K., 1984. Detection of hepatic tumor by means of single photon emission computed tomography, gray scale ultrasonography, and X-ray computed tomography. Nippon Shokakibyo Gakkai Zasshi 81, 1582–1591.

Zhao, Y.Z., Kim, J.Y., Park, E.J., Lee, S.H., Woo, S.W., Ko, G., Sohn, D.H., 2004. Tetrandrine induces apoptosis in hepatic stellate cells. Phytother. Res. 18, 306–309.

Zhou, J., Sun, H.-C., Wang, Z., Cong, W.-M., Wang, J.-H., Zeng, M.-S., Yang, J.-M., Bie, P., Liu, L.-X., Wen, T.-F., 2018. Guidelines for diagnosis and treatment of primary liver cancer in China (2017 Edition). Liver Cancer 7, 235–260.

CHAPTER 7

Chronic liver diseases

Renald Blundell[a,b] and Joseph Ignatius Azzopardi[a]
[a]*Department of Physiology and Biochemistry, Faculty of Medicine, University of Malta, Msida, Malta*
[b]*American University of Malta, Bormla, Malta*

7.1 Introduction

Chronic liver disease (CLD) is an umbrella term that encompasses a spectrum of diseases that affect the liver for at least a period of 6 months (Ladep et al., 2019). The etiology and nature of CLDs varies greatly, ranging from being viral in origin due to hepatitis C infection or hepatic steatosis as a result of alcohol abuse, among others (Ladep et al., 2019; Yao et al., 2016).

CLD is a major public health problem that is often underestimated, with 844 million people worldwide estimated to have a CLD, 2 million of which will die every year (Byass, 2014).

In this chapter, we will discuss some of the entities that fall under the term "chronic liver diseases" and whether naturally occurring chemicals can prove useful leads in the production of treatments for such diseases.

7.2 Primary sclerosing cholangitis

Primary sclerosing cholangitis (PSC) is a CLD characterized by multifocal stenosis and ectasia along the biliary tree as a result of persistent and progressive inflammation and fibrosis in its walls. Owing to the lack of an effective medical treatment, the resultant stenosis and ectasia cause obstruction to the flow of bile into the intestine, eventually leading to hepatic cirrhosis and liver failure. As a result, the median survival from the time of diagnosis is only 12 years. Although the exact etiology of PSC is as of yet unknown, both genetic and environmental risk factors are known to play a role in the development and progression of this condition (Björnsson et al., 2008; Eaton et al., 2013; Lazaridis and LaRusso, 2015, 2016; Tabibian and Lindor, 2013; Warren et al., 1966).

While the extrahepatic and the large intrahepatic bile ducts are the most commonly affected structures, in around 5% of cases, it is the small intrahepatic bile ducts that are exclusively involved in what is known as small duct primary sclerosing cholangitis (Björnsson et al., 2008; Ludwig, 1991).

Influence of Nutrients, Bioactive Compounds, and Plant Extracts in Liver Diseases. https://doi.org/10.1016/B978-0-12-816488-4.00005-X

PSC is asymptomatic in the majority of cases until the disease progresses to biliary cirrhosis leading to liver failure. In the cases where PSC is symptomatic, it may present with a variety of symptoms, including fatigue, jaundice, abdominal pain, recurrent episodes of acute cholangitis, pruritis, fever, and diarrhea (Björnsson et al., 2004; Kaplan et al., 2007; Porayko et al., 1990; Tabibian et al., 2016; Wiesner et al., 1985).

Approximately two-thirds of PSC patients also have, or will develop, ulcerative colitis while PSC occurs in 3%–7% of patients suffering from ulcerative colitis (Olsson et al., 1991). In 2017, a unique case was published in which an 18-year old man presented a triad of PSC, autoimmune hemolytic anemia, and ulcerative colitis (Khalid et al., 2017).

PSC is also associated with Crohn's disease as well as with an increased risk in the occurrence of hepatocellular carcinoma, cholangiocarcinoma, colorectal cancer, and cancer of the gallbladder (Folseraas and Boberg, 2016; Lazaridis and LaRusso, 2016; Mcgarity et al., 1991).

Cholangiography is the gold standard for the diagnosis of PSC, where diffuse involvement with characteristic findings such as multifocal annular structuring within the intra- and/or extrahepatic bile ducts with alternating dilated segments is seen. In contrast, the cholangiogram appears normal in small duct primary sclerosing cholangitis, in which case a liver biopsy may be indicated for diagnosis (Björnsson et al., 2008; MacCarty et al., 1983).

7.3 Hepatic steatosis

Hepatic steatosis, also known as fatty liver disease, occurs when the intrahepatic fat exceeds 5% of the liver weight due to the accumulation of triglyceride-rich droplets within the hepatocyte cytoplasm. The severity of hepatic steatosis can be graded according to the percentage of fat in the liver, with healthy levels being below 5% (grade 0) while levels more than 66% being graded as severe (grade 3) (Nassir et al., 2015).

The term "fatty liver disease" encompasses a spectrum of liver-related diseases, the most important of which are alcoholic fatty liver disease (AFLD) and nonalcoholic fatty liver disease (NAFLD). The latter can be further classified as nonalcoholic fatty liver characterized by the presence of simple steatosis and nonalcoholic steatohepatitis in which hepatic inflammation accompanies steatosis (Iser and Ryan, 2013).

As the name suggests, excessive alcohol consumption is the major risk factor for the development for AFLD, whereas increasing age, obesity, and diabetes are the risk factors associated with NAFLD (Hassan et al., 2014; Iser and Ryan, 2013; Lazo and Mitchell, 2016).

NAFLD is the most common cause of liver disease in the Western world, accounting for 20%–30% of such cases. The incidence of NAFLD is projected to increase due to the current obesity epidemic (Bedogni et al., 2014; Pappachan et al., 2017).

It is not possible to distinguish between AFLD and NAFLD with liver biopsies; instead, their differentiation depends on the evaluation of alcohol (ethanol) consumption. According to the

European Association for the Study of the Liver guidelines, after other causes of fatty liver are excluded, NAFLD is diagnosed when alcohol intake is less or equal to 20 and 30 g/d in women and men, respectively (Bedogni et al., 2014; Ratziu et al., 2010).

Both types of fatty liver disease, if left unchecked, may lead to cirrhosis and death (Tolman and Dalpiaz, 2007).

7.4 Primary biliary cirrhosis

Primary biliary cirrhosis (PBC) is an uncommon autoimmune disease of the liver characterized by the progressive destruction of the intrahepatic bile ducts leading to chronic cholestasis, portal inflammation, and fibrosis, which can eventually lead to cirrhosis, liver failure, and finally, death (Invernizzi et al., 2010; Selmi et al., 2011).

Similar to other autoimmune diseases, PBC occurs more commonly in females than males, at a ratio of 9:1, affecting 1 in 1000 women over 40 years of age (Kaplan, 2013; Lleo et al., 2008).

Although the exact pathogenesis has not been elucidated, both genetic and environmental factors have been implicated, as shown in Fig. 7.1. Strong genetic associations with PBC include HLA DRBI*08, IL1RN-IL 1B, and CTLA4* G haplotypes as well as

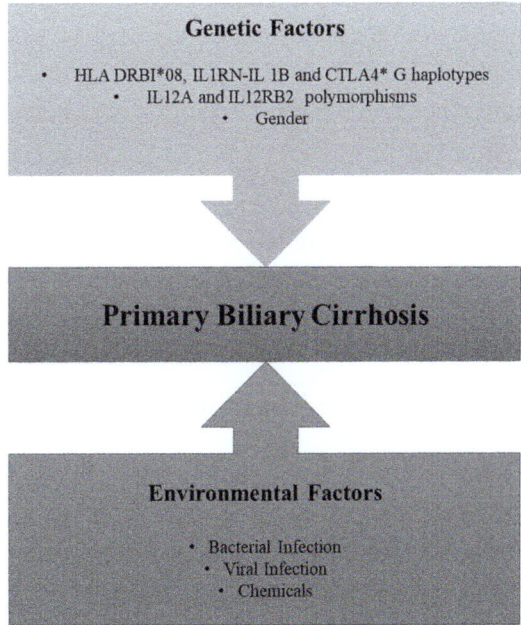

Genetic Factors

- HLA DRBI*08, IL1RN-IL 1B and CTLA4* G haplotypes
- IL12A and IL12RB2 polymorphisms
- Gender

Primary Biliary Cirrhosis

Environmental Factors

- Bacterial Infection
- Viral Infection
- Chemicals

Fig. 7.1

A nonexhaustive list of genetic and environmental factors that are suspected to play a role in the pathogenesis of primary biliary cirrhosis.

polymorphisms in the IL12A and IL12RB2 loci (Jones and Donaldson, 2003; Juran and Lazaridis, 2008; Liu et al., 2012).

In around 95% of cases, antimitochondrial antibodies (AMAs) against the mitochondrial protein PDC-E2 are found in the blood and they are therefore important in the diagnosis of PBC. Although PDC-E2 is broadly expressed in the human body, AMAs target specifically those expressed by the biliary epithelial cells that line the small interlobular bile ducts. It has been theorized that this is the result of molecular mimicry following an environmental exposure with an infective agent or chemical, the nature of which is in many cases not yet elucidated (Invernizzi et al., 2010; Sutton and Neuberger, 2002; Van de Water et al., 1993, 2001).

Clinical features of PBC may include fatigue, pruritus, jaundice, portal hypertension, osteoporosis, xanthomas, and dyslipidemia (Al-Harthy et al., 2010; Cauch-Dudek et al., 1998; Heathcote, 1997; Imam et al., 2012; Leuschner, 2003; Longo et al., 2002; Mounach et al., 2008). Currently, the only available medical therapy is ursodeoxycholic acid (UDCA), which is effective in only around 50% of patients (Corpechot et al., 2008).

7.5 Liver fibrosis

Liver fibrosis occurs in many types of CLD. It consists of excessive accumulation of extracellular matrix proteins such as collagen in the liver. The accumulation of the extracellular matrix proteins forms fibrous scars and nodules that distort the normal architecture of the liver. A crucial event in hepatic fibrogenesis is the conversion of hepatic stellate cells into myofibroblasts. It occurs as a result of chronic damage to the liver, mainly due to chronic alcohol abuse, nonalcoholic steatohepatitis, and chronic hepatitis C infection (Bataller and Brenner, 2005).

Of importance to note is that recent studies have revealed the possibility that liver fibrosis may be reversed if the insulting agents are removed. If left to progress, liver fibrosis results in cirrhosis, portal hypertension, and liver failure, requiring a transplantation as no effective medical therapy is currently available (Sun and Kisseleva, 2015).

7.6 The use of bioactive compounds and plant extracts in chronic liver diseases

Two early studies on the effect of (+)-catechin (a member of the polyphenol group found in many dietary products such as kiwi, strawberries, apples, cocoa, and green tea) on alcohol-induced liver disease showed a marked improvement in liver function, inflammation, and hepatocellular necrosis (Palmas, 1981; Traisac and Borg, 1977; Zanwar et al., 2014). The structure of (+)-catechin illustrated in Fig. 7.2. A similar study has, however, found no change in the course of the disease when patients were administered with (+)-catechin for 3 months

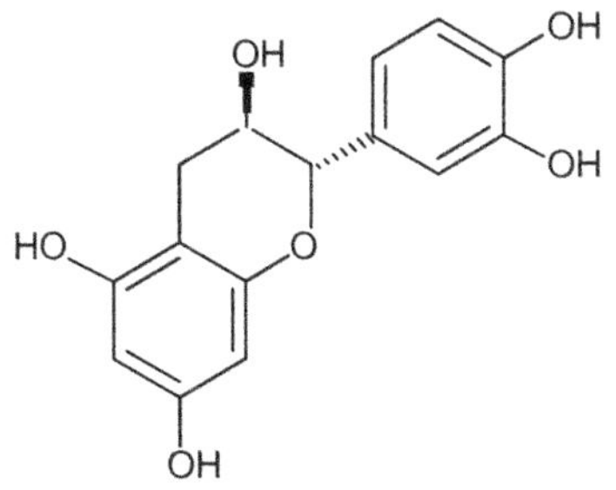

Fig. 7.2
(+)-Catechin.

(Colman et al., 1980). It has been suggested that the results in the latter study are due to the short period of treatment (Thabrew and Robin, 1996).

Recently, the effect of *Rhododendron oldhamii* leaf extract on NAFLD in vitro and in vivo was studied. The results obtained from this study showed that in vitro, the ethanolic extract of *R. oldhamii* leaves had great potential in preventing free fatty acid-induced fat accumulation in the human liver cancer cell line HepG2. In vivo, the ethanolic extract of *R. oldhamii* significantly improved the fatty liver syndrome and the total cholesterol and triglyceride levels in mice with NAFLD by simultaneously stimulating lipid oxidation and inhibiting the lipogenesis pathway. The ethanolic extract was found to contain, through reverse-phase high-performance liquid chromatography, four phytochemicals: hyposide, guaijaverin, (2R, 3R)-astilbin, and quercitrin (Liu et al., 2017).

Milk thistle (*Silybum marianum* Gaertneri) has been used as a remedy for diseases of the liver and gallbladder for at least the last 2000 years. As such, it is the most researched herbal treatment for liver disease (Langmead and Rampton, 2001; Ross, 2008). A major extract obtained from the milk thistle is silymarin. This extract has shown both antioxidative and antifibrotic properties, possibly providing a lead to a useful drug for the treatment of chronic liver diseases such as liver fibrosis (Boigk et al., 1997; Carola et al., 1996).

The evidence for the antifibrotic effect of silymarin has been mostly obtained from animal studies, including cases where the administration of silymarin for 3 years retarded the development of alcohol-induced liver fibrosis in baboons and a reduction in hepatic collagen content by 55% in rats with carbon tetrachloride (CCl_4)-induced liver damage (Abenavoli et al., 2010).

A Cochrane review that analyzed 13 randomized clinical trials that assessed milk thistle in 915 patients with alcoholic and/or hepatitis B or C liver disease found inconclusive evidence due to the lack of high-quality data (Rambaldi et al., 2007).

Curcumin is a phytocompound derived from *Curcuma longa* that has also shown potential to be used as treatment for a variety of hepatobiliary diseases, including PSC and nonalcoholic steatohepatitis (NASH), among others (Hu et al., 2017). In vitro studies have found that curcumin exerts significant antifibrotic effects on different cell lines such as HSC-16 and Hep2G through the transforming growth factor β (TGFβ) signaling (Bassiouny et al., 2011; Lin et al., 2009; Nakayama et al., 2011). Animal studies have also suggested that curcumin has the potential to treat or prevent NASH through its ability to decrease hepatic cholesterol and triglyceride levels and the accumulation of free fatty acids (Rukkumani et al., 2002, 2005).

In a clinical trial that concluded in 2019, the effect of a regimen consisting of 750 mg curcumin given by mouth twice daily for 12 weeks on participants suffering from PSC was studied. This study concluded that although curcumin was well tolerated by the participants, there was no improvement in cholestasis and in the symptoms associated with PSC (Eaton et al., 2019).

The aqueous extract of *Agrimonia eupatoria* has shown hepatoprotective effects against alcohol-induced liver injury, probably due to its ability to supress both oxidative stress and toll-like receptor-mediated inflammatory signaling (Yoon et al., 2012).

A recent study has shown that extracts obtained from *Limonium tetragonum*—a plant known to traditional folk medicine for the treatment of gynecological ailments—exert a hepatoprotective effect in mice with alcohol-induced liver damage (Kim et al., 2018).

The use of antioxidant supplements as a potential treatment for liver diseases has been suggested due to the fact that many liver diseases are associated with oxidative stress. However, a Cochrane review published in 2011 concluded that although antioxidant supplements may increase liver enzyme activity, the use of the antioxidants β-carotene and vitamins A, C, and E cannot be recommended for the treatment of liver diseases such as alcoholic liver disease and liver cirrhosis due to a lack of sufficient evidence (Bjelakovic et al., 2011). As discussed later on, more recent studies have found a positive effect of vitamin E in cases of NAFLD (Cicero et al., 2018).

7.7 Nutritional support in CLD

Through the metabolism of protein, fats, and carbohydrates, the liver is a vital organ in the maintenance of an appropriate nutritional status. As a consequence of this, those who suffer from a CLD are at a higher risk of malnutrition, most commonly protein-calorie malnutrition (Alberino et al., 2001; Merli et al., 1996; Shergill et al., 2018).

Malnutrition in CLD patients can be due to multiple factors, mainly malabsorption, increased metabolic requirements, and a loss of appetite (Shergill et al., 2018).

Patients with CLD or cirrhosis typically have low levels of branched chain amino acids (BCAAs), that is, leucine, isoleucine, and valine. BCAAs are involved in protein synthesis, the proliferation of hepatocytes, and insulin resistance, among others. The decrease in the serum levels of BCAAs coupled with an increase in the levels of aromatic amino acids (AAAs) are thought to result in hepatic encephalopathy (Shergill et al., 2018; Tajiri and Shimizu, 2013). In fact, the correlation between BCAA supplementation in patients with CLD and a better prognosis has been established through several studies, thereby highlighting the importance of using these supplements in the management of patients with CLD (Bianchi et al., 2005; Plauth et al., 2006; Shergill et al., 2018).

CLD patients can have other metabolic changes. For instance, the majority of cirrhotic patients suffer from some degree of insulin resistance or glucose intolerance, with around 14%–40% having type II diabetes mellitus (Merli et al., 1996). Decreased glycogen stores in the liver and muscle cells are also common among these patients, resulting in reduced levels of glucose available for energy production resulting in increased consumption of proteins and fats instead, eventually leading to sarcopenia (Petrides et al., 1994; Rivera Irigoin and Abilés, 2012).

Several studies have shown promising results in the use of plant extracts and other bioactive compounds as nutraceuticals in patients with CLD. For instance, when administered at the correct dose for medium to long periods together with appropriate lifestyle changes, curcumin, silymarin, berberine, and vitamins D and E are all associated with positive effects on NAFLD and its related parameters such as the reduction of insulin resistance and transaminase levels (Cicero et al., 2018).

Therefore, CLD patients should have proper nutritional support as an effort to improve their prognosis because malnutrition has been recognized as an independent predictor of mortality in this group of patients. This should be done through an appropriate history taking, physical examination, and investigations such as serum markers (Alberino et al., 2001; Merli et al., 1996; Shergill et al., 2018).

Management can be either through the form of enteral or parenteral nutrition, the indications for which depend on the patient's characteristics and the severity of their CLD. In the majority of patients, enteral nutrition in oral form together with supplementation is sufficient, whereas more serious conditions might require tube feeding or parenteral nutrition (Shergill et al., 2018).

In conclusion, current research is showing very promising results in the use of extracts and compounds derived from natural sources for the prevention and treatment of diseases affecting the liver, although more research is warranted before these can find their place in the clinical setting.

References

Abenavoli, L., Capasso, R., Milic, N., Capasso, F., 2010. Milk thistle in liver diseases: past, present, future. Phytother. Res. 24, 1423–1432. https://doi.org/10.1002/ptr.3207.

Alberino, F., Gatta, A., Amodio, P., Merkel, C., Di Pascoli, L., Boffo, G., Caregaro, L., 2001. Nutrition and survival in patients with liver cirrhosis. Nutrition 17, 445–450.

Al-Harthy, N., Kumagi, T., Coltescu, C., Hirschfield, G.M., 2010. The specificity of fatigue in primary biliary cirrhosis: evaluation of a large clinic practice. Hepatology 52, 562–570. https://doi.org/10.1002/hep.23683.

Bassiouny, A.R., Zaky, A., Fawky, F., Kandeel, K.M., 2011. Alteration of AP-endonuclease 1 expression in curcumin-treated fibrotic rats. Ann. Hepatol. 10, 516–530. https://doi.org/10.1016/S1665-2681(19)31521-2.

Bataller, R., Brenner, D.A., 2005. Liver fibrosis. J. Clin. Invest. 115, 209–218.

Bedogni, G., Nobili, V., Tiribelli, C., 2014. Epidemiology of fatty liver: an update. World J. Gastroenterol. 20, 9050–9054. https://doi.org/10.3748/wjg.v20.i27.9050.

Bianchi, G., Marzocchi, R., Agostini, F., Marchesini, G., 2005. Update on branched-chain amino acid supplementation in liver diseases. Curr. Opin. Gastroenterol. 21, 197–200. https://doi.org/10.1097/01. mog.0000153353.45738.bf.

Bjelakovic, G., Gluud, L.L., Nikolova, D., Bjelakovic, M., Nagorni, A., Gluud, C., 2011. Antioxidant supplements for liver disease. Cochrane Database Syst. Rev. https://doi.org/10.1002/14651858.CD007749.pub2.

Björnsson, E., Simren, M., Olsson, R., Chapman, R.W., 2004. Fatigue in patients with primary sclerosing cholangitis. Scand. J. Gastroenterol. 39, 961–968. https://doi.org/10.1080/00365520410003434.

Björnsson, E., Olsson, R., Bergquist, A., Lindgren, S., Braden, B., Chapman, R.W., Boberg, K.M., Angulo, P., 2008. The natural history of small-duct primary sclerosing cholangitis. Gastroenterology 134, 975–980. https://doi.org/10.1053/j.gastro.2008.01.042.

Boigk, G., Stroedter, L., Herbst, H., Waldschmidt, J., Riecken, E.O., Schuppan, D., 1997. Silymarin retards collagen accumulation in early and advanced biliary fibrosis secondary to complete bile duct obliteration in rats. Hepatology 26, 643–649. https://doi.org/10.1002/hep.510260316.

Byass, P., 2014. The global burden of liver disease: a challenge for methods and for public health. BMC Med. 12, 1–3. https://doi.org/10.1186/s12916-014-0159-5.

Carola, D., Jochen, E., Herbert, D., 1996. Inhibition of Kupffer cell functions as an explanation for the hepatoprotective properties of silibinin. Hepatology 23, 749–754.

Cauch-Dudek, K., Abbey, S., Stewart, D.E., Heathcote, E.J., 1998. Fatigue in primary biliary cirrhosis. Gut 43, 705–710. https://doi.org/10.1136/gut.43.5.705.

Cicero, A.F.G., Colletti, A., Bellentani, S., 2018. Nutraceutical approach to non-alcoholic fatty liver disease (NAFLD): the available clinical evidence. Nutrients 10, 1153. https://doi.org/10.3390/nu10091153.

Colman, J.C., Morgan, M.Y., Scheuer, P.J., Sherlock, S., 1980. Treatment of alcohol-related liver disease with (+)-cyanidanol-3: a randomised double-blind trial. Gut 21, 965–969. https://doi.org/10.1136/gut.21.11.965.

Corpechot, C., Abenavoli, L., Rabahi, N., Chrétien, Y., Andréani, T., Johanet, C., Chazouillères, O., Poupon, R., 2008. Biochemical response to ursodeoxycholic acid and long-term prognosis in primary biliary cirrhosis. Hepatology 48, 871–877. https://doi.org/10.1002/hep.22428.

Eaton, J.E., Talwalkar, J.A., Lazaridis, K.N., Gores, G.J., Lindor, K.D., 2013. Pathogenesis of primary sclerosing cholangitis and advances in diagnosis and management. Gastroenterology 145, 521–536. https://doi.org/10.1053/j.gastro.2013.06.052.

Eaton, J.E., Nelson, K.M., Gossard, A.A., Carey, E.J., Tabibian, J.H., Lindor, K.D., LaRusso, N.F., 2019. Efficacy and safety of curcumin in primary sclerosing cholangitis: an open label pilot study. Scand. J. Gastroenterol. 54, 633–639. https://doi.org/10.1080/00365521.2019.1611917.

Folseraas, T., Boberg, K.M., 2016. Cancer risk and surveillance in primary sclerosing cholangitis. Clin. Liver Dis. 20, 79–98. https://doi.org/10.1016/j.cld.2015.08.014.

Hassan, K., Bhalla, V., Ezz, M., Regal, E., A-kader, H.H., Hassan, K., Bhalla, V., Ezz, M., Regal, E., 2014. Nonalcoholic fatty liver disease: a comprehensive review of a growing epidemic. World J. Gastroenterol. 20, 12082–12101. https://doi.org/10.3748/wjg.v20.i34.12082.

Heathcote, J., 1997. The clinical expression of primary biliary cirrhosis. Semin. Liver Dis. 17, 23–33. https://doi.org/10.1055/s-2007-1007180.

Hu, R.W., Carey, E.J., Lindor, K.D., Tabibian, J.H., 2017. Curcumin in hepatobiliary disease: pharmacotherapeutic properties and emerging potential clinical applications. Ann. Hepatol. 16. https://doi.org/10.5604/01.3001.0010.5273.

Imam, M.H., Gossard, A.A., Sinakos, E., Lindor, K.D., 2012. Pathogenesis and management of pruritus in cholestatic liver disease. J. Gastroenterol. Hepatol. 27, 1150–1158. https://doi.org/10.1111/j.1440-1746.2012.07109.x.

Invernizzi, P., Selmi, C., Gershwin, M.E., 2010. Update on primary biliary cirrhosis. Dig. Liver Dis. 42, 401–408. https://doi.org/10.1016/j.dld.2010.02.014.

Iser, D., Ryan, M., 2013. Fatty liver disease: a practical guide for GPs. Aust. Fam. Physician 42, 444–447.

Jones, D.E.J., Donaldson, P.T., 2003. Genetic factors in the pathogenesis of primary biliary cirrhosis. Clin. Liver Dis. 7, 841–864. https://doi.org/10.1016/S1089-3261(03)00095-3.

Juran, B.D., Lazaridis, K.N., 2008. Genetics and genomics of primary biliary cirrhosis. Clin. Liver Dis. 12, 349–ix. https://doi.org/10.1016/j.cld.2008.02.007.

Kaplan, M.M., 2013. Primary biliary cirrhosis. Encycl. Biol. Chem. Second Ed., 561–565. https://doi.org/10.1016/B978-0-12-378630-2.00086-4.

Kaplan, G.G., Laupland, K.B., Butzner, D., Urbanski, S.J., Lee, S.S., 2007. The burden of large and small duct primary sclerosing cholangitis in adults and children: a population-based analysis. Am. J. Gastroenterol. 102, 1042–1049.

Khalid, S., Hasan, S.A., Ali, A., Khetpal, N., Idrisov, E., Burt, J.R., Ward, D., Albors-Mora, M., 2017. A unique triad of ulcerative colitis with autoimmune hemolytic anemia and primary sclerosing cholangitis. Am. J. Gastroenterol. 112, S1109–S1110. https://doi.org/10.14309/00000434-201710001-02015.

Kim, N.-H., Heo, J.-D., Rho, J.-R., Yang, M.H., Jeong, E.J., 2018. The standardized extract of *Limonium tetragonum* alleviates chronic alcoholic liver injury in C57Bl/6J mice. Pharmacogn. Mag. 14, 58–63. https://doi.org/10.4103/pm.pm_44_17.

Ladep, N.G., Akbar, S.M.F., Al Mahtab, M., 2019. Clinical Epidemiology of Chronic Liver Diseases, first ed. Springer International Publishing, Cham, https://doi.org/10.1007/978-3-319-94355-8.

Langmead, L., Rampton, D.S., 2001. Review article: herbal treatment in gastrointestinal and liver disease—benefits and dangers. Aliment. Pharmacol. Ther. 15 (9), 1239–1252.

Lazaridis, K.N., LaRusso, N.F., 2015. The cholangiopathies. Mayo Clin. Proc. 90, 791–800. https://doi.org/10.1016/j.mayocp.2015.03.017.

Lazaridis, K.N., LaRusso, N.F., 2016. Primary sclerosing cholangitis. N. Engl. J. Med. 375, 1161–1170. https://doi.org/10.1056/NEJMra1506330.

Lazo, M., Mitchell, M.C., 2016. Epidemiology and risk factors for alcoholic liver disease. In: Chalasani, N., Szabo, G. (Eds.), Alcoholic and Non-Alcoholic Fatty Liver Disease: Bench to Bedside. Springer, pp. 1–20.

Leuschner, U., 2003. Primary biliary cirrhosis—presentation and diagnosis. Clin. Liver Dis. 7, 741–758. https://doi.org/10.1016/S1089-3261(03)00101-6.

Lin, Y.-L., Lin, C.-Y., Chi, C.-W., Huang, Y.-T., 2009. Study on antifibrotic effects of curcumin in rat hepatic stellate cells. Phytother. Res. 23, 927–932. https://doi.org/10.1002/ptr.2764.

Liu, J.Z., Almarri, M.A., Gaffney, D.J., Mells, G.F., Jostins, L., Cordell, H.J., Ducker, S.J., Day, D.B., Heneghan, M.A., Neuberger, J.M., Donaldson, P.T., Bathgate, A.J., Burroughs, A., Davies, M.H., Jones, D.E., Alexander, G.J., Barrett, J.C., Sandford, R.N., Anderson, C.A., UK Primary Biliary Cirrhosis (PBC) Consortium, Wellcome Trust Case Control Consortium, 2012. Dense fine-mapping study identifies new susceptibility loci for primary biliary cirrhosis. Nat. Genet. 44, 1137–1141. https://doi.org/10.1038/ng.2395.

Liu, Y.-L., Lin, L.-C., Tung, Y.-T., Ho, S.-T., Chen, Y.-L., Lin, C.-C., Wu, J.-H., 2017. *Rhododendron oldhamii* leaf extract improves fatty liver syndrome by increasing lipid oxidation and decreasing the lipogenesis pathway in mice. Int. J. Med. Sci. 14, 862–870. https://doi.org/10.7150/ijms.19553.

Lleo, A., Battezzati, P.M., Selmi, C., Gershwin, M.E., Podda, M., 2008. Is autoimmunity a matter of sex? Autoimmun. Rev. 7, 626–630. https://doi.org/10.1016/j.autrev.2008.06.009.

Longo, M., Crosignani, A., Battezzati, P.M., Squarcia Giussani, C., Invernizzi, P., Zuin, M., Podda, M., 2002. Hyperlipidaemic state and cardiovascular risk in primary biliary cirrhosis. Gut 51, 265–269. https://doi.org/10.1136/gut.51.2.265.

Ludwig, J., 1991. Small-duct primary sclerosing cholangitis. Semin. Liver Dis. 11, 11–17. https://doi.org/10.1055/s-2008-1040417.

MacCarty, R.L., LaRusso, N.F., Wiesner, R.H., Ludwig, J., 1983. Primary sclerosing cholangitis: findings on cholangiography and pancreatography. Radiology 149, 39–44. https://doi.org/10.1148/radiology.149.1.6412283.

Mcgarity, B., Bansi, D.S., Robertson, D.F., Millward-Sadler, G.H., Shepherd, H.A., 1991. Primary sclerosing cholangitis: an important and prevalent complication of Crohn's disease. Eur. J. Gastroenterol. Hepatol., 361–364.

Merli, M., Riggio, O., Dally, L., 1996. Does malnutrition affect survival in cirrhosis? PINC (Policentrica Italiana Nutrizione Cirrosi). Hepatology 23, 1041–1046. https://doi.org/10.1002/hep.510230516.

Mounach, A., Ouzzif, Z., Wariaghli, G., Achemlal, L., Benbaghdadi, I., Aouragh, A., Bezza, A., El Maghraoui, A., 2008. Primary biliary cirrhosis and osteoporosis: a case-control study. J. Bone Miner. Metab. 26, 379. https://doi.org/10.1007/s00774-007-0833-1.

Nakayama, N., Nakamura, T., Okada, H., Iwaki, S., Sobel, B.E., Fujii, S., 2011. Modulators of induction of plasminogen activator inhibitor type-1 in HepG2 cells by transforming growth factor-β. Coron. Artery Dis. 22.

Nassir, F., Rector, R.S., Hammoud, G.M., Ibdah, J.A., 2015. Pathogenesis and prevention of hepatic steatosis. Gastroenterol. Hepatol. 11, 167–175. https://doi.org/10.3109/00365521.2015.1030687.

Olsson, R., Danielsson, A., Järnerot, G., Lindström, E., Lööf, L., Rolny, P., Rydén, B.O., Tysk, C., Wallerstedt, S., 1991. Prevalence of primary sclerosing cholangitis in patients with ulcerative colitis. Gastroenterology 100, 1319–1323. https://doi.org/10.1016/0016-5085(91)70019-T.

Palmas, S., 1981. Treatment of alcoholic cirrhosis with (+)-cyanidanol-3. In: Conn, H.O. (Ed.), International Workshop on (+)-Cyanidanol-3 in Diseases of the Liver. The Royal Society of Medicine, London, pp. 167–171.

Pappachan, J.M., Babu, S., Krishnan, B., Ravindran, N.C., 2017. Non-alcoholic fatty liver disease: a clinical update. J. Clin. Transl. Hepatol. 5, 384–393. https://doi.org/10.14218/JCTH.2017.00013.

Petrides, A.S., Vogt, C., Schulze-Berge, D., Matthews, D., Strohmeyer, G., 1994. Pathogenesis of glucose intolerance and diabetes mellitus in cirrhosis. Hepatology 19, 616–627. https://doi.org/10.1002/hep.1840190312.

Plauth, M., Cabré, E., Riggio, O., Assis-Camilo, M., Pirlich, M., Kondrup, J., Ferenci, P., Holm, E., vom Dahl, S., Müller, M.J., Nolte, W., 2006. ESPEN guidelines on enteral nutrition: liver disease. Clin. Nutr. 25, 285–294. https://doi.org/10.1016/j.clnu.2006.01.018.

Porayko, M.K., Wiesner, R.H., LaRusso, N.F., Ludwig, J., MacCarty, R.L., Steiner, B.L., Twomey, C.K., Zinsmeister, A.R., 1990. Patients with asymptomatic primary sclerosing cholangitis frequently have progressive disease. Gastroenterology 98, 1594–1602. https://doi.org/10.5555/uri:pii:0016508590910960.

Rambaldi, A., Jacobs, B.P., Gluud, C., 2007. Milk thistle for alcoholic and/or hepatitis B or C virus liver diseases. Cochrane Database Syst. Rev. https://doi.org/10.1002/14651858.CD003620.pub3.

Ratziu, V., Bellentani, S., Cortez-Pinto, H., Day, C., Marchesini, G., 2010. A position statement on NAFLD/NASH based on the EASL 2009 special conference. J. Hepatol. 53, 372–384. https://doi.org/10.1016/j.jhep.2010.04.008.

Rivera Irigoin, R., Abilés, J., 2012. Soporte nutricional en el paciente con cirrosis hepática. Gastroenterol. Hepatol. 35, 594–601. https://doi.org/10.1016/j.gastrohep.2012.03.001.

Ross, S.M., 2008. Milk thistle (*Silybum marianum*): an ancient botanical medicine for modern times. Holist. Nurs. Pract. 22.

Rukkumani, R., Sri Balasubashini, M., Vishwanathan, P., Menon, V.P., 2002. Comparative effects of curcumin and photo-irradiated curcumin on alcohol- and polyunsaturated fatty acid-induced hyperlipidemia. Pharmacol. Res. 46, 257–264. https://doi.org/10.1016/S1043-6618(02)00149-4.

Rukkumani, R., Aruna, K., Varma, P.S., Viswanathan, P., Rajasekaran, K.N., Menon, V.P., 2005. Protective role of a novel curcuminoid on alcohol and PUFA-induced hyperlipidemia. Toxicol. Mech. Methods 15, 227–234. https://doi.org/10.1080/15376520590945658.

Selmi, C., Bowlus, C.L., Gershwin, M.E., Coppel, R.L., 2011. Primary biliary cirrhosis. Lancet 377, 1600–1609. https://doi.org/10.1016/S0140-6736(10)61965-4.

Shergill, R., Syed, W., Rizvi, S.A., Singh, I., Syed, W., Rizvi, S.A., Singh, I., 2018. Nutritional support in chronic liver disease and cirrhotics. World J. Hepatol. 10, 685–694. https://doi.org/10.4254/wjh.v10.i10.685.

Sun, M., Kisseleva, T., 2015. Reversibility of liver fibrosis. Clin. Res. Hepatol. Gastroenterol. 39 (Suppl. 1), S60–S63. https://doi.org/10.1016/j.clinre.2015.06.015.

Sutton, I., Neuberger, J., 2002. Primary biliary cirrhosis: seeking the silent partner of autoimmunity. Gut 50, 743–746. https://doi.org/10.1136/gut.50.6.743.

Tabibian, J.H., Lindor, K.D., 2013. Primary sclerosing cholangitis: a review and update on therapeutic developments. Expert Rev. Gastroenterol. Hepatol. 7, 103–114. https://doi.org/10.1016/j.livres.2017.12.002.

Tabibian, J.H., Yang, J.D., Baron, T.H., Kane, S.V., Enders, F.B., Gostout, C.J., 2016. Weekend admission for acute cholangitis does not adversely impact clinical or endoscopic outcomes. Dig. Dis. Sci. 61, 53–61. https://doi.org/10.1007/s10620-015-3853-z.

Tajiri, K., Shimizu, Y., 2013. Branched-chain amino acids in liver diseases. World J. Gastroenterol. 19, 7620–7629. https://doi.org/10.3748/wjg.v19.i43.7620.

Thabrew, M.I., Robin, D., 1996. Phytogenic Agents in the Therapy of Liver Disease.

Tolman, K.G., Dalpiaz, A.S., 2007. Treatment of non-alcoholic fatty liver disease. Ther. Clin. Risk Manage. 3, 1153–1163.

Traisac, F.J., Borg, R., 1977. Una nuova tereapia dell'insufficienza epatica. Sperimentazione del (+)-cyanidanot-3. Suo interesse nel trattamento dell'epatite alcoholica. Minerva Diet. e. Gastroent., 237–242.

Van de Water, J., Turchany, J., Leung, P.S., Lake, J., Munoz, S., Surh, C.D., Coppel, R., Ansari, A., Nakanuma, Y., Gershwin, M.E., 1993. Molecular mimicry in primary biliary cirrhosis. Evidence for biliary epithelial expression of a molecule cross-reactive with pyruvate dehydrogenase complex-E2. J. Clin. Invest. 91, 2653–2664. https://doi.org/10.1172/JCI116504.

Van de Water, J., Ishibashi, H., Coppel, R.L., Gershwin, M.E., 2001. Molecular mimicry and primary biliary cirrhosis: premises not promises. Hepatology 33, 771–775. https://doi.org/10.1053/jhep.2001.23902.

Warren, K.W., Athanassiades, S., Monge, J.I., 1966. Primary sclerosing cholangitis: a study of forty-two cases. Am. J. Surg. 111, 23–38. https://doi.org/10.1016/0002-9610(66)90339-4.

Wiesner, R.H., Larusso, N.F., Ludwig, J., Rolland Dickson, E., 1985. Comparison of the clinicopathologic features of primary sclerosing cholangitis and primary biliary cirrhosis. Gastroenterology 88, 108–114. https://doi.org/10.1016/S0016-5085(85)80141-4.

Yao, H., Qiao, Y., Zhao, Y., Tao, X., Xu, L., Yin, L., Qi, Y., Peng, J., 2016. Herbal medicines and nonalcoholic fatty liver disease. World J. Gastroenterol. 22, 6890–6905. https://doi.org/10.3748/wjg.v22.i30.6890.

Yoon, S.-J., Koh, E.-J., Kim, C.-S., Zee, O.-P., Kwak, J.-H., Jeong, W.-J., Kim, J.-H., Lee, S.-M., 2012. *Agrimonia eupatoria* protects against chronic ethanol-induced liver injury in rats. Food Chem. Toxicol. 50, 2335–2341. https://doi.org/10.1016/j.fct.2012.04.005.

Zanwar, A.A., Badole, S.L., Shende, P.S., Hegde, M.V., Bodhankar, S.L., 2014. Antioxidant role of catechin in health and disease. In: Watson, R.R., Preedy, V.R., Zibadi, S. (Eds.), Polyphenols in Human Health and Disease. Academic Press, San Diego, pp. 267–271, https://doi.org/10.1016/B978-0-12-398456-2.00021-9.

Drug-induced hepatotoxicity

Amandeep Singh[a], Sneha Joshi[b], Ashima Joshi[c], Pooja Patni[d], and Devesh Tewari[e]

[a]Department of Pharmacognosy, Khalsa College of Pharmacy, Amritsar, Punjab, India [b]Department of Pharmaceutical Chemistry, PCTE Group of Institutions, Ludhiana, Punjab, India [c]MojoLab Foundation, New Delhi, India [d]Department of Pharmaceutics, School of Pharmaceutical Sciences, Lovely Professional University, Phagwara, Punjab, India [e]Department of Pharmacognosy, School of Pharmaceutical Sciences, Lovely Professional University, Phagwara, Punjab, India

8.1 Background

The term "iatrogenesis" is derived from the Greek, with "iatros" meaning "physician" and "gennan" meaning 'to produce." Hence, iatrogenic diseases are those harmful effects that occur due to the administration of drugs and chemicals intended for diagnostic and therapeutic treatment. Such diseases are independent of the medical condition for which the diagnostic and therapeutic treatment is initially given (Bachmann et al., 2018). Iatrogenic diseases may be of various types that include drug-induced cutenaceous manifestations, drug-induced hematological conditions, drug-producing neutropenia, drug-induced thrombocytopenia, and drug-induced gastrointestinal diseases, among others (Krishnan and Kasthuri, 2005).

The liver plays a key role in most metabolic processes occurring in the body, including detoxification, the breakdown of amino acids, bile production, etc. The most important factor affecting the vulnerability of the liver to drug-induced hepatotoxicity (DIH) is its vital involvement in the process of metabolism. A variety of prescription drugs are associated with liver toxicity, including antimicrobials such as antituberculous compounds, antibacterials, and more rarely antifungals (with an exception being isoniazid). DIH is an important reason for acute liver failure. It is usually the primary cause as to why therapeutically active drugs are withdrawn from the drug market (Björnsson, 2016; Njoku, 2014; Polson, 2007).

The mechanisms through which DIH may occur are (a) reactive species formation, (b) immune system reactions, (c) apoptosis, and (d) mitochondrial dysfunction, among others. In clinical situations, however, more than one mechanism seems to take place collectively (Shehu et al., 2017). One of the major functions of the liver is to detoxify the body by converting lipid soluble metabolites into hydrophilic metabolites. During the phase I

Influence of Nutrients, Bioactive Compounds, and Plant Extracts in Liver Diseases. https://doi.org/10.1016/B978-0-12-816488-4.00001-2

metabolism, CYP450 enzymes accelerate the process of oxidation, reduction, and/or hydrolysis and result in the formation of hydrophilic metabolites of lipophilic drugs. These polar metabolites are then excreted by the phase II metabolism (Njoku, 2014). But sometimes, the drug metabolism may result in the formation of toxic and chemically reactive metabolites such as reactive oxygen species (ROS) and/or reactive nitrogen species (RNS). These metabolites generally have the potential to bind irreversibly and modify cellular macromolecules, causing a loss of protein function, DNA damage, and lipid peroxidation (Antoine et al., 2008; Shehu et al., 2017; Shuhendler et al., 2014). Another mechanism involves permeability changes in the mitochondria, finally leading to cell death.

Increased concentrations of two liver enzymes, serum alanine aminotransferase (ALT) and aspartate aminotransferase (AST), with or without an increase in bilirubin are the biomarkers linked with DIH genomic biomarkers for short-term studies. Techniques such as toxicogenomics for predictive toxicology of the liver may be used to develop in vitro testing of liver toxicity (Blomme et al., 2009). Toxicogenomics is a branch of toxicology that uses genomics methodology and tools to study the side effects of xenobiotics. Such studies deal with the analysis of gene expression throughout the world to identify changes in gene expression that help in defining drug toxicity. Despite the various advantages and disadvantages of conventional hepatotoxicity models, the three-dimensional (3D) dynamic flow systems for an in vitro cell culture may be the best for toxicological studies (Soldatow et al., 2013; Suter et al., 2004).

Contemporary development aimed at in vitro assays for screening hepatotoxicity is generally centered around the hepatocyte. But, according to recent studies, a secondary response to primary damage to hepatocytes also has immune cells or nonparenchyma cells and may intensify the initial damage (Godoy et al., 2013). The most important cell categories involved in drug-induced hepatotoxicity are liver sinusoidal endothelial cells (LSEC), hepatic stellate cells (HSC), and hepatocytes.

8.2 Hepatotoxicity: An overview

The liver is positioned at the upper abdominal cavity on the right side. Cells present in the liver are called hepatocytes. These are involved in various functions such as the synthesis of proteins and bile; the storage of glycogen, vitamins, and iron; and the metabolism of toxic chemicals and drugs (Bhaargavi et al., 2014). It is an essential organ and its strategic location and mutifaceted tasks support nearly every other organ in the body. It is also considered to be the chief organ that performs the biotransformation and excretion of drugs. However, the liver is susceptible to many diseases such as allergies to food and it involves the immune system as well. The unclad area of the liver is a site that is unfortified to the passing of infection from the abdominal cavity to the thorax. Different causes of hepatitis include lead poisoning, viruses, and autoimmunity and it can also be the out turn from nonalcoholic fatty liver disease (NAFLD) which is associated with obesity and steatosis. Hepatic encephalopathy is caused by the assembly of toxins in the bloodstream that are detached by the liver (Gulati et al., 2018).

The liver performs astounding vital functions to control body homeostasis. It is also analogous with nearly all the biochemical pathways that take place in the liver that are responsible for growth, reproduction, antibody synthesis, and nutrient supply. The essential role of the liver is the metabolism of fats, proteins, and carbohydrates along with the removal of toxins, bile secretion, and vitamin storage. Hence, to sustain a healthy life, the liver is considered a key element for comprehensive health and welfare.

Consumption of specific formulation in a higher quantity or even if taken with the sanative ranges can also injure liver. Different medicinal agents that can induce hepatotoxicity are natural and herbal agents, which are used in industries and laboratories. The most familiar cause for a drug to be dropped from the market is that it causes liver injury. More than 900 drugs have been involved in promoting serious hepatic injury. Medicinal agents or chemicals are usually responsible for causing liver injury, which shows as abnormal values of liver enzymes. Liver injury caused by drugs is around 5% of the total patients admitted to the hospital and is 50% with respect to acute liver failure. Idiosyncratic drug reactions cause liver transplantation or death in more than 75% of cases (Pandit et al., 2012).

Liver damage can be generally caused by drugs, particularly antitubercular, paracetamol, general anesthetics, and some anticancer drugs. Toxic hepatitis is the most common severe adverse reaction caused by antituberculosis drugs. It mostly starts in the first few weeks of treatment accompanying liver necrosis, which may unfold to neurological disorders and death. Due to the excessive consumption of alcohol, alcoholic liver disease with cirrhosis (formation of fibrous tissue in the liver) can occur. Liver injury can sometime be induced by some chemicals called hepatotoxins, such as chloroform and galactosamine (Gulati et al., 2018).

Due to the growing risk of hepatic disease and the low effectiveness of modern medicine, plant-based preparations are chiefly employed to treat liver diseases. In recent years, these formulations have gained immense popularity and importance as they are safe, effortlessly accessible, and cheap. In India, out of many plants, more than 87 plants are utilized, among which 33 are patented and exclusive mixed-ingredient plant formulations. For different types of hepatic toxicity, about 40 polyherbal formulations are used that have hepatoprotective activity. It has been reported that around 160 phytoconstituents were isolated from 101 medicinal plants that possessed hepatoprotective action (Handa, 1986). Various herbs have been used to reduce different types of hepatic toxicity, with the most popular being curcumin extracted from *Curcuma longa*; picroside and kutkoside extracted from *Picrorrhiza kurroa*; Silymarin extracted from *Silybum marianum*; andrographolide and neoandrographolide extracted from *Andrographis paniculata*; glycyrrhizin extracted from *Glycyrrhiza glabra*; phyllanthin and hypophyllanthin from *Phyllanthus niruri*; etc. (Bhaargavi et al., 2014).

8.3 Drug metabolic pathways of the liver and hepatotoxicity

Biotransformation, also known as drug metabolism, is a process under which detoxification takes place. During this procedure, a substance is chemically reformed under the influence of certain enzymatic reactions into a less-toxic form. The high cellular content of cytochrome P4501 enables the liver to accomplish various oxidative metabolisms. The liver is the central organ for metabolism, and it is highly prone to injuries caused by drugs and chemicals. The symptomless elevation of liver enzymes leading to uncontrollable hepatic injury or failure (Bhaargavi et al., 2014).

Being the most important digestive gland, the liver performs the function of metabolism via hydrolysis, condensation, hydration, oxidation, reduction, conjugation, condensation, or isomerization. To convert a pharmaceutical product into a conjugated water-soluble substance, P450 enzymes are involved via two stages of hepatic drug metabolism; after that, they are excreted via urine or bile. Because the liver is accountable for drug metabolism, any disturbance in these processes can lead to hepatotoxicity. There are innumerable mechanisms for the occurrence of hepatotoxicity: apoptosis of hepatocytes, injury to the bile duct, disassembly of hepatocytes, cytolytic T-cell activation, and inhibition of mitochondria (Thompson et al., 2017). The intimation hepatotoxicity arises with a number of illnesses such as jaundice, blood coagulation, dyspepsia, pruritus, and edema. At one point when hepatotoxicity is initiated, patients exhibit the following symptoms: liver cirrhosis, swelling of the legs and feet, elevated serum transaminases, bilirubin, cholestasis, liver failure, hepatic veno-occlusive disease, hepatic necrosis, and fibrosis (Thompson et al., 2017).

The liver plays a fundamental role in the metabolism of various complex compounds. As a result of this, varied liver complications such as hindrances in signal transduction pathways, imbalance of ions, and the emergence of reactive metabolic species (RMS) take place that cause oxidative stress, translational constraints at various levels, a Ca^{2+} shift, and the deterioration of the mitochondrial respiratory chain (Dey et al., 2013).

Hepatotoxicity is generally classified into three different categories. The separation is based on the level of different enzymes, for instance, if there is a threefold increase in the level of enzyme alanine amino transferase (ALT) along with a twofold increase in the level of alkaline phosphatase (ALP) and serum bilirubin (SBLN), respectively. An increase in the level of ALT or ALP in this condition is termed hepatocellular or hepatic injury. An elevation in the ALP and bilirubin levels is termed cholestatic injury, and lastly when both the ALP and ALT levels are increased, the condition is termed mixed injury. Table 8.1 shows the drugs associated with various types of hepatotoxicity (Thompson et al., 2017).

Table 8.1: Association of different drugs with various modes of hepatotoxicity.

Hepatocellular injury	Cholestatic injury	Mixed injury
Acetaminophen	Amoxicillin	Amitriptyline
Allopurinol	Anabolic steroids	Azathioprine
Baclofen	Chlorpromazine	Captopril
Fluoxetine	Oral contraceptives	Clindamycin
Isoniazid	Erythromycins	Cyproheptadine
Ketoconazole	Estrogens	Enalapril
Losartan	Mirtazapine	Nitrofurantoin
Methotrexate	Phenothiazines	Phenobarbital
Omeprazole	Terbinafine	Phenytoin
Pyrazinamide	Tricyclics	Sulfonamides
Rifampin		Trazodone
Risperidone		Verapamil
Tetracyclines		
Valproic acid		

8.4 Drug-induced hepatotoxicity: Mechanisms and risk factors

Drug-induced hepatotoxicity generally occurs whenever there is an increased level of liver enzymes, which can be calculated by liver function tests irrespective of elevated or constant values of bilirubin. In the case of ALT, the range is five times above the normal limit while ALP is two times above the normal limit. Considering the combination factor, the ALT range is three times above the normal limit and bilirubin is two times above the normal limit. Further, the elevation pattern of liver enzymes is categorized into three different subcategories, and this depends on the value of R. The value of R is determined as the ratio between ALT and ALP. When the value of R is more than 5, it is a hepatocellular or hepatic injury. If it is between 2 and 5, it is said to be mixed, and if the value is less than 2, it is a cholestatic injury. Hepatocellular or hepatic injury is generally represented as cell death or inflammation in which a slightly increased or no increased level of bilirubin take place. In this type of injury, the levels of ALT and AST are already high and the ALP levels slowly elevate, which may lead to discomfort and weariness. In the cholestatic type of injury, bile agglomeration occurs in the hepatocytes, which leads to an increased level of bilirubin and ALP, followed by skin itching and jaundice. The last category is usually a combination of the first two, that is, hepatic and cholestatic injury. Due to the augmented level of ALT and ALP, the accumulation of bile takes place, which leads to itching and enervation in patients (Shehu et al., 2017). The chemical structures of some drugs that produce hepatotoxicity are presented in Fig. 8.1.

The chemical structures of some drugs that produce hepatotoxicity are presented in Fig. 8.1.

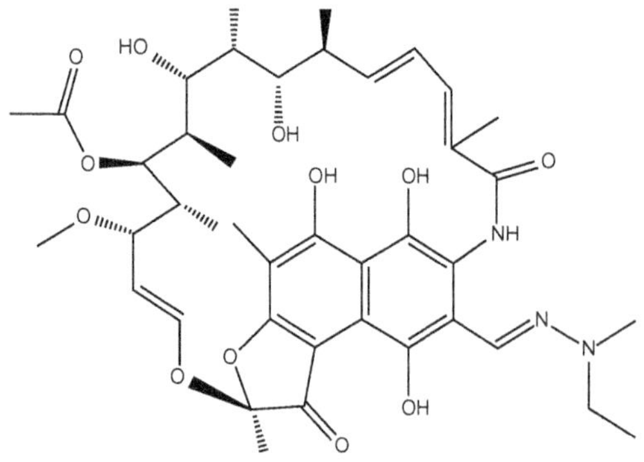

Rifampicin

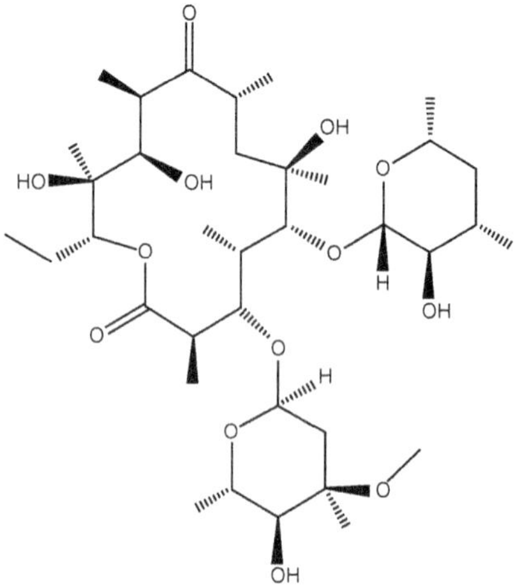

Erythromycin

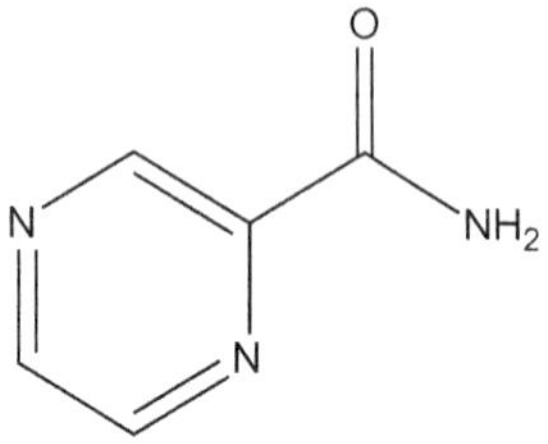

Pyrazinamide

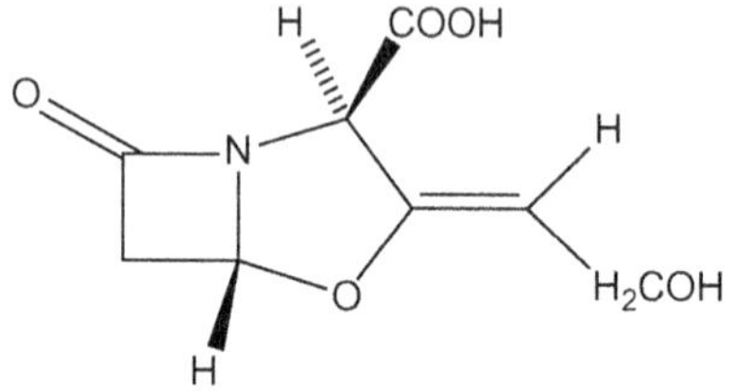

Clavulanic acid

Fig. 8.1
Structures of some reported hepatotoxic agents.

The mechanism of drug-induced hepatotoxicity involves cell death, formation of reactive metabolite and mitochondrial myopathies (Shehu et al., 2017). Many oral drugs and xenobiotics are lipophilic in nature, and are certainly absorbed across the membranes of intestines. They tend to be hydrophilic via the hepatic metabolism, and due to which, they are easily excreted. The metabolism of exogenous products in the liver generally occurs through phase I and phase II reactions. The phase I and II reactions are involved in the metabolism of exogenous products present in the liver. The prime enzyme involved in the phase I reactions, which include oxidation, reduction, hydroxylation, and demethylation pathways, is cytochrome P450. It is located in the endoplasmic reticulum and is considered to be the vital metabolizing enzyme (Gulati et al., 2018).

By detoxification pathways, the toxic intermediates that are produced by phase I reactions are transformed into nontoxic compounds by phase II reactions. These phase II reactions lead to the formation of water-soluble metabolites by chemical conjugation with different hydrophilic moieties such as glucuronide, amino acids, or sulfate. These water-soluble metabolites are excreted easily. Moreover, phase II reactions involve glutathione, which noncovalently binds to the toxic intermediates with the help of the enzyme glutathione *S* transferase. However, this phase can form unstable precursors of reactive species that might lead to hepatotoxicity (Gulati et al., 2018).

There are various factors that can affect the drug metabolism such as the age of the patient, the genetic make-up, diet, causal liver disease, and the use of other drugs. In prescribing any hepatotoxic drugs, these factors must be strongly considered. Table 8.2 depicts examples of drugs, and the toxicity of which can be predisposed by several factors.

8.5 Epidemiological aspects

Drug-induced hepatotoxicity is presumed to be unpublicized and to a great extent its frequency is underemphasized in society (Pugh et al., 2009). The sole recurrent drugs related to drug-induced liver injury are paracetamol (PCM) and acetaminophen (APAP). In Australia, the United States, and the United Kingdom, acetaminophen is the only drug that causes acute injuries to the liver. More than 80,000 annual emergency visits occur that are related to a PCM overdose in the United States, which reflects an incidence of emergency visits at around 27 per 100,000. Another important point is that, the highest incidences are seen is age like 3 and 4-years-old as well as 15–30-years-old reaching more than 40/1000,000. Interestingly, a risk factor associated with mortality from PCM is weight loss (Pugh et al., 2009).

Table 8.2: External/environmental factors and risk for DILI (Pugh et al., 2009).

Factor	Factor modifier	Examples
Gender	Men, hepatotoxicity ↑ Women, hepatotoxicity ↑	Halothane, nitrofurantoin, azathioprine
Age	Children, hepatotoxicity ↑ >60 y, hepatotoxicity ↑	Valproic acid, halothane, salicylates, isoniazid
Dose	Blood levels ↑ → Hepatotoxicity ↑ Exposure dose, duration Hepatotoxicity ↑	Methotrexate, aspirin, acetaminophen, vitamin A
Nutrition	Obesity, hepatotoxicity ↑ Fasting, hepatotoxicity ↑	Acetaminophen, methotrexate
Other drugs	Hepatotoxicity ↑ Hepatotoxicity ↑	Rifampicin, isoniazid, and pyrazinamide, valproic acid, and other antiepileptics
Excessive ethyl alcohol	Hepatotoxicity ↑	Isoniazid, acetaminophen

Abbreviations: ↑ (increased); → (leads to).

8.6 Hepatoprotective activity of natural compounds and plant extracts in drug-induced hepatotoxicity

Indian medicinal plants have been traditionally utilized as powerful antioxidants that also exhibit a hepatoprotective effect against liver intoxication. The rich chemical diversity of Indian medicinal plants of folklore has further convinced global researchers to explore the potential hepatocurative therapeutic agents from these plants. The literature highlights the significant hepatoprotective response of plant molecules against liver damage induced by different drugs. Alcohol consumption is considered an aggravating factor in liver damage. It was observed that the simultaneous administration of the crude alcoholic extract of *Phyllanthus emblica* L. (Amla) along with alcohol may reduce the level of hepatic necrosis. The crude alcoholic extract and one of its active metabolite quercetin was found significantly effective in exhibiting hepatoprotection (Gulati et al., 1995).

In another in vitro study, amla extracts also demonstrated a significant reduction in alcohol-induced cell death. Further, a biochemical investigation showed that the pretreatment of rats with 25, 50, and 75 mg/kg of amla extracts before administering ethanol caused a decline in AST, ALT, and interleukin-1β level in serum at a dose-dependant level. Moreover, the alcoholic extract of amla at a dose of 75 mg/kg displayed an equivalent effect to that of the standard hepatoprotective agent silymarin (Pramyothin et al., 2006). In addition to this, amla also showed a significant hepatoprotective effect against liver injury caused by isoniazid, heavy metals, carbon tetrachloride, paracetamol, thioacetamide, D-galactosamine, and some mycotoxins (Deori et al., 2017; Sharma et al., 2009; Kaisar et al., 2005).

Psidium guajava is a tropical fruit of India that belongs to the family Myrtaceae. It has been reported to have antiplasmodial, antioxidant, antidiarrheal, antimicrobial, and antispasmodic activities (Gutiérrez et al., 2008). Traditionally, the fruits and leaf extracts of this plant have been recommended for their hepatoprotective properties (Gutiérrez et al., 2008). In recent investigations, the dried aqueous extract of guava leaves was preclinically examined for its hepatoprotective role in acute and chronic liver injury induced by CCl_4, paracetamol, and thioacetamide. The simultaneous administration of guava leaf extracts (250 and 500 mg/kg) with selective hepatotoxins to animals in experiments significantly depleted the elevated serum level of AST, ALT, and alkaline phosphate (Gutiérrez et al., 2008).

The protective effect of the aqueous leaf extracts of *Abutilon indicum* were also inspected against the hepatic damage caused by CCl_4 and paracetamol. The biochemical estimation of SGOT, SGPT, ALKP, T Bil, D Bil, and GSH suggested that the plant exhibited a significant reduction in the elevated serum concentration of these enzymes in comparison to standard silymarin (Porchezhian and Ansari, 2005). The use of another important plant, *Asparagus racemosus* (AR), also known as Shatavari, is described in traditional medical scriptures for the treatment of diseases associated with bile imbalance. Thus, various authors have reported the hepatoprotective role of this plant in a variety of animal models. The crude hydroalcoholic extract of the roots of A. racemosus and its various biofractions were evaluated for a hepatoprotective effect against liver toxicity raised by CCl_4 in rats. CCl_4 successfully induced liver injury as was indicative from the elevated levels of SGPT, SGOT, ALP, T bil, and D Bil in the serum. The coadministration of plant extract and its fractions along with CCl_4 at different doses to the selective group of animals showed a significant decline in elevated levels of all the serum enzymes in comparison to the negative and positive control groups. Histological investigations of CCl_4-treated rats showed profound necrotic lesions and extensive vacuolization of the cytoplasm in comparison to the normal group of rats. On the contrary, no evidence of any vacuolization, necrosis, or distortion in the size of the liver was observed in the livers of rats simultaneously held on CCl_4 and plant treatment (Palanisamy and Manian, 2012). In another study, the hepatoprotective activity of *Asparagus racemosus* was also evaluated against isoniazid-induced hepatotoxicity in male albino rats. Isoniazid significantly caused hepato injury as indicated from the alteration in serum enzyme concentration. The hepatoprotective activity of AR was observed by examining the body weight of rats and the serum levels of a variety of enzymes such as aspartate aminotransferase, g-glutamyl transferase, alanine aminotransferase, alkaline phosphatase, albumin, total protein, hepatic malondialdehyde content, catalase, cytochrome P450 2E1 (CYP2E1), superoxide dismutase, and glutathione (GSH). No significant effect of isoniazid was observed in the group of rats pretreated with *A. racemosus* extract, as was indicated from the biochemical estimation of serum enzyme concentration. These results revealed that the hepatoprotective effect of *A. racemosus* extract was by free radical inhibition and the free radical generation was inhibited through hepatic CYP2E1 activity inhibition and the induction of antioxidant enzymes (Palanisamy and Manian, 2012).

Butea monosperma is one of the most highly traded medicinal plants of the family Fabaceae, and is commonly known as "Palash." The flowers of *B. monosperma* have been represented as traditional medicine due to their rich pharmacological effects and chemical diversity. The plant has been utilized in traditional medicinal practices due to its antistress, antiestrogenic, and hepatoprotective role in the human physiological system (Kasture et al., 2002; Shah and Baxi, 1990; Wagner et al., 1986). Considering the modern aspects of the preclinical evaluation of plant drugs, the dried aqueous flower extract of *B. monosperma* has been examined for its possible hepatoprotective role in adult albino swiss mice and rats against hepatotoxicty induced by CCl_4. Both blood and tissue biochemical assays were carried out to determine the serum AST, ALT, lipid peroxidation, reduced glutathione, adenosine tri-phosphate, and glucose-6- phosphatase levels, respectively. The preliminary results showed that the groups of animals orally treated with CCl_4 had a significant increase in all the enzymatic activities as well as oxidative stress, which may be considered as leading causes of liver injury. The concurrent administration of *B. monosperma* extract at different doses along with CCl_4 showed a significant reduction in the elevated concentration of all enzymes compared to the positive control groups. Similarly, a significant decline in lipid peroxidation and reduced glutathione in comparison to the control groups can be considered an important factor in protecting the liver from the impact of CCl_4. Further restoration of all the histopathological lesions induced by CCl_4 to the animals also confirms the great potential of BM having therapeutically effective hepatocurative agents (Sharma and Shukla, 2011). Comprehensive details on the plants utilized for hepatoprotective effects are presented in Table 8.3.

Similar results were also observed in rabbits intoxicated with paracetamol (Ahmad et al., 2010). *Cassia fistula,* commonly known in India by the name of the amaltas tree, belongs to the family Fabaceae. The plant is cultivated throughout India due to its ornamental values as well as for its preventive role in various physiological disorders. The pharmacological aspects of *C. fistula* have been widely explored by traditional medicinal healers.

In Ayurvedic medicine, the different parts of plants have been recommended to human patients suffering from diabetes, allergies, and skin and certain liver ailments (Rahmani, 2015). Based on the rich therapeutic significance, a variety of studies on its hepatoprotective role are available in the literature. Bhakta et al., (1999, 2001) reported that the lipophillic fraction of the hydroalocholic matrix of the leaves of *C. fistula* displayed significant hepatocurative action against the hepatotoxicity induced by CCl_4 and paracetamol (Bhakta et al., 2001). In both studies, the plant extract profoundly reduced the increased serum levels of biomarkers such as SGOT, SGPT, bilirubin, and ALP. Jehangir et al. (2010) further evaluated the role of *C. fistula* leaves in controlling hepatitis in rats induced with isoniazid (INH) and rifampicin (RIF) administration. The oral administration of INH and RIF experimentally raised the serum ALT, AST, ALP, and T bilirubin level in the animals compared to the positive control group. The concurrent treatment of a group of animals with ethanolic extract along with INH and RIF abrogated the elevated level of all serum enzymes by displaying significant hepatoprotective activity in a dose-dependant manner compared to the control group. Histopathological investigations further showed evidence of vascular congestion, normal liver appearance, and regeneration of hepatocytes (Jehangir et al., 2010). Moreover, the ethanolic leaf extract of *C. fistula* also showed significant hepatoprotective activity against liver injury induced by diethylnitrosamine (Pradeep et al., 2007). Such studies declared *C. fistula* as a potential resource to be investigated for hepatoprotective agents.

Several other Indian medicinal plants have shown hepatoprotective activity against the different hepatotoxic animal models induced by various drugs; these are displayed in Table 8.3. Most of them have been utilized by traditional medicinal healers as folklore medicine in the treatment of liver disorders. Moreover, all these plants have been mentioned in the Ayurvedic Pharmacopeia of India and also included in the list of highly traded Indian medicinal plants. Despite the effective utilization of these plants as hepatoprotective agents, their biochemical aspects and mechanism of action in liver protection remain unexplored.

Table 8.3: Plants investigated as hepatoprotective agents.

Plant/part used	Family	Hepatoxic agents	Biochemical parameters investigated	Maximum safe effective dose (mg/kg)	References
Acacia nilotica	Mimosoideae	Scetaminophen	ALT, AST, ALP, T Bilirubin, LPO, GSH, histopathological changes	250 mg/kg	Kannan et al. (2013)
Adhatoda vasica/leaves	Acanthaceae	D-Galactosamine	SGOT, SGPT, LPO, protein concentration	100 mg/kg	Bhattacharyya et al. (2005)
Aegle marmelos/whole plant	Rutaceae	CCl_4	Lipid peroxidation (LPO), xanthine oxidase (XO), SGOT, LDH, SGPT, reduced glutathione (GSH), glutathione reductase (GR), glutathione peroxidase (GPx), quinone reductase (QR), catalase (CAT), ornithine decarboxylase (ODC)	50 mg/kg	Khan and Sultana (2009)
Allium cepa/fresh bulbs	Liliaceae	Ethanol	ALT, ALP, AST, TB	600 mg/kg	Kumar et al. (2013)
Apium graveolens/seeds	Apiaceae	CCl_4	SGOT, SGPT, ALP, TP, GSH, ALT, CHL	250 mg/kg	Ahmed et al. (2002)
Bauhinia racemosa/bark	Fabaceae	CCl_4	SGOT, SGPT, SOD, GSH, TBARS	500 mg/kg	Gupta et al. (2004)
Bauhinia variegata/stem bark	Fabaceae	CCl_4	AST, ALP, GGT, ALT, TBARS	100 mg/kg	Ajay and Neelam (2006)
Bidens pilosa/aerial parts	Asteraceae	CCl_4	AST, ALT, LDH	15 mg/kg	Kviecinski et al. (2011)
Boerhavia diffusa/roots	Nyctaginaceae	Local liquor	SGPT, SAP, TG, SGPT, TB, ALP, SGOT	400 mg/kg	Mishra et al. (2014)
Calendula officinalis/whole plant	Asteraceae	Acetaminophen	ALT, AST, LDH	500 mg/kg	Singh et al. (2011)
Cassia fistula/seeds	Fabaceae	Paracetamol	SGPT, SGOT, ALP, TB, DB	400 mg/kg	Chaudhari et al. (2009)
Cichorium intybus/leaves	Asteraceae	CCl_4	ALT, AST, ALP	100 mg/kg	Jamshidzadeh et al. (2010)
Cinnamomum cassia/bark	Lauraceae	Dimethylnitrosamine	TP, TB, DB, GOT, GPT, ALP	40 mg/kg	Lim et al. (2010)

Continued

Table 8.3: Plants investigated as hepatoprotective agents—cont'd

Plant/part used	Family	Hepatoxic agents	Biochemical parameters investigated	Maximum safe effective dose (mg/kg)	References
Convolvulus arvensis/whole plant	Convolvulaceae	Paracetamol	ALP, AST, TB	500 mg/kg	Ali et al. (2013)
Corylus avellana/leaves	Betulaceae	CCl$_4$	GPT, GOT	NA	Rusu et al. (1999)
Cucurbita maxima/aerial parts	Cucurbitaceae	CCl$_4$	SGOT, SGPT, ALP, TP, TB	500 mg/kg	Saha et al. (2011)
Curcuma longa/roots	Zingiberaceae	Paracetamol	ALT, ALP, AST	600 mg/kg	Hsieh et al. (2008)
Cynara scolymus/roots	Apiaceae	CCl$_4$	ALT, ALP, AST, GSH	900 mg/kg	Fallah Huseini et al. (2011)
Ficus cordata/roots	Moraceae	CCl$_4$	LDH	400 mg/kg	Donfack et al. (2011)
Ficus indica/leaves	Moraceae	CCl$_4$	AST, ALT	2 mL/kg	Djerrou et al. (2015)
Galium aparine/whole plants	Rubiaceae	CCl$_4$	ALT, AST, ALP	2 mL/kg	Khan et al. (2011)
Glycyrrhiza glabra/roots	Fabaceae	CCl$_4$	SOD, GST, CAT, GSH	2 mg/kg	Al-Razzuqi et al. (2012)
Hibiscus miltiorrhiza/roots	Malvaceae	Cholesterol:cholic acid	AST, ALT, ALP	240 mg/kg	Biswas et al. (2014)
Ipomoea staphylina/leaves	Convolvulaceae	CCl$_4$	ALP, SGOT, SGPT, AST, CHL, ALT	200 mg/kg	Bag and Mumtaz (2013)
Mimosa pudica/leaves	Mimosaceae	CCl$_4$	AST, SGOT, SGPT, ALT, TB, TP, ALP	200 mg/kg	Sohil and Sundaram (2009)
Nigella sativa/seeds	Ranunculaceae	Galactosamine	ALP, ALT, TB, AST, TP	NA	Gani and John (2013)
Pandanus odorifer/roots	Pandanaceae	Paracetamol	SGOT, SGPT, ALP, TB	400 mg/kg	Mishra et al. (2015)
Phyllanthus emplica/fruits	Euphorbiaceae	CCl$_4$	GSH	100 mg/kg	Haque et al. (2001)
Phyllanthus muellarianus/leaves	Euphorbiaceae	Acetaminophen	ALP, ALT, AST, ALB, TB, CAT	400 mg/kg	Ajiboye et al. (2017)

Plant/part	Family	Toxicant	Parameters	Dose	Reference
Phyllanthus urinaria/whole plants	Euphorbiaceae	Acetaminophen	Cytochrome P450, CYP2E1 protein	200 mg/kg	Hau et al. (2009)
Picorrhiza kurroa/Roots	Scrophulariaceae	CCl_4	SGOT, SGPT, ALP, CHL, TB, TP	2060 mL/kg	Arsul et al. (2011)
Punica granatum/seed juice	Lythraceae	INH and RIF	AST, ALT, LDH	400 mg/kg	Yogeeta et al. (2007)
Rheum palmatum/roots	Polygonaceae	CCl_4	ALT, AST	400 mg/kg	Wang et al. (2011)
Rosa damascena/flower	Rosaceae	Acetaminophen	AST, ALT, ALP, LDH, TBARS, GSH	1000 mg/kg	Sharma et al. (2012)
Tecomella undulata/aerial parts	Bignoniaceae	Paracetamol	AST, GSH, SGOT, SGPT, SOD, CAT, GST, ALP, ALT	200 mg/kg	Singh and Gupta (2011)
Tephrosia purpurea/aerial parts	Fabaceae	TAA	AST, GSH, ALT, ALP, TB, GGT	500 mg/kg	Khatri et al. (2009)
Thymus linearis/leaves	Lamiaceae	Paracetamol	SGOT, SGPT, ALT, TB, ALP, AST	500 mg/kg	Nawaz et al. (2014)
Trigonella foenum leaves	Fabaceae	CCl_4	ALT, AST, ALP, GGT	100 mg/kg	Meera et al. (2009)
Vitis venifera/leaves	Vitaceae	CCl_4	AST, ALT	125 mg/kg	Orhan et al. (2007)
Vitis venifera/roots	Vitaceae	CCl_4	SGOT, SGPT, ALP, TB	200 mg/kg	Sharma and Vasudeva (2012)
Ziziphus mucronata leaves	Rhamnaceae	Dimethoate	SGPT, SGOT, TBARS, GSH, SOD, CHL, TGA	200 mg/kg	Kwape et al. (2013)
Ziziphus oenoplia/roots	Rhamnaceae	INH and RIF	SGOT, SGPT, ALP, SB, CAT, GST	300 mg/kg	Rao et al. (2012)

8.7 Conclusion

Hepatotoxicity from a range of drugs is a common drawback of many synthetic drugs. Many antitubercular and anticancer drugs have been attributed to drug-induced hepatotoxicity. Apart from synthetic drugs, many agents such as alcohol consumption also play a significant role in liver damage. Although many of the synthetic drugs are available to treat hepatotoxicity, natural product-based drugs such as silymarin are among the favorable choices for hepatotoxicity. Many medicinal plants have been evaluated for their potential effect against hepatotoxicity induced by many of synthetic drugs such as acetaminophen, rifampicin, and others. Still, there is a substantial need to evaluate some of the prominent plants clinically as well.

References

Ahmad, M., Bhatti, A.S.A., Maryam, S., Afzal, S., Ahmad, M., Gillani, A.N., 2010. Hepatoprotective evaluation of *Butea monosperma* against liver damage by paracetamol in rabbits. Ann. King Edward Med. Univ. 16.

Ahmed, B., Alam, T., Varshney, M., Khan, S.A., 2002. Hepatoprotective activity of two plants belonging to the Apiaceae and the Euphorbiaceae family. J. Ethnopharmacol. 79, 313–316.

Ajay, K.G., Neelam, M., 2006. Hepatoprotective activity of aqueous and ethanolic extract of *Boerhaavia erecta.* in carbontetrachloride intoxicated albino rats. Am. J. Pharmacol. Toxicol. 1, 17–20.

Ajiboye, T.O., Ahmad, F.M., Daisi, A.O., Yahaya, A.A., Ibitoye, O.B., Muritala, H.F., Sunmonu, T.O., 2017. Hepatoprotective potential of *Phyllanthus muellarianus* leaf extract: studies on hepatic, oxidative stress and inflammatory biomarkers. Pharm. Biol. 55, 1662–1670.

Ali, M., Qadir, M.I., Saleem, M., Janbaz, K.H., Gul, H., Hussain, L., Ahmad, B., 2013. Hepatoprotective potential of *Convolvulus arvensis* against paracetamol-induced hepatotoxicity. Bangladesh J. Pharmacol. 8, 300–304.

Al-Razzuqi, R., Al-Jawad, F.H., Al-Hussaini, J.A., Al-Jeboori, A., 2012. Hepatoprotective effect of *Glycyrrhiza glabra* in carbon tetrachloride-induced model of acute liver injury. J. Phys. Pharm. Adv. 2, 259–263.

Antoine, D.J., Williams, D.P., Park, B.K., 2008. Understanding the role of reactive metabolites in drug-induced hepatotoxicity: state of the science. Expert Opin. Drug Metab. Toxicol. 4, 1415–1427.

Arsul, V.A., Wagh, S.R., Mayee, R.V., 2011. Hepatoprotective activity of livergen, a polyherbal formulation against carbon tetrachloride induced hepatotoxicity in rats. Int. J. Pharm. Pharm. Sci. 3, 228–231.

Bachmann, G., Bakris, G.L., Barone, J.A., Baumann, S., Becher, T., Behnes, M., Birati, E.Y., Boutari, C., Cao, H., Dimitriadis, K., 2018. Iatrogenicity: Causes and Consequences of Iatrogenesis in Cardiovascular Medicine. Rutgers University Press.

Bag, A.K., Mumtaz, S.M.F., 2013. Hepatoprotective and nephroprotective activity of hydroalcoholic extract of *Ipomoea staphylina* leaves. Bangladesh J. Pharmacol. 8, 263–268.

Bhaargavi, V., Jyotsna, G.S.L., Tripurana, R., 2014. A review on hepatoprotective activity. Int. J. Pharm. Sci. Res. 5, 690.

Bhakta, T., Banerjee, S., Mandal, S.C., Maity, T.K., Saha, B.P., Pal, M., 2001. Hepatoprotective activity of *Cassia fistula* leaf extract. Phytomedicine 8, 220–224.

Bhakta, T., Mukherjee, P.K., Mukherjee, K., Banerjee, S., Mandal, S.C., Maity, T.K., Pal, M., Saha, B.P., 1999. Evaluation of hepatoprotective activity of *Cassia fistula* leaf extract. J. Ethnopharmacol. 66, 277–282.

Bhattacharyya, D., Pandit, S., Jana, U., Sen, S., Sur, T.K., 2005. Hepatoprotective activity of *Adhatoda vasica* aqueous leaf extract on D-galactosamine-induced liver damage in rats. Fitoterapia 76, 223–225.

Biswas, A., D'Souza, U.J., Bhat, S., Damodar, D., 2014. The hepatoprotective effect of *Hibiscus rosa sinensis* flower extract on diet-induced hypercholesterolemia in male albino wister rats. Int. J. Med. Pharm. Sci. 4, 1–10.

Björnsson, E., 2016. Hepatotoxicity by drugs: the most common implicated agents. Int. J. Mol. Sci. 17, 224.

Blomme, E.A.G., Yang, Y., Waring, J.F., 2009. Use of toxicogenomics to understand mechanisms of drug-induced hepatotoxicity during drug discovery and development. Toxicol. Lett. 186, 22–31.

Chaudhari, N.B., Chittam, K.P., Patil, V.R., 2009. Hepatoprotective activity of *Cassia fistula* seeds against paracetamol-induced hepatic injury in rats. Arch. Pharm. Sci. Res. 1 (2), 218–221.

Deori, C., Das, S., Bordoloi, S.K., 2017. Study of hepatoprotective activity of *Emblica officinalis* (AMLA) in albino rats. J. Evid. Based Med. Heal. 4, 3298–3301.

Dey, P., Saha, M.R., Sen, A., 2013. An overview on drug-induced hepatotoxicity. Asian J. Pharm. Clin. Res. 6, 1–4.

Djerrou, Z., Maameri, Z., Halmi, S., Djaalab, H., Riachi, F., Benmaiza, L., Hamdipacha, Y., 2015. Hepatoprotective effect of *Opuntia ficus-indica* aqueous extract against carbon tetrachloride-induced toxicity in rats. Online J. Biol. Sci. 15, 36.

Donfack, H.J., Kengap, R.T., Ngameni, B., Chuisseu, P.D.D., Tchana, A.N., Buonocore, D., Ngadjui, B.T., Moundipa, P.F., Marzatico, F., 2011. *Ficus cordata* Thunb (Moraceae) is a potential source of some hepatoprotective and antioxidant compounds. Pharmacologia 2, 137–145.

Fallah Huseini, H., Zareei Mahmoudabady, A., Ziai, S.A., Mehrazma, M., Alavian, S.M., Mehdizadeh, M., Radjabian, T., 2011. The effects of *Cynara scolymus* L. leaf and *Cichorium intybus* L. root extracts on carbon tetrachloride induced liver toxicity in rats. J. Med. Plants 1, 33–40.

Gani, M.S., John, S.A., 2013. Evaluation of hepatoprotective effect of *Nigella sativa* L. Int. J. Pharm. Pharm. Sci. 5, 428–430.

Godoy, P., Hewitt, N.J., Albrecht, U., Andersen, M.E., Ansari, N., Bhattacharya, S., Bode, J.G., Bolleyn, J., Borner, C., Boettger, J., 2013. Recent advances in 2D and 3D in vitro systems using primary hepatocytes, alternative hepatocyte sources and non-parenchymal liver cells and their use in investigating mechanisms of hepatotoxicity, cell signaling and ADME. Arch. Toxicol. 87, 1315–1530.

Gulati, R.K., Agarwal, S., Agrawal, S.S., 1995. Hepatoprotective studies on *Phyllanthus emblica* Linn. and quercetin. Indian J. Exp. Biol. 33, 261–268.

Gulati, K., Reshi, M.R., Rai, N., Ray, A., 2018. Hepatotoxicity: its mechanisms, experimental evaluation and protective strategies. Am. J. Pharmacol. 1, 1004.

Gupta, M., Mazumder, U.K., Kumar, T.S., Gomathi, P., Kumar, R.S., 2004. Antioxidant and hepatoprotective effects of *Bauhinia racemosa* against paracetamol and carbon tetrachloride induced liver damage in rats. Iran. J. Pharmacol. Ther. 3, 10–12.

Gutiérrez, R.M.P., Mitchell, S., Solis, R.V., 2008. *Psidium guajava*: a review of its traditional uses, phytochemistry and pharmacology. J. Ethnopharmacol. 117.

Handa, S.S., 1986. Natural products and plants as liver protecting drugs. Fitoterapia 57, 307–351.

Haque, R., Bin-Hafeez, B., Ahmad, I., Parvez, S., Pandey, S., Raisuddin, S., 2001. Protective effects of *Emblica officinalis* Gaertn. in cyclophosphamide-treated mice. Hum. Exp. Toxicol. 20, 643–650.

Hau, D.K.P., Gambari, R., Wong, R.S.M., Yuen, M.C.W., Cheng, G.Y.M., Tong, C.S.W., Zhu, G.Y., Leung, A.K.M., San Lai, P.B., Lau, F.Y., 2009. *Phyllanthus urinaria* extract attenuates acetaminophen induced hepatotoxicity: involvement of cytochrome P450 CYP2E1. Phytomedicine 16, 751–760.

Hsieh, C.-C., Fang, H.-L., Lina, W.-C., 2008. Inhibitory effect of *Solanum nigrum* on thioacetamide-induced liver fibrosis in mice. J. Ethnopharmacol. 119, 117–121.

Jamshidzadeh, A., Khoshnood, M.J., Dehghani, Z., Niknahad, H., 2010. Hepatoprotective activity of *Cichorium intybus* L. leaves extract against carbon tetrachloride induced toxicity. Iran. J. Pharm. Res., 41–46.

Jehangir, A., Nagi, A.H., Shahzad, M., Zia, A., 2010. The hepatoprotective effect of *Cassia fistula* (amaltas) leaves in isoniazid and rifampicin induced hepatotoxicity in rodents. Biomedica 26, 25–29.

Kannan, N., Sakthivel, K.M., Guruvayoorappan, C., 2013. Protective effect of *Acacia nilotica* (L.) against acetaminophen-induced hepatocellular damage in wistar rats. Adv. Pharmacol. Sci. 2013.

Kasture, V.S., Kasture, S.B., Chopde, C.T., 2002. Anticonvulsive activity of *Butea monosperma* flowers in laboratory animals. Pharmacol. Biochem. Behav. 72, 965–972.

Khan, T.H., Sultana, S., 2009. Antioxidant and hepatoprotective potential of *Aegle marmelos* Correa. against CCl_4-induced oxidative stress and early tumor events. J. Enzyme Inhib. Med. Chem. 24, 320–327.

Khan, M.U., Rohilla, A., Bhatt, D., Afrin, S., Rohilla, S., Ansari, S.H., 2011. Diverse belongings of *Calendula officinalis*: an overview. Int. J. Pharm. Sci. Drug Res. 3, 173–177.

Khatri, A., Garg, A., Agrawal, S.S., 2009. Evaluation of hepatoprotective activity of aerial parts of *Tephrosia purpurea* L. and stem bark of *Tecomella undulata*. J. Ethnopharmacol. 122, 1–5.

Krishnan, N.R., Kasthuri, A.S., 2005. Iatrogenic disorders. Med. J. Armed Forces India 61, 2.

Kumar, K.E., Harsha, K.N., Sudheer, V., 2013. In vitro antioxidant activity and in vivo hepatoprotective activity of aqueous extract of *Allium cepa* bulb in ethanol induced liver damage in Wistar rats. Food Sci. Human Wellness 2, 132–138.

Kviecinski, M.R., Felipe, K.B., Gomes Correia, J.F., Ferreira, E.A., Rossi, M.H., de Moura Gatti, F., Filho, D.W., Curi Pedrosa, R., 2011. Brazilian *Bidens pilosa* Linné yields fraction containing quercetin-derived flavonoid with free radical scavenger activity and hepatoprotective effects. Libyan J. Med. 6, 5651.

Kwape, T.E., Chaturvedi, P., Kamau, J.M., George, S., 2013. Hepato-protective potential of methanol extract of leaf of *Ziziphus mucronata* (ZMLM) against dimethoate toxicity: biochemical and histological approach. Ghana Med. J. 47, 112–120.

Lim, C.-S., Kim, E.-Y., Lee, H.-S., Soh, Y., Sohn, Y., Kim, S.Y., Sohn, N.-W., Jung, H.-S., Kim, Y.-B., 2010. Protective effects of *Cinnamomum cassia* Blume in the fibrogenesis of activated HSC-T6 cells and dimethylnitrosamine-induced acute liver injury in SD rats. Biosci. Biotechnol. Biochem. https://doi.org/10.1271/bbb.90435.

Meera, R., Devi, P., Kameswari, B., Madhumitha, B., Merlin, N.J., 2009. Antioxidant and hepatoprotective activities of *Ocimum basilicum* Linn. and *Trigonella foenum-graecum* Linn. against H_2O_2 and CCl_4 induced hepatotoxicity in goat liver. Indian J. Exp. Biol. 47 (7), 584–590.

Mishra, G., Khosa, R.L., Singh, P., Jha, K.K., 2014. Hepatoprotective potential of ethanolic extract of *Caesalpenia crista* leaves against paracetamol induced hepatotoxicity in rats. J. Coast Life Med. 2, 575–579.

Mishra, G., Khosa, R.L., Singh, P., Jha, K.K., 2015. Hepatoprotective potential of ethanolic extract of *Pandanus odoratissimus* root against paracetamol-induced hepatotoxicity in rats. J. Pharm. Bioallied Sci. 7, 45.

Nawaz, M., Ahmad, T., Mushtaq, M.N., Batool, A., 2014. Hepatoprotective activity of *Thymus linearis* against paracetamol and carbon tetrachloride-induced hepatotoxicity in albino mice. Bangladesh J. Pharmacol. 9, 230–234.

Njoku, D., 2014. Drug-induced hepatotoxicity: metabolic, genetic and immunological basis. Int. J. Mol. Sci. 15, 6990–7003.

Orhan, D.D., Orhan, N., Ergun, E., Ergun, F., 2007. Hepatoprotective effect of *Vitis vinifera* L. leaves on carbon tetrachloride-induced acute liver damage in rats. J. Ethnopharmacol. 112, 145–151.

Palanisamy, N., Manian, S., 2012. Protective effects of *Asparagus racemosus* on oxidative damage in isoniazid-induced hepatotoxic rats: an in vivo study. Toxicol. Ind. Health 28, 238–244.

Pandit, A., Sachdeva, T., Bafna, P., 2012. Drug-induced hepatotoxicity: a review. J. Appl. Pharm. Sci. 2, 233–243.

Polson, J.E., 2007. Hepatotoxicity due to antibiotics. Clin. Liver Dis. 11, 549–561.

Porchezhian, E., Ansari, S.H., 2005. Hepatoprotective activity of *Abutilon indicum* on experimental liver damage in rats. Phytomedicine 12, 62–64.

Pradeep, K., Mohan, C.V.R., Gobianand, K., Karthikeyan, S., 2007. Effect of *Cassia fistula* Linn. leaf extract on diethylnitrosamine induced hepatic injury in rats. Chem. Biol. Interact. 167, 12–18.

Pramyothin, P., Samosorn, P., Poungshompoo, S., Chaichantipyuth, C., 2006. The protective effects of *Phyllanthus emblica* Linn. extract on ethanol induced rat hepatic injury. J. Ethnopharmacol. 107, 361–364.

Pugh, A.J., Barve, A.J., Falkner, K., Patel, M., McClain, C.J., 2009. Drug-induced hepatotoxicity or drug-induced liver injury. Clin. Liver Dis. 13, 277–294.

Rahmani, A.H., 2015. *Cassia fistula* Linn: potential candidate in the health management. Pharmacogn. Res. 7, 217.

Rao, C.V., Rawat, A.K.S., Singh, A.P., Singh, A., Verma, N., 2012. Hepatoprotective potential of ethanolic extract of *Ziziphus oenoplia* (L.) Mill roots against antitubercular drugs induced hepatotoxicity in experimental models. Asian Pac. J. Trop. Med. 5, 283–288.

Rusu, M.A., Bucur, N., Puică, C., Tămaş, M., 1999. Effects of *Corylus avellana* in acetaminophen and CCl_4 induced toxicosis. Phyther. Res. 13, 120–123.

Saha, P., Mazumder, U.K., Haldar, P.K., Bala, A., Kar, B., Naskar, S., 2011. Evaluation of hepatoprotective activity of *Cucurbita maxima* aerial parts. J. Herb. Med. Toxicol. 5, 17–22.

Shah, K.G., Baxi, A.J., 1990. Phytochemical studies and antioestrogenic activity of butea frondosa flowers. Indian J. Pharm. Sci. 52, 272.

Sharma, N., Shukla, S., 2011. Hepatoprotective potential of aqueous extract of *Butea monosperma* against CCl$_4$ induced damage in rats. Exp. Toxicol. Pathol. 63, 671–676.

Sharma, S.K., Vasudeva, N., 2012. Hepatoprotective activity of *Vitis vinifera* root extract against carbon tetrachloride-induced liver damage in rats. Acta Pol. Pharm. 69, 933–937.

Sharma, A., Sharma, M.K., Kumar, M., 2009. Modulatory role of *Emblica officinalis* fruit extract against arsenic induced oxidative stress in Swiss albino mice. Chem. Biol. Interact. 180, 20–30.

Sharma, M., Shakya, A., Sharma, N., Shrivastava, S., Shukla, S., 2012. Therapeutic efficacy of *Rosa damascena* Mill. on acetaminophen-induced oxidative stress in albino rats. J. Environ. Pathol. Toxicol. Oncol. 31.

Shehu, A.I., Ma, X., Venkataramanan, R., 2017. Mechanisms of drug-induced hepatotoxicity. Clin. Liver Dis. 21, 35–54. https://doi.org/10.1016/j.cld.2016.08.002.

Shuhendler, A.J., Pu, K., Cui, L., Uetrecht, J.P., Rao, J., 2014. Real-time imaging of oxidative and nitrosative stress in the liver of live animals for drug-toxicity testing. Nat. Biotechnol. 32, 373–380. https://doi.org/10.1038/nbt.2838.

Singh, D., Gupta, R.S., 2011. Hepatoprotective activity of methanol extract of *Tecomella undulata* against alcohol and paracetamol induced hepatotoxicity in rats. Life Sci. Med. Res. 26, 1–8.

Singh, M.K., Sahu, P., Nagori, K., Dewangan, D., Kumar, T., Alexander, A., Badwaik, H., Tripathi, D.K., 2011. Organoleptic properties in-vitro and in-vivo pharmacological activities of *Calendula officinalis* Linn: an over review. J. Chem. Pharm. Res. 3, 655–663.

Sohil, V., Sundaram, R.M., 2009. Hepatoprotective activity of *Mimosa pudica* leaves against carbontetrachloride induced toxicity. J. Nat. Prod. 2.

Soldatow, V.Y., LeCluyse, E.L., Griffith, L.G., Rusyn, I., 2013. In vitro models for liver toxicity testing. Toxicol. Res. (Camb.) 2, 23–39.

Suter, L., Babiss, L.E., Wheeldon, E.B., 2004. Toxicogenomics in predictive toxicology in drug development. Chem. Biol. 11, 161–171.

Tasduq, S.A., Kaisar, P., Gupta, D.K., Kapahi, B.K., Jyotsna, S., Maheshwari, H.S., Johri, R.K., 2005. Protective effect of a 50% hydroalcoholic fruit extract of *Emblica officinalis* against anti-tuberculosis drugs induced liver toxicity. Phyther. Res. 19, 193–197.

Thompson, M., Jaiswal, Y., Wang, I., Williams, L., 2017. Hepatotoxicity: treatment, causes and applications of medicinal plants as therapeutic agents. J. Phytopharm. 6, 186–193.

Wagner, H., Geyer, B., Fiebig, M., Kiso, Y., Hikino, H., 1986. Isoputrin and butrin, the antihepatotoxic principles of *Butea monosperma* flowers. Planta Med. 52, 77–79.

Wang, J., Zhao, H., Zhao, Y., Jin, C., Liu, D., Kong, W., Fang, F., Zhang, L., Wang, H., Xiao, X., 2011. Hepatotoxicity or hepatoprotection? Pattern recognition for the paradoxical effect of the Chinese herb *Rheum palmatum* L. in treating rat liver injury. PLoS One 6, e24498.

Yogeeta, S., Ragavender, H.R.B., Devaki, T., 2007. Antihepatotoxic effect of *Punica granatum* acetone extract against isoniazid-and rifampicin-induced hepatotoxicity. Pharm. Biol. 45, 631–637.

Influence of nutrients, plant extracts and natural compounds in liver diseases

CHAPTER 9

Influence of omega-3 fatty acids and monounsaturated fats in liver diseases

Abdullah[a], Maqsood Ur Rehman[a], Fazlullah Khan[b], and Kamal Niaz[c]

[a]Department of Pharmacy, University of Malakand, Chakdara, Pakistan [b]Department of Allied Health Sciences, Bashir Institute of Health Sciences, Bhara Kahu, Islamabad, Pakistan [c]Department of Pharmacology and Toxicology, Faculty of Bio-Sciences, Cholistan University of Veterinary and Animal Sciences (CUVAS), Bahawalpur, Pakistan

9.1 Introduction

Fatty acids are composed of carboxylic acid with a long aliphatic chain that may be saturated or unsaturated (Moss et al., 1995). Chemically, fatty acids are composed of carbon atoms in the form of chains with hydrogen atoms attached to the carbon atoms. Naturally occurring fatty acids may contain 4–28 carbons. Fatty acids may be saturated, monounsaturated, or polyunsaturated (Lands et al., 1990). A fatty acid is considered saturated when it has a maximum number of H-atoms attached to almost all carbon atoms. A fatty acid with a couple of H-atoms absent in the middle of a chain that leaves two carbon atoms with a double bond (=) is a monounsaturated fatty acid. A fatty acid with two or more double bonds is called polyunsaturated (Johnson and Shoolery, 1962).

Omega-3 fatty acids, also known as n-3 fatty acids, are polyunsaturated fatty acids that are categorized by the first double bond at the third position considered from the methyl group. The description of a polyunsaturated fatty acid as an Ω-3 fatty acid, for example, defines the position of the first location of unsaturation relative to the Ω end of that fatty acid (Bourre, 2004). Thus, a Ω-3 fatty acid such as α-linolenic acid (ALA), which has three double bonds, has a location of unsaturation between the third and fourth carbons from the Ω end. Furthermore, to the position of the first spot of unsaturation relative to the Ω end of an unsaturated fatty acid, the correct use of the Ω nomenclature can only be pragmatic to unsaturated fatty acids whose double bonds among the carbon atoms are all in the *cis*-orientation (Roach et al., 2004).

Omega-3 fatty acids cannot be synthesized within the human body; therefore, they are called essential fatty acids. Thus, it is essential for humans to have sufficient intake from food or other sources (Simopoulos, 2002). The omega-3 (Ω-3) fatty acids are generally divided into

Influence of Nutrients, Bioactive Compounds, and Plant Extracts in Liver Diseases. https://doi.org/10.1016/B978-0-12-816488-4.00013-9

short chain omega-3 fatty acids, that is, alpha-linolenic acid (ALA), and very long chain omega-3 fatty acids, that is, eicosapentaenoic acid (EPA). ALA has 18 carbon molecules and three double bonds, and is denoted as (C18:3 n-3). ALA is chiefly present in vegetable oils and nuts, among others. The omega-3 fatty acids of a very long chain are largely found in fish and other sea products. A long chain Ω-3 fatty acid has at least 20 carbons with five or more than five unsaturated carbon double bonds. The two important long chain omega-3 fatty acids are eicosapentaenoic acid, (EPA) denoted as C20:5 n-3, and docosahexaenoic acid (DHA), denoted as C22:6 n-3.

Monounsaturated fatty acids (MUFA) are the unsaturated fatty acids with only one double bond between the carbon atoms in the fatty acid chain with the rest of the carbon atoms being saturated or bonded with a single bond. MUFA-containing oils are naturally in a liquid form at room temperature, but at a low temperature, they are converted into a solid (Gillingham et al., 2011; Chatgilialoglu et al., 2002). The typical example of oil that contains monounsaturated fatty acid is olive oil (Schwingshackl and Hoffmann, 2014). MUFA has been found effective in decreasing the risk of cardiovascular diseases and stroke by reducing the level of bad cholesterol in the bloodstream (Kris-Etherton, 1999). MUFA also provides nutrients to maintain and form body cells (Siriwardhana et al., 2013). Oils rich with MUFA also provide vitamin E, an important antioxidant of the body. In this chapter, we aim to discuss the influence of omega-3 fatty acids and monounsaturated fats in liver diseases.

9.2 Chemistry and classification of omega fatty acids

Omega fatty acids are polyunsaturated fatty acids. If the first double bond is located at position 3 while counting from the omega carbon, they are known as omega-3 (or ω-3) fatty acids. The chemical structures of fatty acids such as saturated, monounsaturated, and polyunsaturated are shown in Fig. 9.1.

Although there are many omega-3 fatty acids, the most important Ω-3 fatty acids synthesized from the precursor, consumed as part of the diet, and then utilized by the body are eicosapentaenoic acid (EPA), alpha-linolenic acid (ALA), docosahexaenoic (DHA), and docosapentaenoic acid (DPA). Inside the body through an enzymatic process, ALA changes to EPA, EPA changes to DPA, and lastly to DHA (Fig. 9.2). The basic unit of a fatty acid is a shorter chain omega-3 fatty acid, ALA. It is found in several plants such as canola oil, walnuts, flaxseed, and soybeans (Doughman et al., 2007). ALA may give protection against cardiovascular diseases by inhibiting the formation of proinflammatory eicosanoids (McCowen et al., 2004; De Lorgeril et al., 2002). Substituting the double bond of ALA at the third carbon will produce omega-3 fatty acid or at the sixth carbon will produce omega-6 fatty acid. The conversion of ALA to EPA (omega-3 fatty acid) occurs in a very small quantity, that is, 2%–5%, while its conversion to DHA (an omega-6 fatty acid) is less than 1% in the human body (Van Horn et al., 2008). ALA (an essential fatty acid) cannot be synthesized by the

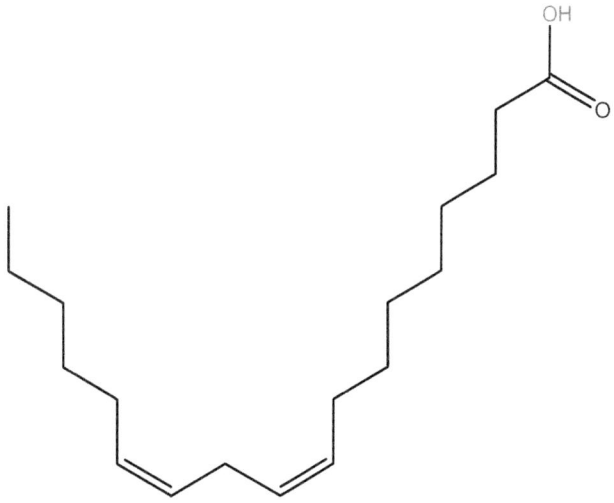

(A)   Saturated fatty acid (Behenic acid)

(B)   b.   Saturated fatty acid (Caprylic acid)

(C)   Monounsaturated fatty acid (Oleic acid)

(D)   Polyunsaturated fatty acid (Linoleic acid)

Fig. 9.1
Chemical structures of (A) and (B) saturated fatty acid (behenic acid and caprylic acid),
(C) monounsaturated fatty (oleic acid), and (D) polyunsaturated fatty acid (linoleic acid).

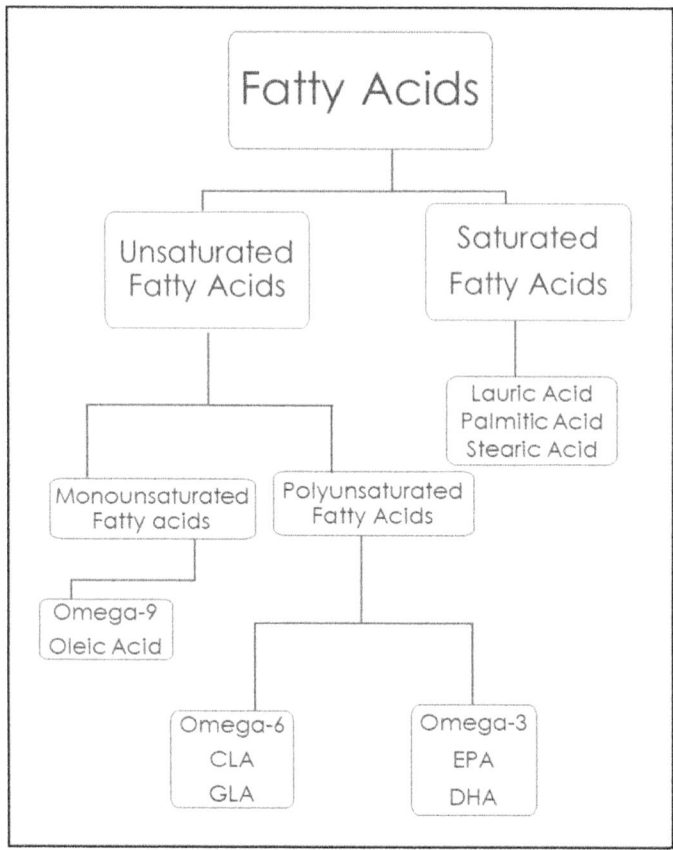

Fig. 9.2
Classification of fatty acids.

human body due to the absence of the enzymes needed to act on double bonds at the omega-3 or 6 positions (Simopoulos, 2002; Wallis et al., 2002).

a. **Alpha-linolenic acid (ALA):** The word "lino" is a derivative of the Greek word that means "linon" (flax) while the word oleic means "of or relating to oleic acid" because saturating linoleic acid's omega-6 double bond produces oleic acid. ALA is an essential omega-3 fatty acid that must be taken through food. The main dietary sources of ALA are seeds (flaxseed, chia, hemp), nuts (walnuts), and some common vegetable oils. ALA undergoes rancidity more rapidly than other types of oils. This is one of the reasons that producers choose to partly hydrogenate oils with ALA, for example, soybean oil, the prime source of edible oils (Balestrasse et al., 2010).

b. **Eicosapentaenoic acid (EPA):** EPA is another example of omega-3 fatty acid. EPA is a precursor for prostaglandin-III, thromboxane-III, and leukotriene-V eicosanoids (Keten, 2019). EPA is obtained from oily fish or fish oil, for example salmon, cod liver, menhaden, herring, mackerel, sardine, and several edible algae. Mother's breast milk also has some quantity of EPA (Helland et al., 1998).

c.   **Docosahexaenoic acid (DHA)**: This is a type of omega-3 fatty acid that is a key structural constituent of the brain, cerebral cortex, retina, and skin of the human body (Connor and Neuringer, 1988). DHA can be synthesized from ALA or may be gained from mother's milk, edible algae oil, or fish oil (Duragkar, 2014). The DHA in mother's milk is essential for the developing toddler (Jørgensen et al., 2001). Generally, DHA is obtained from the diet directly, but some DHA may be obtained through enzymatic conversion of EPA. But the rate of this conversion is 15% less in men in comparison with women (Kitson et al., 2010). The human brain contains 40% of the total DHA while the retina has 60% of the DHA (Singh, 2005). The plasma membrane of the neuron is composed of almost 50% of DHA. Cognitive decline, depression in some patients, and even Alzheimer's disease are related to DHA (Yurko-Mauro et al., 2010).

9.3 Conversion of ALA to EPA and DHA

Alpha-linolenic acid (ALA) is transformed to the Ω-3 polyunsaturated fatty acids (PUFA), that is, EPA, DPA, and DHA, through several microsomal enzymatic actions in the endoplasmic reticulum, as shown in Fig. 9.3 (Brenna et al., 2009). This conversion involves D5D and D6D, the desaturases encoded by the FAD-S1 and FAD-S2 genes, respectively. All steps of microsomal elongation are performed by four important enzymes.

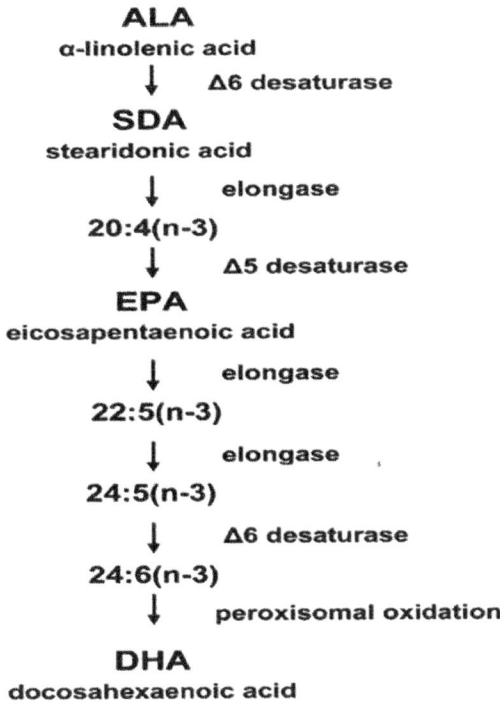

Fig. 9.3
Synthesis of omega-3 fatty acids.

9.4 Chemistry and classification of MUFA

As stated earlier, MUFA has only one double bond, which can be present in diverse positions. The majority of MUFAs have a chain length of 16–22 (carbons) and one *cis*-configurated double bond (Rustan and Drevon, 2001). However, the *trans*-isomers can be manufactured through an industrial hydrogenation process (Hauff and Vetter, 2009). This double bond restricts the movement of the whole molecule (acyl chain) (Maccarone et al., 2014). The *cis*-configuration gives a twist to the chain. The *trans*-molecule is thermodynamically more stable than the *cis* form of MUFA. Similarly, *trans* MUFAs have a higher melting point than *cis* MUFA (Lewis et al., 1988).

9.5 Sources of omega-3 fatty acids and MUFAs

The main sources of Ω-3 fatty acids are fish and other seafood (e.g., salmon, cold-water fatty fish, herring, mackerel, cod liver, tuna, and sardines), nuts and seeds (chia seeds, walnuts, and flaxseeds), vegetable oils (canola, flaxseed, and soybean oils), and fortified foods (soy beverages, eggs, milk, yogurt, juices, and infant formulas) (Tur et al., 2012).

Some foods contain higher amounts of healthy fats than others, but most of them contain a combination of all types of fats. Foods and oils containing higher quantities of monounsaturated fats include nuts and seeds (peanuts, almonds, sesame seeds, and cashews), avocados (both avocados and their oil), canola oil, sunflower oil, sesame oil, peanut oil, olive oil, safflower oil, fatty fish, such as salmon and mackerel, and butter (Latreille et al., 2012).

9.6 Metabolism of omega-3 fatty acids and monounsaturated fats

When taken up by cells, fatty acids may perform three important roles. The first is as precursors to synthesize other essential compounds. The second is to provide fuels to produce energy, and the third is to act as substrates for ketone body synthesis (McGarry and Foster, 1980). The ketone bodies may then be distributed to other body tissues where more ATPs are produced as a source of energy. Regarding the metabolism, free fatty acids (FFA) get into cells mostly by protein carriers located in the plasma membrane and then are intracellularly transported through fatty acid binding proteins (FABP). First, the FFA is activated in the form of acyl-CoA. The acyl-CoA travels to the mitochondria or peroxisomes through the acyl-CoA binding protein (ACBP) for beta-oxidation, resulting in the production of energy as ATPs and heat. Some of the activated FFA (acyl-CoA) move to the endoplasmic reticulum, which results in the esterification of diverse lipid types.

The acyl-CoA or some FFAs may bind with transcription factors, which further controls gene expression. Some acyl-CoA when attached to the transcription factor may be converted to eicosanoids (signaling molecules) (Fig. 9.4). This is also important as spare glucose in the cells that may also be converted into fatty acids may be similarly metabolized (Ballard et al., 1960).

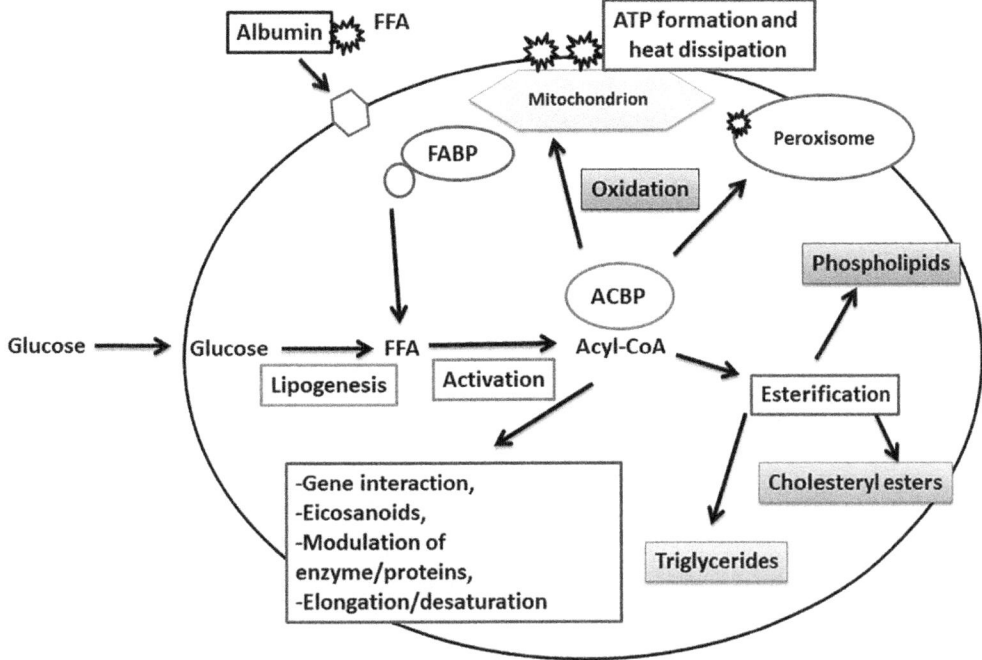

Fig. 9.4

Metabolism of fatty acids (Rustan and Drevon, 2001).*From Rustan, A.C., Drevon, C.A., 2005. Fatty Acids: Structures and Properties. https://doi.org/10.1038/npg.els.0003894.*

9.7 Role of omega-3 fatty acids and monounsaturated fats in various liver diseases

9.7.1 Nonalcoholic fatty liver disease (NAFLD)

The term NAFLD is used for chronic hepatic diseases that include benign hepatosteatosis, nonalcoholic steatohepatitis (NASH), primary hepatocellular cancer, and cirrhosis (Lauby-Secretan et al., 2016). NAFLD is the most prevalent fatty liver disease in developing countries (Bellentani et al., 2010). According to an estimate, the number of obese (BMI ≥ 30) adults in the United States is 80 million with 13 million of them children; all are at high risk of developing NAFLD. There is a strong correlation between NAFLD and obesity, which is why NAFLD is going to become a major public health problem across the globe (Chalasani et al., 2012; Loomba and Sanyal, 2013). A diet that is deficient in omega-3 polyunsaturated fatty acids (PUFAs) and has an excess of omega-6 fatty acids is believed to be associated with NAFLD (Promrat et al., 2010). Currently, there is no drug treatment for NAFLD. Omega-3 fatty acids are useful to reduce hypertriglyceridemia and inflammation while enhancing insulin sensitivity (Alwayn et al., 2005).

ALA, DHA, and EPA affect the transcription of the peroxisome proliferator-activated receptor, the carbohydrate regulatory element gene, and the sterol regulatory element binding protein-1. These transcription factors are the key determinants of the carbohydrates and lipid metabolism, which causes the alteration of lipid storage (Jump, 2008). PUFA decreases the plasma lipid levels, increasing lipoprotein breakdown. It reduces the uptake of lipids by hepatocytes. PUFA has been found to protect the liver from fatty degeneration in animals (Table 9.1) (Le Yu and Wang, 2017). Studies have shown different effects on the role of monounsaturated fatty acids (MUFA) in NAFLD due to different methodologies and different sources of MUFA. Virgin olive oil-derived MUFA has been shown to improve NAFLD. A

Table 9.1: Sources and roles of PUFA and MUFA in liver diseases.

	Examples	Sources	Role in liver disease	References
Omega-3 fatty acid metabolite	EPA (eicosapentaenoic acid)	Oily fish, fish oil, certain seaweeds, human breast milk	High dietary intake of EPA blocks the metabolites of AA and prevents inflammation, antiangiogenic.	Della Pepa et al. (2017), Figueras et al. (2011), Kohashi, (2014), and Iketani et al. (2013)
	DHA (docosahexaenoic acid)	Cold-water fish, metabolic synthesis from EPA	High dietary intake of DHA blocks the metabolites of AA and prevents inflammation, reduces NASH, antifibrotic.	Lytle et al. (2017), Della Pepa et al. (2017), Ryan et al. (2009), and Bazan et al. (2011)
	ALA (α-linoleic acid)	Plant oils, linseed oil, kiwifruit oil, chia seed oil, flaxseed oil, canola (rapeseed) oil, soybean, purslane, walnuts	Antioxidant, antiinflammatory, hypolipidemic, prevents steatohepatitis.	Rodriguez-Leyva et al. (2010), Jang et al. (2014), and Jeyapal et al. (2018)
Omega-6 fatty acid metabolite	AA (arachidonic acid)	Meat, eggs, dairy products	AA metabolites (PG2, TX2 and LT4) are prothrombotic and proinflammatory, causing high production of IL-1, IL-6, NF-KB, and TNF resulting in inflammation and NASH.	Jeyapal et al. (2018), Chawengsub et al. (2009), and Frelinger et al. (2006)
	LA (linoleic acid)	Corn, peanut, soybean, cottonseed, other plant oils	Antiinflammatory and hypolipidimic, reduces NAFLD.	IBD in EPIC Study Investigators (2009), Dichtl et al. (2002), and Bjermo et al. (2012)
MUFA	Oleic acid	Canola, sunflower, olive, and nut oils	It activates peroxisome proliferator-activated receptor-alpha (PPAR-α) and PPAR and reduces liver fat content.	Varela et al. (2013), DeLany et al. (2000), and Ferramosca et al. (2008)

randomized control trial in patients with DM2 showed that an isocaloric diet enriched with MUFA significantly reduced NAFLD (Bozzetto et al., 2012).

9.7.2 Nonalcoholic steatohepatitis (NASH)

NASH is characterized by oxidative stress, hepatic inflammation, injury, and fibrosis. Patients suffering from NASH have a disturbed cholesterol metabolism and high blood lipid level (dyslipidemia) (Kerr and Davidson, 2012; Lonardo et al., 2016). It has been observed that about 10%–30% of patients suffering from benign steatosis progress to NASH while 20%–30% of patients suffering from NASH develop cirrhosis over a period of 10 years (Fig. 9.5); this is a risk factor for hepatocellular carcinoma (Heimbach, 2014; Cohen et al., 2011).

EPA and DHA (omega-3 fatty acids) inhibit inflammation via (1) competing with omega-6 fatty acids for the COX and LOX-mediated production of inflammatory eicosanoids, (2) forming antiinflammatory ω3-PUFA derived oxylipins such as maresins, protectins, and resolvins, and (3) forming ω3 eicosanoids generated by COX that weakly bind to eicosanoid receptors (Lytle et al., 2017; Calder, 2015).

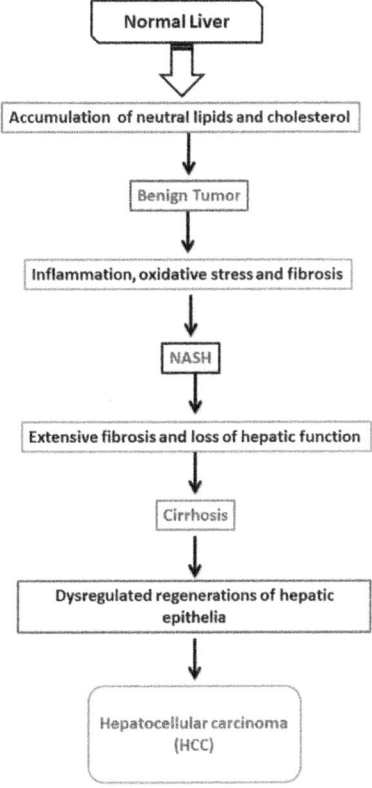

Fig. 9.5
Transition from a normal liver to HCC.

9.7.3 Fibrosis

Fibrosis induced by the Western diet is ameliorated by DHA by targeting the TGFβ-Smad3 pathway (Lytle et al., 2015). DHA suppresses the accumulation of phospho-smad3 in the hepatic nuclei, which is an important mediator of TGFβ induction of ECM production. DHA also ameliorates the expression of many transcripts related to fibrosis, including ECM remodeling, collagen subtypes, matrix metalloproteases (MMPs), tissue inhibitors of metalloproteases, and lysyl oxidases. Furthermore, DHA has multiple effects on signaling pathways that control fibrosis, inflammation, and the lipid metabolism. Similarly, C20–22 ω3 PUFA proved to be an efficacious and safe agent used in the treatment of severe hypertriglyceridemia (Barter and Ginsberg, 2008; Pratt et al., 2009).

9.7.4 Hepatocellular carcinoma (HCC)

NAFLD is one of the reasons for HCC (Sherman, 2014). When chronic liver damage progresses to cirrhosis, the risk of HCC is enhanced (Llovet et al., 2003). Several investigators have described the usefulness of omega-3 fatty acids to suppress HCC development in animals (Inoue-Yamauchi et al., 2018; Weylandt et al., 2011) and humans (Wen et al., 2016; Gao et al., 2015). The mechanism of the hepatoprotective effect exerted by DHA is the inhibition of metastasis and tumor growth. Moreover, the epoxy metabolites derived from EPA and DHA have shown antiangiogenic activity (Zhang et al., 2013, 2014).

9.8 Conclusion

Omega-3 fatty acids decrease the lipid content of the liver and alleviate inflammation and fibrosis. DHA (omega-3 fatty acid) attenuates the expression of proteins that promote fibrosis. In preclinical studies, DHA has inhibited TGFβ signaling in the liver, but this activity may be indirect and involve the control of other factors by DHA such as circulating cytokines that affect TGFβ signaling. Similarly, another omega-3 fatty acid (α-linolenic acid) decreases plasma and liver lipid levels and is used in the prevention of NASH. The protective activity of omega-3 PUFA has been mediated by the reduction of proinflammatory cytokines and hepatic oxidative stress. MUFA administration has also resulted in the reduction of hepatic steatosis and improved insulin sensitivity. The role of ω3 PUFA in the reduction of liver lipids and the attenuation of inflammation is well known, but its mechanism in fibrosis amelioration is not fully elucidated (Lytle et al., 2017; Calder, 2015). Therefore, future studies need to explore the in vivo mechanism for DHA suppression of TGFβ signaling and hepatic fibrosis.

Conflict of interest

The authors declare that no conflict of interest exists.

References

Alwayn, I.P., et al., 2005. Omega-3 fatty acids improve hepatic steatosis in a murine model: potential implications for the marginal steatotic liver donor. Transplantation 79 (5), 606–608.

Balestrasse, K.B., et al., 2010. The role of 5-aminolevulinic acid in the response to cold stress in soybean plants. Phytochemistry 71 (17–18), 2038–2045.

Ballard, F.B., et al., 1960. Myocardial metabolism of fatty acids. J. Clin. Invest. 39 (5), 717–723.

Barter, P., Ginsberg, H.N., 2008. Effectiveness of combined statin plus omega-3 fatty acid therapy for mixed dyslipidemia. Am. J. Cardiol. 102 (8), 1040–1045.

Bazan, N.G., Molina, M.F., Gordon, W.C., 2011. Docosahexaenoic acid signalolipidomics in nutrition: significance in aging, neuroinflammation, macular degeneration, Alzheimer's, and other neurodegenerative diseases. Annu. Rev. Nutr. 31, 321–351.

Bellentani, S., et al., 2010. Epidemiology of non-alcoholic fatty liver disease. Dig. Dis. 28 (1), 155–161.

Bjermo, H., et al., 2012. Effects of n-6 PUFAs compared with SFAs on liver fat, lipoproteins, and inflammation in abdominal obesity: a randomized controlled trial. Am. J. Clin. Nutr. 95 (5), 1003–1012.

Bourre, J., 2004. Roles of unsaturated fatty acids (especially omega-3 fatty acids) in the brain at various ages and during ageing. J. Nutr. 8, 163–174.

Bozzetto, L., et al., 2012. Liver fat is reduced by an isoenergetic MUFA diet in a controlled randomized study in type 2 diabetic patients. Diabetes Care 35 (7), 1429–1435.

Brenna, J.T., et al., 2009. α-Linolenic acid supplementation and conversion to n-3 long-chain polyunsaturated fatty acids in humans. Prostaglandins Leukot. Essent. Fatty Acids 80 (2–3), 85–91.

Calder, P.C., 2015. Marine omega-3 fatty acids and inflammatory processes: effects, mechanisms and clinical relevance. Biochim. Biophys. Acta 1851 (4), 469–484.

Chalasani, N., et al., 2012. The diagnosis and management of non-alcoholic fatty liver disease: practice guideline by the American Association for the Study of Liver Diseases, American College of Gastroenterology, and the American Gastroenterological Association. Hepatology 55 (6), 2005–2023.

Chatgilialoglu, C., Altieri, A., Fischer, H., 2002. The kinetics of thiyl radical-induced reactions of monounsaturated fatty acid esters. J. Am. Chem. Soc. 124 (43), 12816–12823.

Chawengsub, Y., Gauthier, K.M., Campbell, W.B., 2009. Role of arachidonic acid lipoxygenase metabolites in the regulation of vascular tone. Am. J. Physiol. Heart Circ. Physiol. 297 (2), H495–H507.

Cohen, J.C., Horton, J.D., Hobbs, H.H., 2011. Human fatty liver disease: old questions and new insights. Science 332 (6037), 1519–1523.

Connor, W.E., Neuringer, M., 1988. The effects of n-3 fatty acid deficiency and repletion upon the fatty acid composition and function of the brain and retina. Prog. Clin. Biol. Res. 282, 275–294.

De Lorgeril, M., et al., 2002. Mediterranean diet and the French paradox: two distinct biogeographic concepts for one consolidated scientific theory on the role of nutrition in coronary heart disease. Cardiovasc. Res. 54 (3), 503–515.

DeLany, J.P., et al., 2000. Differential oxidation of individual dietary fatty acids in humans. Am. J. Clin. Nutr. 72 (4), 905–911.

Della Pepa, G., et al., 2017. Isocaloric dietary changes and non-alcoholic fatty liver disease in high cardiometabolic risk individuals. Nutrients 9 (10), 1065.

Dichtl, W., et al., 2002. Linoleic acid-stimulated vascular adhesion molecule-1 expression in endothelial cells depends on nuclear factor-[kappa] B activation. Metab. Clin. Exp. 51 (3), 327–333.

Doughman, S.D., Krupanidhi, S., Sanjeevi, C.B., 2007. Omega-3 fatty acids for nutrition and medicine: considering microalgae oil as a vegetarian source of EPA and DHA. Curr. Diabetes Rev. 3 (3), 198–203.

Duragkar, N.J., 2014. Docosahexaenoic acid (DHA) as polyunsaturated free fatty acid in its directly compressible powder form and method of isolation thereof. Google Patents.

Ferramosca, A., Savy, V., Zara, V., 2008. Olive oil increases the hepatic triacylglycerol content in mice by a distinct influence on the synthesis and oxidation of fatty acids. Biosci. Biotechnol. Biochem. 72 (1), 62–69.

Figueras, M., et al., 2011. Effects of eicosapentaenoic acid (EPA) treatment on insulin sensitivity in an animal model of diabetes: improvement of the inflammatory status. Obesity 19 (2), 362–369.

Frelinger 3rd, A., Furman, M.I., Linden, M.D., Li, Y., Fox, M.L., Barnard, M.R., et al., 2006. Residual arachidonic acid-induced platelet activation via an adenosine diphosphate-dependent but cyclooxygenase-1-and cyclooxygenase-2-independent pathway: a 700-patient study of aspirin resistance. Circulation 113 (25), 2888–2896.

Gao, M., et al., 2015. Fish consumption and n-3 polyunsaturated fatty acids, and risk of hepatocellular carcinoma: systematic review and meta-analysis. Cancer Causes Control 26 (3), 367–376.

Gillingham, L.G., Harris-Janz, S., Jones, P.J., 2011. Dietary monounsaturated fatty acids are protective against metabolic syndrome and cardiovascular disease risk factors. Lipids 46 (3), 209–228.

Hauff, S., Vetter, W., 2009. Quantitation of cis-and trans-monounsaturated fatty acids in dairy products and cod liver oil by mass spectrometry in the selected ion monitoring mode. J. Agric. Food Chem. 57 (9), 3423–3430.

Heimbach, J., 2014. Debate: a bridge too far—liver transplantation for nonalcoholic steatohepatitis will overwhelm the organ supply. Liver Transpl. 20 (S2), S32–S37.

Helland, I., et al., 1998. Fatty acid composition in maternal milk and plasma during supplementation with cod liver oil. Eur. J. Clin. Nutr. 52 (11), 839–845.

IBD in EPIC Study Investigators, 2009. Linoleic acid, a dietary n-6 polyunsaturated fatty acid, and the aetiology of ulcerative colitis: a nested case–control study within a European prospective cohort study. Gut **58** (12), 1606–1611.

Iketani, T., Takazawa, K., Yamashina, A., 2013. Effect of eicosapentaenoic acid on central systolic blood pressure. Prostaglandins Leukot. Essent. Fatty Acids 88 (2), 191–195.

Inoue-Yamauchi, A., Itagaki, H., Oda, H., 2018. Eicosapentaenoic acid attenuates obesity-related hepatocellular carcinogenesis. Carcinogenesis 39 (1), 28–35.

Jang, J.-Y., et al., 2014. Perilla oil improves blood flow through inhibition of platelet aggregation and thrombus formation. Lab. Anim. Res. 30 (1), 21–27.

Jeyapal, S., et al., 2018. Substitution of linoleic acid with α-linolenic acid or long chain n-3 polyunsaturated fatty acid prevents Western diet induced nonalcoholic steatohepatitis. Sci. Rep. 8 (1), 1–14.

Johnson, L.F., Shoolery, J., 1962. Determination of unsaturation and average molecular weight of natural fats by nuclear magnetic resonance. Anal. Chem. 34 (9), 1136–1139.

Jørgensen, M.H., et al., 2001. Is there a relation between docosahexaenoic acid concentration in mothers' milk and visual development in term infants? J. Pediatr. Gastroenterol. Nutr. 32 (3), 293–296.

Jump, D.B., 2008. N-3 polyunsaturated fatty acid regulation of hepatic gene transcription. Curr. Opin. Lipidol. 19 (3), 242.

Kerr, T.A., Davidson, N.O., 2012. Cholesterol and NAFLD: renewed focus on an old villain. Hepatology **56** (5), 1995.

Keten, M., 2019. Review on the beneficial effects of omega-3 enriched eggs by dietary flaxseed oil supplementation. J. Istanbul Vet. Sci. 3 (3), 89–94.

Kitson, A.P., Stroud, C.K., Stark, K.D., 2010. Elevated production of docosahexaenoic acid in females: potential molecular mechanisms. Lipids 45 (3), 209–224.

Kohashi, K., et al., 2014. Effects of eicosapentaenoic acid on the levels of inflammatory markers, cardiac function and long-term prognosis in chronic heart failure patients with dyslipidemia. J. Atheroscler. Thromb. 21 (7), 712–729. https://doi.org/10.5551/jat.21022.

Kris-Etherton, P.M., 1999. Monounsaturated fatty acids and risk of cardiovascular disease. Circulation 100 (11), 1253–1258.

Lands, W.E., Morris, A., Libelt, B., 1990. Quantitative effects of dietary polyunsaturated fats on the composition of fatty acids in rat tissues. Lipids 25 (9), 505–516.

Latreille, J., et al., 2012. Dietary monounsaturated fatty acids intake and risk of skin photoaging. PLoS One 7 (9), e44490.

Lauby-Secretan, B., et al., 2016. Body fatness and cancer—viewpoint of the IARC Working Group. N. Engl. J. Med. 375 (8), 794–798.

Le Yu, M.Y., Wang, L., 2017. The effect of omega-3 unsaturated fatty acids on non-alcoholic fatty liver disease: a systematic review and meta-analysis of RCTs. Pak. J. Med. Sci. 33 (4), 1022.

Lewis, R.N., Sykes, B.D., McElhaney, R.N., 1988. Thermotropic phase behavior of model membranes composed of phosphatidylcholines containing cis-monounsaturated acyl chain homologs of oleic acid: differential scanning calorimetric and phosphorus-31 NMR spectroscopic studies. Biochemistry 27 (3), 880–887.

Llovet, J.M., Burroughs, A., Bruix, J., 2003. Hepatocellular carcinoma. Lancet **362** (9399), 1907–1917.

Lonardo, A., et al., 2016. Non-alcoholic fatty liver disease and risk of cardiovascular disease. Metabolism 65 (8), 1136–1150.

Loomba, R., Sanyal, A.J., 2013. The global NAFLD epidemic. Nat. Rev. Gastroenterol. Hepatol. 10 (11), 686–690.

Lytle, K.A., et al., 2015. Docosahexaenoic acid attenuates Western diet-induced hepatic fibrosis in Ldlr$^{-/-}$ mice by targeting the TGFβ-Smad3 pathway. J. Lipid Res. 56 (10), 1936–1946.

Lytle, K.A., Wong, C.P., Jump, D.B., 2017. Docosahexaenoic acid blocks progression of western diet-induced nonalcoholic steatohepatitis in obese Ldlr$^{-/-}$ mice. PLoS One 12 (4), e0173376.

Maccarone, A.T., et al., 2014. Characterization of acyl chain position in unsaturated phosphatidylcholines using differential mobility-mass spectrometry. J. Lipid Res. 55 (8), 1668–1677.

McCowen, K.C., et al., 2004. Abnormal regulation of serum lipid fatty acid profiles in short gut rats fed parenteral nutrition with lipid. Metabolism 53 (3), 273–277.

McGarry, J., Foster, D., 1980. Regulation of hepatic fatty acid oxidation and ketone body production. Annu. Rev. Biochem. 49 (1), 395–420.

Moss, G., Smith, P., Tavernier, D., 1995. Glossary of class names of organic compounds and reactivity intermediates based on structure (IUPAC Recommendations 1995). Pure Appl. Chem. 67 (8–9), 1307–1375.

Pratt, C.M., et al., 2009. Efficacy and safety of prescription omega-3-acid ethyl esters for the prevention of recurrent symptomatic atrial fibrillation: a prospective study. Am. Heart J. **158** (2), 163–169. e3.

Promrat, K., et al., 2010. Randomized controlled trial testing the effects of weight loss on nonalcoholic steatohepatitis. Hepatology 51 (1), 121–129.

Roach, C., et al., 2004. Comparison of cis and trans fatty acid containing phosphatidylcholines on membrane properties. Biochemistry 43 (20), 6344–6351.

Rodriguez-Leyva, D., et al., 2010. The cardiovascular effects of flaxseed and its omega-3 fatty acid, alpha-linolenic acid. Can. J. Cardiol. 26 (9), 489–496.

Rustan, A.C., Drevon, C.A., 2001. Fatty Acids: Structures and Properties. eLS.

Ryan, A.S., et al., 2009. The hypolipidemic effect of an ethyl ester of algal-docosahexaenoic acid in rats fed a high-fructose diet. Lipids 44 (9), 817–826.

Schwingshackl, L., Hoffmann, G., 2014. Monounsaturated fatty acids, olive oil and health status: a systematic review and meta-analysis of cohort studies. Lipids Health Dis. 13 (1), 154.

Sherman, M., 2014. Surveillance for hepatocellular carcinoma. Best Pract. Res. Clin. Gastroenterol. 28 (5), 783–793.

Simopoulos, A.P., 2002. The importance of the ratio of omega-6/omega-3 essential fatty acids. Biomed. Pharmacother. 56 (8), 365–379.

Singh, M., 2005. Essential fatty acids, DHA and human brain. Indian J. Pediatr. 72 (3), 239–242.

Siriwardhana, N., et al., 2013. Modulation of adipose tissue inflammation by bioactive food compounds. J. Nutr. Biochem. 24 (4), 613–623.

Tur, J., et al., 2012. Dietary sources of omega 3 fatty acids: public health risks and benefits. Br. J. Nutr. 107 (S2), S23–S52.

Van Horn, L., et al., 2008. The evidence for dietary prevention and treatment of cardiovascular disease. J. Am. Diet. Assoc. 108 (2), 287–331.

Varela, L.M., et al., 2013. The effects of dietary fatty acids on the postprandial triglyceride-rich lipoprotein/apoB48 receptor axis in human monocyte/macrophage cells. J. Nutr. Biochem. 24 (12), 2031–2039.

Wallis, J.G., Watts, J.L., Browse, J., 2002. Polyunsaturated fatty acid synthesis: what will they think of next? Trends Biochem. Sci. 27 (9), 467–473.

Wen, X., et al., 2016. Hepatic arterial infusion of low-density lipoprotein docosahexaenoic acid nanoparticles selectively disrupts redox balance in hepatoma cells and reduces growth of orthotopic liver tumors in rats. Gastroenterology 150 (2), 488–498.

Weylandt, K.H., et al., 2011. Suppressed liver tumorigenesis in fat-1 mice with elevated omega-3 fatty acids is associated with increased omega-3 derived lipid mediators and reduced TNF-α. Carcinogenesis 32 (6), 897–903.

Yurko-Mauro, K., et al., 2010. Beneficial effects of docosahexaenoic acid on cognition in age-related cognitive decline. Alzheimers Dement. 6 (6), 456–464.

Zhang, G., et al., 2013. Epoxy metabolites of docosahexaenoic acid (DHA) inhibit angiogenesis, tumor growth, and metastasis. Proc. Natl. Acad. Sci. U. S. A. 110 (16), 6530–6535.

Zhang, G., Kodani, S., Hammock, B.D., 2014. Stabilized epoxygenated fatty acids regulate inflammation, pain, angiogenesis and cancer. Prog. Lipid Res. 53, 108–123.

CHAPTER 10

Influence of vitamins (C, B₃, D, and E) in liver health

H.G. Ağalar

Pharmacognosy Department, Faculty of Pharmacy, Anadolu University, Eskişehir, Turkey

10.1 Introduction

The liver is a prime organ for maintaining the body's internal environment through the processing of nutrients and the metabolism of carbohydrates, proteins, and fats, among others. It is also responsible for the detoxification of xenobiotics to maintain the homeostasis of the body. Therefore, this organ is critical for processing metabolites, which are key to whole body nutrient/energy homeostasis. Hence, it is essential to maintain a healthy liver for the overall health and well-being of an individual (Wahlang et al., 2018; Simon et al., 2019). Disorders of the liver develop due to a plethora of pathogenic mechanisms, including a high-calorie diet, drugs/alcohol, viral infections, genetics, and environmental stimuli (Wahlang et al., 2018). Interestingly, reactive oxygen species (ROS) is a primary contributor to liver complications. Previous studies have shown that ROS may be the link between chronic liver injury and hepatic fibrosis. Reports have shown that viruses or excessive alcohol consumption alter etheno-modified DNA via lipid peroxidation. Conversely, multiple enzymatic/nonenzymatic mechanisms can protect cells against ROS, including glutathione (GSH) and vitamins A, C, and E (Oliveira et al., 2003; Ha et al., 2010; Okamura et al., 2018).

Vitamins are essential for everyday cell functions and maintenance. They are involved in intermediary and specialized metabolism, and are commonly derivatives to more complex coenzymatic compounds. In this chapter, the influence of some vitamins in liver diseases will be critically reviewed. The focus will be on vitamins C, B₃ (niacin), D, and E and the combinations, which are widely studied by researchers.

10.2 Vitamin C

Vitamin C (ascorbic acid) is water soluble and is critical for optimal health. Most mammals have the ability to synthesize vitamin C on their own and are not prone to the effects of its deficiency. Humans, however, rely on dietary sources to get vitamin C (Aumailley et al., 2016).

Influence of Nutrients, Bioactive Compounds, and Plant Extracts in Liver Diseases. https://doi.org/10.1016/B978-0-12-816488-4.00009-7

Vitamin C has been linked to tissue healing and key signaling functions for neurotransmitters. This potent antioxidant helps to strengthen the immune system (Su et al., 2019a).

Vitamin C can regulate iron levels/function and has been documented in the amelioration of ALD. Vitamin C can correct iron-metabolic complications due to excessive alcohol intake. Vitamin C has been shown to result in increased liver hepcidin and decreased TfR1 levels. It also has been shown to regulate the expression of intestinal Fpn1 and DMT1. A sufficient supplementation with vitamin C (50–100 mg/kg) has been shown to prevent liver damage resulting from autoimmune or chronic inflammation (Xiaoqiang et al., 2010). Vitamin C was also shown to regulate immunoactivation as well as the maintenance of IL-22Ra signaling cascades (Bae et al., 2013).

Vitamin C regulates both circulating and hepatic lipid levels, and may be important in the progression of NAFLD. Vitamin C deficiency has been shown to result in increased plasma and hepatic lipids, ROS, fibrosis, and inflammation. Vitamin C has been shown to decrease liver ROS markers in animal models (Grajeda-Cota et al., 2004; Abdulkhaleq et al., 2018; Xu et al., 2019). The role of vitamin C deficiency and NAFLD is not well understood and the studies have led to conflicting results. Few reports have studied vitamin C levels in NAFLD patient plasma (Ipsen et al., 2014). A moderate inverse correlation between vitamin C intake and NAFLD in middle-aged and older males has been suggested (Wei et al., 2016). Some studies have reported low levels of vitamin C in NAFLD subjects while others found no significant differences (Ipsen et al., 2014). These conflicting findings may be due to a lack of plasma concentration measurement and only an estimation of dietary intake. Vitamin C in NAFLD subjects has only been studied in two RCTs (Del Ben et al., 2017). A 6-month therapy with vitamin C at a 1000 mg/daily dose improved liver fibrosis scores in NASH patients (Harrison et al., 2003).

Vitamin C was investigated using L-gulono-γ-lactone oxidase knockout mice for its role in liver fibrosis. The gulo-knockout mice cannot synthesize vitamin C, so, in the loss of vitamin C synthesis augmented liver fibrosis and ROS in mice. It was significantly increased in low-dose vitamin C (Bae et al., 2013). Vitamin C has also been shown to suppress cell proliferation and H_2O_2 stimulated COL1A1 levels (Kim et al., 2014). Vitamin C has also been shown to have antifibrotic properties by blocking ROS. Vitamin C has been shown to alter lipid peroxidation in alcohol-treated male guinea pigs and rats while catalase, superoxide dismutase, and glutathione peroxidase were increased (Abhilash et al., 2012; Prathibha et al., 2013).

The pretreatment of mice with vitamin C against oxidative liver damage is more beneficial than posttreatment (Ha et al., 2010).

Perfluorooctane sulfonate-exposed mice treated with vitamin C displayed a smaller liver size/mass and improved liver structure as determined morphologically. The pharmacological nature of vitamin C has been underscored in the cyto-architecture of the liver. Vitamin C has improved functional/morphological changes in hepatocytes and may act to protect hepatocyte growth/proliferation by increasing FGF21 expression and lowering inflammatory cytokines involved in liver cell dysfunction (Su et al., 2019b). Treatment with vitamin C also blocked liver injury through aspartate transaminase and alanine aminotransferase reduction in mice while restoring total superoxide dismutase and glutathione. These findings suggest that vitamin C is protective against injury via regulation of ROS (Xu et al., 2019; Zhong et al., 2017). Vitamin C ameliorated severe liver injury caused by azathioprine in rabbits. The study suggested that vitamin C may be prescribed to patients taking azathioprine as a prophylactic therapy to prevent liver injury (Talpur et al., 2017). One study demonstrated the ability of ascorbic acid to reduce antibiotic-induced hepatotoxicity. This proves that it can be used as an adjuvant offering a hepatoprotective effect against antibiotics such as sulfamethoxazole, tetracycline, and clavulanic acid. Based on the findings, an approximate dose of a 3 g equivalent vitamin C-rich diet per day for a healthy adult (1.5 kg liver) during antibiotic therapy was recommended. This may be sufficient to produce a significant protective effect because of its greater bioavailability (70%–90%) (Simon et al., 2019). An in vivo study showed that vitamin C could block cypermethrin damage (up to 90%). Vitamin C may have been shown to be a primary hepatoprotector in rats (Grajeda-Cota et al., 2004). Vitamin C lowered ROS and blocked methionine choline diet-induced liver steatosis in Wistar rats (Oliveira et al., 2003). Vitamin C has been linked to the protection of mitochondria and DNA from ROS damage associated with arsenic trioxide. It has a protective role against arsenic trioxide-induced liver injury (Singh and Rana, 2010).

10.3 Vitamin B$_3$ (niacin)

Niacin, commonly known as nicotinic acid, is an important therapeutic option for the treatment of atherosclerosis and dyslipidemia. It has lipid-regulating effects via lowering blood triglycerides (TGs) and reducing low-density lipoproteins (LDL). Niacin altered key pathways in the regulation of TG and LDL synthesis while increasing high-density lipoprotein (HDL) levels. Clinical evidence has concluded that niacin can be used as a therapeutic option for heart disease. These findings suggest that niacin may be important in the treatment of atherogenic disease (Cooper et al., 2015).

Niacin has been shown to inhibit fat deposits in hepatocytes, ROS, and IL-8 expression, which are important in the progression of NAFLD and NASH (Ganji et al., 2015). In vivo data supported the HDL-C lowering effect of niacin, which was mediated via GPR109A in hepatocytes (Li et al., 2010). Another in vivo study using a mouse model of ALD suggested that niacin might be effective in the prevention of oxidative stress in liver disease. Niacin can protect hepatocytes from H_2O_2-induced cell death, which involves the prevention of glutathione depletion. A better understanding of the role of niacin in ROS inhibition will help to improve our knowledge of the mechanisms associated with liver disease (Dou et al., 2013).

The predominant side effect of niacin is flushing while other side effects (e.g., nausea, gastrointestinal complications, and hepatotoxicity) have been documented. Hepatic stress can present in as little as 1 week following the start of niacin treatment (Cooper et al., 2015). Irregular SR niacin product consumption has been associated with hepatotoxicity. But, the rapid-acting formulations of niacin are less hepatotoxic when compared to time-release formulations (McCarty, 2000; Cooper et al., 2015).

10.4 Vitamin D

Vitamin D is an essential hormone for calcium homeostasis. Even though the key functions of vitamin D are mineral and skeletal homeostasis, most studies have shown that its status is also related to cancer, autoimmune, diabetes, infectious, and cardiovascular diseases (Tavakoli et al., 2019).

The endogenous form of vitamin D obtained from skin exposure to UV-B radiation or ingested vitamin D is converted to 25-hydroxyvitamin D (25-OHD) by hepatic microsomal vitamin D hydroxylases. 25-OHD's active form, calcitriol, 1,25-dihydroxyvitamin D, is subsequently converted in the kidney. Owing to its longer half-life (2–3 weeks), the 25-OHD level is the best measure of storage. The Endocrine Society Clinical Practice Guidelines recently defined serum levels < 30 ng/mL as insufficient and levels < 20 ng/mL as deficient (Backstedt et al., 2017).

Animal models have demonstrated 1,25-dihydroxyvitamin D's contribution in the regulation of oxidative stress, the production of proinflammatory cytokines, hepatocytes, apoptosis, and liver fibrosis (Zhang et al., 2007; George et al., 2012; Roth et al., 2012).

The status of vitamin D was found to be associated with some liver enzymes such as alanine aminotransferase (ALT), aspartate transaminase (AST), γ-glutamyl transferase (GGT), etc. The lower vitamin D status (serum 25-OHD level) leads to slightly higher liver enzymes (Skaaby et al., 2014).

The specific receptor of vitamin D called VDR is expressed in all hepatic cell populations. Vitamin D exerts its direct action on the liver through its receptor. VDR expression was found to be negatively correlated with the inflammatory damage in chronic hepatic diseases. These findings concluded that the VD/VDR system plays a role in the progression of metabolic and viral chronic liver damage (Barchetta et al., 2012). A recent study has shown that the critical role of the vitamin D/VDR axis was the modulation of both autophagy and apoptosis in HCV infection. It was suggested that VDR-targeted therapy in addition to vitamin D supplementation might be a great option to restore the vital biological functions of vitamin D (Abdel-Mohsen et al., 2018).

The common problem among patients with chronic liver diseases is vitamin D deficiency (Arteh et al., 2010; Buonomo et al., 2017; Sriram et al., 2018; Ebadi et al., 2019). Studies have suggested that reduced vitamin D in the serum is linked to liver fibrosis chronic liver disease patients, including hepatitis B and C as well as NAFLD and ALD, among others (Backstedt et al., 2017). In 2010, Arteh et al. reported that vitamin D insufficiency or deficiency was seen in up to 92% of patients with chronic liver disease. A recent clinical study reported that severe vitamin D deficiency was a prognostic biomarker for autoimmune hepatitis patients (Ebadi et al., 2019). In patients with chronic hepatitis C infection, the prevalence of vitamin D deficiency (10–20 ng/mL) and severe deficiency (< 10 ng/mL) was found to be significantly high, but vitamin D did not change during the course of direct-acting antiviral therapy (Backstedt et al., 2017). The risk for specific cancers, liver cancer, and hepatitis C-related hepatocellular carcinoma has been linked to lower circulating 25-hydroxyvitamin D, which is the major circulating metabolite (Abdel-Mohsen et al., 2018; Budhathoki et al., 2018).

Some previous studies have shown a relationship between vitamin D deficiency and the metabolic syndrome's components such as insulin resistance and dyslipidemia. Based on this relationship, a new hypothesis on vitamin D deficiency and NAFLD was proposed. As known, NAFLD occurs via triglyceride accumulation in hepatic cells. Simple steatosis, NASH, and liver cirrhosis are included in the spectrum of the disease. Clinical data revealed that the common findings among NAFLD patients are the vitamin D deficiency (in the majority group) or insufficiency (average). The findings of many clinical studies regarding the association between vitamin D deficiency and NAFLD have come out (Barchetta et al., 2012; Black et al., 2014; Bril et al., 2015; Agrwal et al., 2017; Wimalawansa, 2018). Vitamin D was also found to have beneficial effects on NAFLD through the modulation of adipokines (Abenavoli et al., 2016). Vitamin D supplementation (50,000 IU/biweekly) for 16 weeks significantly improved the serum levels of both inflammation and lipid peroxidation biomarkers in patients with NAFLD (Sharifi et al., 2014). In a double-blind, placebo-controlled trial, to assess the beneficial effects of vitamin D3 (2000 IU/d) or a placebo for 6 months in type 2 diabetic patients with NAFLD were applied. It was concluded that high dose oral vitamin D supplementation over 24 weeks did not improve hepatic steatosis and metabolic parameters in patients (Barchetta et al., 2016). A recent and randomized clinical study on the effects of vitamin D supplementation on liver fibrogenic factors in NAFLD patients with steatohepatitis was published. The authors showed that vitamin D could control liver fibrosis in NAFLD patients with NASH (Ebrahimpour-Koujan et al., 2019). Clinical data based on limited data has suggested that vitamin D might be a potential therapeutic option for liver damage in NAFLD and NASH.

In Table 10.1, current clinical studies on vitamin D's effects on liver health are summarized.

Table 10.1: Clinical trials on vitamin D's effects on liver health.

Aim of the study/country	Subjects/results	Reference
Vitamin D (VD) deficiency Canada	– 209 Patients with probable or definitive autoimmune hepatitis (AIH) – 20% of the patients had severe VD deficiency. Treatment nonresponse was more common in patients with severe VD deficiency than in patients without. – Severe VD deficiency is a prognostic biomarker in AIH	Ebadi et al. (2019)
Association between serum 25-OHD deficiency and hepatic encephalopathy India	– A retroperspective study, 250 patients with chronic liver disease – Moderate to severe 25-OHD deficiency in 160 patients – 25-OHD deficiency was observed in the majority of patients with chronic liver disease	Sriram et al. (2018)
VD deficiency in HCV-related liver cirrhosis Italy	– 291 Patients affected by HCV-related liver cirrhosis – VD deficiency (< 20 ng/mL) diagnosed in 68.3% – VD may play a role in the development of infections in patients affected by liver cirrhosis	Buonomo et al. (2017)
VD deficiency in chronic liver disease (CLD) United States	– 118 Consecutive patients with CLD – VD deficiency defined in 92.4% of patients – African American females are at highest risk of VD deficiency	Arteh et al. (2010)
Plasma VD concentration and risk of specific cancers Japan	– A large case-cohort study, 3301 incident cases of cancer and 4044 randomly selected subcohort participants – 25-OHD conc. showed a significant inverse association with the risk of liver cancer – Higher circulating VD lowered the risk of subsequent cancer	Budhathoki et al. (2018)
VD and VD receptor (VDR) association with hepatocellular carcinoma (HCC) Egypt	– Cross-sectional study – Deficiency of VD and decreased levels of its receptors were observed in hepatitis C viral infection (HCV) and HCV-HCC patients – The perturbation in VD/VDR axis, which modulates both autophagy and apoptosis in HCV infection, may point to its involvement and implication in the pathogenesis of HCV infection and the development of HCV-related HCC	Abdel-Mohsen et al. (2018)
25-OHD levels in chronic hepatitis infection	– 218 Patients with chronic hepatitis C – Prevalence of VD deficiency (10–20 ng/mL) and severe deficiency (< 10 ng/mL) significantly high, VD did not change during the course of direct-acting antiviral therapy – The prevalence of VD deficiency is higher in HC-related cirrhotic cohorts compared to noncirrhotic patients and correlates with components of hepatic function	Backstedt et al. (2017)

Table 10.1: Clinical trials on vitamin D's effects on liver health—cont'd

Aim of the study/country	Subjects/results	Reference
25-OHD association with alcoholic steatohepatitis (ASH) France	- A cohort study with 101 patients - A severe deficiency in 25-OHD in 60.4% of patients - In alcoholic patients, severe deficiency in 25-OHD independently associated with the occurrence of ASH	Anty et al. (2015)
VD level association with insulin resistance and disease severity in nonalcoholic fatty liver disease (NAFLD)	- A cohort study with 239 patients - VD deficiency 47%, insufficiency 31% - Plasma VD levels are not associated with insulin resistance, the amount of liver fat accumulation, or the severity of NASH	Bril et al. (2015)
25-OHD levels associated with cirrhosis France	- A prospective and randomized study with 50 patients - Severe deficiency in VD in 56.8% of patients and more frequent infections - Low levels of 25-OHD were independently associated with bacterial infections in cirrhotic patients	Anty et al. (2014)
25-OHD levels association with NAFLD Australia	- A prospective population-based study - The majority of participants with NAFLD had either insufficient (51%) or deficient (17%) VD status. Lower 25-OHD concentrations at 17 years were significantly associated with increased risk of NAFLD - Lower 25-OHD concentrations are significantly associated with NAFLD, independent of adiposity and IR	Black et al. (2014)
VD status in chronic HCV-1 infected patients Germany	- 191 Patients infected chronically with HCV-1 - Decreased 25-OHD and increased ferritin serum levels indicate the severity of hepatic inflammation and fibrosis in patients infected chronically with HCV-1 - Eradication of HCV was found to coincide with a significant increase in serum 25-OHD and a reduction in serum ferritin concentrations	Amanzada et al. (2013)
VD3 levels in nonalcoholic steatohepatitis (NASH) or HCV patients Italy	- 61 (25 NASH, 36 CHC) patients underwent liver biopsy - VDR is widely expressed in the liver and inflammatory cells of chronic liver disease patients and its expression is negatively associated with the severity of liver - VD/VDR system plays a role in the progression of metabolic and viral chronic liver damage	Barchetta et al. (2012)
25-OHD supplementation India	- 50 NAFLD patients, 50 control group - NAFLD patients had markedly reduced circulating levels of 25-OHD compared with controls - Low VD level can contribute to alterations in mineral metabolism as well as risk factors in NAFLD patients	Agrwal et al. (2017)

Continued

Table 10.1: Clinical trials on vitamin D's effects on liver health—cont'd

Aim of the study/country	Subjects/results	Reference
VD supplementation (Cholecalciferol), 2000 IU/d dose Italy	– Randomized, double-blind, placebo-controlled, 65 patients – High-dose VD oral supplementation has no effect on hepatic fat content in T2D patients affected by NAFLD – 24-week cholecalciferol suppl. Did not improve either transaminases levels or the serum levels of biomarkers specific for hepatic injury and fibrogenesis such as CK18-M30 and P3NP – Oral high-dose VD supplementation over 24 weeks did not improve HS or metabolic/cardiovascular parameters in T2D patients with NAFLD	Barchetta et al. (2016)
VD3 (Vitamidyne D), 2000 IU/d dose Israel	– Randomized study, 72 consecutive patients with chronic HCV-1 – Addition of a VD suppl. to current standard therapy can significantly improve the rate of rapid viral response, early viral response, and sustained virologic response – VD + Peg-α-2b/Ribavirin therapy significantly improves the viral response	Abu-Mouch et al. (2011)

10.5 Vitamin E

Vitamin E is an essential lipid-soluble antioxidant that breaks lipid chains and reduces oxidation by scavenging ROS (Liebler, 1993; Papandreou and Andreou, 2015). ROS has been shown to be involved in liver damage and the progression of steatosis to steatohepatitis. Enhanced ROS generation can cause lipid peroxidation, resulting in the activation of stellate cells that are involved in inflammation and fibrogenesis, which ultimately leads to nonalcoholic fatty liver disease (NAFLD) (Papandreou and Andreou, 2015; Del Ben et al., 2017).

Vitamin E administered at 50 IU/kg body weight was shown to protect against heavy metal-induced liver injury in albino mice (Al-Attar, 2011). It can also modify phoxim-induced liver toxicity via the reduction of serum gamma-glutamyl transferase, liver malondialdehyde, and the CYP2E1 expression in rats (Zhang et al., 2017).

Past reports have demonstrated that liver cell vitamin E content is inversely proportional to ROS damage and protects against DNA damage in hepatocellular carcinoma cultures (Fantappie et al., 2004). In mouse models of NASH, dietary vitamin E supplementation blocked the effects of lipopolysaccharide-induced liver injury and inhibited methionine-choline diet-induced ROS-related complications such as steatosis and inflammation. Moreover, vitamin E has been shown to downregulate ROS-induce TGF-β expression, which is associated with fibrosis. Another report using an experimental model of NASH showed the ability of vitamin E to restore glutathione levels and diminish oxidative stress markers, stellate cell activation, and fibrosis.

Vitamin E is protective against liver steatosis and it has been shown to significantly reduce body weight. Treatment with vitamin E effectively prevented steatosis to steatohepatitis in mice deficient in an enzyme that converts phosphatidylethanolamine to phospatidylcholine. These are the two main phospholipids in plasma membranes in mammalian cells (Presa et al., 2019). In addition, it has also been documented to improve glucose tolerance and insulin sensitivity (He et al., 2019). Vitamin E reduces biomarkers of liver injury and oxidative stress induced by a high fat diet but not TNF-α. Vitamin E was partially effective in inhibiting liver dysfunction (Ellatif et al., 2018).

Vitamin E has also been documented for its improvement of NAFLD patients. In pediatric patients, vitamin E was shown to improve steatosis scores, but with marginal effects that were not statistically significant. Clinical trials, including PIVENS (Sanyal et al., 2010) and TONIC (Lavine et al., 2011) studies, used vitamin E to assess the efficacy in large numbers of adult and pediatric NASH patients. The PIVENS trial concluded that vitamin E therapy (800 IU daily) led to a clinical improvement, but pioglitazone at 30 mg daily had no effect. Both compounds improved hepatic steatosis severity, inflammation, and hepatocellular ballooning; however, fibrosis was not improved. Interestingly, both metformin at 1000 mg/d and vitamin E at 800 IU/d improved hepatocellular ballooning and NAFLD activity scores in the TONIC trial. Yet, neither were able to decrease alanine aminotransferase levels or resolve inflammation, steatosis, or fibrosis (Sanyal et al., 2010; Lavine et al., 2011; Stellavato et al., 2018). On the other hand, vitamin E therapy for 1 year improved fibrosis scores and liver plasticity in the NAFLD subject cohort (Fukui et al., 2015).

Vitamin E has been shown to reduce the harmful effects of hepatic steatosis via the suppression of hepatic lipid peroxidation/accumulation. Moreover, vitamin E resulted in a reduction of inflammation via decreased M1 macrophages and concomitant augmentation of M2 macrophages in NASH patients. It is known that the suppression of T cell recruitment and Th1 and CD8 + T cell infiltration precedes M1 macrophage recruitment in obese subjects. Lipid peroxidation was shown to increase the recruitment of T cells to the liver and enhance M1 macrophage activation in a mouse mode of NASH. Therefore, vitamin E benefits are, at least in part, associated with reduced T cell recruitment and increased M2 macrophages, which block fibrosis and inflammation. Vitamin E may be effective in preventing NASH through both antioxidant and nonantioxidant effects (Nagashimada and Ota, 2019).

Clinical trials evaluating vitamin E efficacy (mono- or combination) in NASH treatment have been debatable. One study showed that vitamin E (800 mg/d for 24 weeks) reduced transaminase levels and steatosis; however, no effects were observed on inflammation or fibrosis. Lower doses (300 mg) and a year's treatment were shown to reduce both transaminase levels and steatosis as well as improve inflammation and fibrosis in a cohort of 12 NASH patients (Perumpail et al., 2018).

Multiple reports have demonstrated that vitamin E serum levels are diminished in alcoholic liver disease (ALD) patients. Levels are negatively associated with ROS and are directly proportional to liver damage severity. For this reason, normal vitamin E levels may be necessary for lipid peroxidation prevention and even reducing mitochondrial damage (Ha et al., 2010).

The role of vitamin E in chronic hepatitis B virus (HBV) treatment has also been studied. Two out of three published trials have documented serum hepatitis B e-antigen clearance, antibody production, and antiangiogenesis therapy normalization in the majority of patients treated with vitamin E. The role of vitamin E in the epigenetic regulation of the HBV life cycle in patients with HBV-related chronic hepatitis was investigated (Andreone et al., 2001; Dikici et al., 2007; Gerner et al., 2008). It was determined that vitamin E inhibited the viral-induced epigenetic regulation in patients (Fiorino et al., 2014).

Vitamin E has been shown to have gene-regulatory activities at the transcriptional/posttranscriptional level (Ha et al., 2010; Fiorino et al., 2014). It has been determined to prevent fibrotic phenotypes and decrease NF-κB-induced inflammatory pathways. Preclinical studies have documented that vitamin E can enhance liver injury and inhibit apoptotic pathways as well as mitochondrial damage (Hardy et al., 2015).

The treatment of β-thalassemic patients with vitamin E has benefits in promoting antioxidant status and may improve liver function (Hashemian et al., 2012). Vitamin E has been used for first-line therapy in nondiabetic NASH patients. Experimental reports have somewhat explained the role of vitamin E administration in animal models (Nan et al., 2009; Hadi et al., 2018; Presa et al., 2019). The methionine-choline diet mouse model was used to show that vitamin E reduced ROS, apoptosis, and inflammation as well as resolved fibrosis (Nan et al., 2009).

There have been concerns about the adverse effects linked to chronic vitamin E usage. Vitamin E has been linked to the development of prostate cancer, hemorrhagic stroke, and in some cases patient mortality. The side effects and complications must be taken into account before starting this treatment (Mouzaki and Allard, 2012).

Vitamin E pretreatment lowered the degree of ROS, although only slight changes in liver injury were observed. Interestingly, vitamin E rescued the effects of alcohol on the redox state and apoptosis. In addition, vitamin E suppressed HBV replication and normalized alanine aminotransferase in several infected patients with chronic liver disease (Ha et al., 2010).

10.6 Vitamin combinations and liver health

The individual roles of vitamins were mentioned above. Current studies have been focused on potential effects of vitamins in combinations with other vitamins or therapeutic agents in liver health.

The combination of vitamin C and E had hepatoprotective effects against bendiocarb-induced toxicity (Apaydin et al., 2017), methyl parathion-induced hepatotoxicity (Uzunhisarcikli and Kalender, 2011), and hepatotoxicity caused by chronic arsenic exposure (Mondal et al., 2016) in rats. The combination of vitamins C and E was found to be protective against injury in rat livers. The combination was effective against alcohol-mediated toxic effects during liver regeneration. It affected liver regeneration by enhancing the functional role of hepatocytes (Okamura et al., 2018).

Pretreatment using vitamins C, E, and B$_{12}$ was shown to prevent hepatic ROS induced by acetaminophen (APAP) overdose. Vitamin C monotherapy demonstrated protection from APAP-induced liver injury in rats and the protection against APAP-intoxicated proliferation was maximum when a combination was used (Abdulkhaleq et al., 2018; Bashandy et al., 2018). Simultaneous treatment with selenium and vitamin E has a protective effect against sodium azide-induced hepatic damage (Hamza et al., 2017).

A combination of vitamin E + quercetin was found to reduce the cyclosporine-induced ROS in HepG-2 cells (Mostafavi-Pour et al., 2019).

Treatment with two tablets per day of silymarin + vitamin E (Eurosil 85) and a low-calorie diet ameliorated the hepatic test and NAFLD index (Aller et al., 2015). Eurosil 85 has been shown to have beneficial effects on toxicity in mouse liver primary cells (Faedmaleki et al., 2016). Lead-exposed mice treated with Eurosil 85 showed improvement of biochemical and histopathological findings. These data suggest a protective role for Eurosil 85 on liver toxicity (Shalan et al., 2005). Silybin-phospholipids and vitamin E together exert hepatoprotective, antiinflammatory, and antifibrotic effects. It can be beneficial in patients with hepatitis C (Falasca et al., 2008).

A regimen of allopurinol, metformin, and vitamin E significantly blocked fatty changes in comparison to monotherapy. Allopurinol was shown to enhance the protective abilities of metformin and vitamin E by way of inducible nitric oxide synthase (iNOS) expression and uric acid reduction (Khalaf et al., 2019).

A previous report demonstrates that the simultaneous supplementation of vitamin E (400 IU/d) and a symbiotic (Protexin, 2×10^8 CFU/g) may confer advantageous therapeutic outcomes for patients with NAFLD (Ekhlasi et al., 2017). In a randomized, double-blind, placebo-controlled clinical trial, supplementation with vitamin E (400 IU/d) + symbiotic capsule (twice daily) (8 weeks) was shown to be effective in reducing serum liver enzymes and leptin, lipid profiles, fasting blood sugar, and insulin in NAFLD. No adverse effects were seen among patients (Ekhlasi et al., 2019).

10.7 Conclusion

The current findings have clearly shown that dietary vitamin supplementation at suitable doses protects against hepatic oxidative damage. Generally, vitamins can protect cells from free radical-mediated damage by ROS scavenging well before the radicals interact with the cellular compartments. Moreover, the improvement of the activities of the glutathione system by vitamins may have an additional role in eliminating the deleterious radicals. This can be summarized by saying that the antioxidant abilities of the vitamins may protect the liver from the radicals. Also, vitamins are known to exert antiinflammatory, antifibrotic, and reductive effects on lipid peroxidation. The vitamins and/or their combinations with other agents are found to be effective in liver health. On the other hand, clinical trials should be extended to understand the whole mechanisms of the vitamins' effects on the liver.

References

Abdel-Mohsen, M.A., El-Braky, A.A.-A., Ghazal, A.A.E.-R., Shamseya, M.M., 2018. Autophagy, apoptosis, vitamin D, and vitamin D receptor in hepatocellular carcinoma associated with hepatitis C virus. Medicine 97 (12). https://doi.org/10.1097/MD.0000000000010172.

Abdulkhaleq, F.M., Alhussainy, T.M., Badr, M.M., Gammoh, O., Ghanim, B.Y., Qinna, N.A., 2018. Antioxidative stress effects of vitamins C, E, and B12, and their combination can protect the liver against acetaminophen-induced hepatotoxicity in rats. Drug Des. Dev. Ther. 12, 3525–3533.

Abenavoli, L., Milic, N., Di Renzo, L., Preveden, T., Medic-Stojanoska, M., De Lorenzo, A., 2016. Metabolic aspects of adult patients with non-alcoholic fatty liver disease. World J. Gastroenterol. 22, 7006–7016.

Abhilash, P.A., Harikrishnan, R., Indira, M., 2012. Ascorbic acid supplementation down-regulates the alcohol induced oxidative stress, hepatic stellate cell activation, cytotoxicity and mRNA levels of selected fibrotic genes in Guinea pigs. Free Radic. Res. 46 (2), 204–213.

Abu-Mouch, S., Jarchovsky, J., Zeina, A.-R., Assy, N., 2011. Vitamin D supplementation improves sustained virologic response in chronic hepatitis C (genotype 1)-naïve patients. World J. Gastroenterol. 21 (47), 5184–5190.

Agrwal, S.K., Dixit, V.K., Shukla, S.K., Yadav, D., Sachan, S., Kumar, R., 2017. Vitamin D status in non-alcoholic fatty liver patients in north Indian population. J. Clin. Exp. Hepatol. 7 (S2), S37.

Al-Attar, A.M., 2011. Vitamin E attenuates liver injury induced by exposure to lead, mercury, cadminum and copper in albino mice. Saudi J. Biol. Sci. 18, 395–401.

Aller, R., Izaola, O., Gomez, S., Tafur, C., Gonzalez, G., Berroa, E., Mora, N., Gonzalez, J.M., De Luis, D.A., 2015. Effect of silymarin plus vitamin E in patients with non-alcoholic fatty liver disease. A randomized clinical pilot study. Eur. Rev. Med. Pharmacol. Sci. 19, 3118–3124.

Amanzada, A., Goralczyk, A.D., Moriconi, F., van Thiel, D.H., Ramadori, G., Mihm, S., 2013. Vitamin D status and serum ferritin concentration in chronic hepatitis C virus type 1 infection. J. Med. Virol. 85, 1534–1541.

Andreone, P., Fiorino, S., Cursaro, C., Gramenzi, A., Margotti, M., Giammorino, L.D., Biselli, M., Miniero, R., Gasbarrini, G., Bernardi, M., 2001. Vitamin E as treatment for chronic hepatitis B: results of a randomized controlled pilot trial. Antivir. Res. 49 (2), 75–81.

Anty, R., Tonohouan, M., Ferrari-Panaia, P., Piche, T., Pariente, A., Anstee, Q.M., Gual, P., Tran, A., 2014. Low levels of 25-hydroxy vitamin D are independently associated with the risk of bacterial infection in cirrhotic patients. Clin. Transl. Gastroenterol. https://doi.org/10.1038/ctg.2014.6.

Anty, R., Canivet, C.M., Patouraux, S., Ferrari-Panaia, P., Saint-Paul, M.C., Huet, P.-M., Lebeaupin, C., Iannelli, A., Gual, P., Tran, A., 2015. Severe vitamin D deficiency may be an additional cofactor for the occurrence of alcoholic steatohepatitis. Alcohol. Clin. Exp. Res. 39 (6), 1027–1033.

Apaydin, F.G., Baş, H., Kalender, S., Kalender, Y., 2017. Bendiocarb induced histopathological and biochemical alterations in rat liver and preventive role of vitamins C and E. Environ. Toxicol. Pharmacol. 49, 148–155.

Arteh, J., Narra, S., Nair, S., 2010. Prevalence of vitamin D deficiency in chronic liver disease. Dig. Dis. Sci. 55, 2624–2628.

Aumailley, L., Warren, A., Garand, C., Dubois, M.J., Paquet, E.R., Le Couteur, D.G., Marette, A., Cogger, V.C., Lebel, M., 2016. Vitamin C modulates the metabolic and cytokine profiles, alleviates hepatic endoplasmic reticulum stress, and increases the life span of Gulo$^{-/-}$ mice. Aging 8 (3), 458–483.

Backstedt, D., Pedersen, M., Choi, M., Seetharam, A., 2017. 25-Vitamin D levels in chronic hepatitis C infection: association with cirrhosis and sustained virologic response. Ann. Gastroenterol. 30, 344–348.

Bae, S., Cho, C.H., Kim, H., Kim, H.R., Hwang, Y., Yoon, J.H., Kang, J.S., Lee, W.J., 2013. In vivo consequence of vitamin C insufficiency in liver injury: vitamin C ameliorate T-cell mediated acute liver injury in Gulo(−/−) mice. Antioxid. Redox Signal. 19 (17), 2040–2053.

Barchetta, I., Carotti, S., Lbbadia, G., Gentilucci, U.V., Muda, A.O., Angelico, F., Silecchia, G., Leonetti, F., Fraioli, A., Picardi, A., Morini, S., Cavallo, M.G., 2012. Expression: relationship with liver histology and vitamin D$_3$ levels in patients with nonalcoholic steatohepatitis or hepatitis C virus. Hepatology 56 (6), 2018–2187.

Barchetta, I., Ben, M.D., Angelico, F., Martino, M.D., Fraioli, A., La Torre, G., Saulle, R., Perri, L., Morini, S., Tiberti, C., Bertoccini, L., Cimini, F.A., Panimolle, F., Catalano, C., Baroni, M.G., Cavallo, M.G., 2016. No effects of oral vitamin D supplementation on non-alcoholic fatty liver disease in patients with type 2 diabetes: a randomized, double-blind, placebo-controlled trial. BMC Med. 14 (92). https://doi.org/10.1186/s12916-016-0638-y.

Bashandy, S.A.E., Ebaid, H., Moussa, S.A.A., Alhazza, I.M., Hassan, I., Alaamer, A., Al Tamimi, J., 2018. Potential effects of the combination of nicotinamide, vitamin B$_2$ and vitamin C on oxidative-mediated hepatotoxicity induced by thioacctamide. Lipids Health Dis. 17 (29). https://doi.org/10.1186/s12944-018-0674-z.

Black, L.J., Jacoby, P., She Ping-Delfos, W.C., Mori, T.A., Beilin, L.J., Olynyk, J.K., Ayonrinde, O.T., Huang, R.C., Holt, P.G., Hart, P.H., Oddy, W.H., Adams, L.A., 2014. Low serum 25-hydroxyvitamin D concentrations associate with non-alcoholic fatty liver disease in adolescents independent of adiposity. J. Gastroenterol. Hepatol. 29, 1215–1222.

Bril, F., Maximos, M., Portillo-Sanchez, P., Biernacki, D., Lomonaco, R., Subbarayan, S., Correa, M., Lo, M., Suman, A., Cusi, K., 2015. Relationship of vitamin D with insulin resistance and disease severity in non-alcoholic steatohepatitis. J. Hepatol. 62, 405–411.

Budhathoki, S., Hidaka, A., Yamaji, T., Sawada, N., Tanaka-Mizuno, S., Kuchiba, A., Charvat, H., Goto, A., Kojima, S., Sudo, N., Shimazu, T., Sasazuki, S., Inoue, M., Tsugane, S., Iwasaki, M., 2018. Plasma 25-hydroxyvitamin D concentration and subsequent risk of total and site specific cancers in Japanese population: large case-cohort study within Japan Public Health Center-based prospective study cohort. BMJ 360, k671.

Buonomo, A.R., Zappulo, E., Scotto, R., Pinchera, B., Perruolo, G., Formisano, P., Borgia, G., Gentile, I., 2017. Vitamin D deficiency is a risk factor for infections in patients affected by HCV-related liver cirrhosis. Int. J. Infect. Dis. 63, 23–29.

Cooper, D.L., Murrell, D.E., Roane, D.S., Harirforoosh, S., 2015. Effects of formulation design on niacin therapeutics: mechanism of action, metabolism and drug delivery. Int. J. Pharm. 490, 55–64.

Del Ben, M., Polimeni, L., Baratta, F., Pastori, D., Angelico, F., 2017. The role of nutraceuticals for the treatment of non-alcoholic fatty liver disease. Br. J. Clin. Pharmacol. 83, 88–95.

Dikici, B., Dagli, A., Ucmak, H., Bilici, M., Ece, A., 2007. Efficacy of vitamin E in children with immunotolerant-phase chronic hepatitis B infection. Pediatr. Int. 49 (5), 603–607.

Dou, X., Shen, C., Wang, Z., Li, S., Zhang, X., Song, Z., 2013. Protection of nicotinic acid against oxidative stress-induced cell death in hepatocytes contributes to its beneficial effect on alcohol-induced liver injury in mice. J. Nutr. Biochem. 24, 1520–1528.

Ebadi, M., Bhanji, R.A., Mazurak, V.C., Lytvyak, E., Mason, A., Czaja, A.J., Montano-Loza, A.J., 2019. Severe vitamin D deficiency is a prognostic biomarker in autoimmune hepatitis. Aliment. Pharmacol. Ther. 49, 173–182.

Ebrahimpour-Koujan, S., Sohrabpour, A.A., Foroughi, F., Alvandi, E., Esmaillzadeh, A., 2019. Effects of vitamin D supplementation on liver fibrogenic factors in non-alcoholic fatty liver patients with steatohepatitis: study protocol for a randomized clinical trial. Trials 20, 153. https://doi.org/10.1186/s13063-019-3241-7.

Ekhlasi, G., Zarrati, M., Agah, S., Hosseini, A.F., Hosseini, S., Shidfar, S., Arabshahi, S.S.S., Razmpoosh, E., Shidfar, F., 2017. Effects of symbiotic and vitamin E supplementation on blood pressure, nitric oxide and inflammatory factors in non-alcoholic fatty liver disease. EXCLI J. 16, 278–290.

Ekhlasi, G., Mohammadi, R.K., Agah, S., Zarrati, M., Hosseini, A.F., Arabshahi, S.S.S., Shidfar, F., 2019. Do symbiotic and vitamin E supplementation have favorite effects in nonalcoholic fatty liver disease? A randomized, dobule-blind, placebo-controlled trial. J. Res. Med. Sci. 21 (98), 10.

Ellatif, M.A., El Karib, A.O., Dallak, M., Eid, R.A., Al-Ani, R., Haidara, M.A., 2018. Vitamin E protects against hepatocyte ultrastructural damage induced by high fat diet in a rat model of pre-diabetes. Int. J. Morphol. 36 (4), 1350–1355.

Faedmaleki, F., Shirazi, F.H., Ejtemaeimehr, S., Anjarani, S., Salarian, A.-A., Ashtiani, H.A., Rastegar, H., 2016. Study of silymarin and vitamin E protective effects on silver nanoparticle toxicity on mice liver primary cell culture. Acta Med. Iran. 54 (2), 85–95.

Falasca, K., Ucciferri, C., Mancino, P., Vitacolonna, E., De Tullio, D., Pizzigallo, E., Conti, P., Vecchiet, J., 2008. Treatment with silybin-vitamin E-phospholipid complex in patients with hepatitis C infection. J. Med. Virol. 80, 1900–1906.

Fantappie, O., Lodovici, M., Fabrizio, P., Marchetti, S., Fabbroni, V., Solazzo, M., Lasagna, N., Pantaleo, P., Mazzanti, R., 2004. Vitamin E protects DNA from oxidative damage in human hepatocellular carcinoma cell lines. Free Radic. Res. 38 (7), 751–759.

Fiorino, S., Bacchi-Reggiani, L., Sabbbatani, S., Grizzi, F., di Tommaso, L., Masetti, M., Fornelli, A., Bondi, A., de Biase, D., Visani, M., Cuppini, A., Jovine, E., Pession, A., 2014. Possible role of tocopherols in the modulation of host microRNA with potential antiviral activity in patients with hepatitis B virus-related persistent infection: a systematic review. Br. J. Nutr. 112, 1751–1768.

Fukui, A., Kawabe, N., Hashimoto, S., Murao, M., Nakano, T., Shimazaki, H., Kan, T., Nakaoka, K., Ohki, M., Takagawa, Y., Takamura, T., Kamei, H., Yoshioka, K., 2015. Vitamin E reduces liver stiffness in nonalcoholic fatty liver disease. World J. Hepatol. 7 (27), 2749–2756.

Ganji, S.H., Kashyap, M.L., Kamanna, V.S., 2015. Niacin inhibits fat accumulation, oxidative stress, and inflammatory cytokine IL-8 in cultured hepatocytes: impact on non-alcoholic fatty liver disease. Metab. Clin. Exp. 64, 982–990.

George, N., Kumar, T.P., Antony, S., Jayanarayanan, S., Paulose, C., 2012. Effect of vitamin D3 in reducing metabolic and oxidative stress in the liver of streptozotocin-induced diabetic rats. Br. J. Nutr. 108, 1410–1418.

Gerner, P., Posselt, H.-G., Krahl, A., Ballauf, A., Innerhofer, A., Binder, C., Wenzl, T.G., Zense, M., Hector, A., Dockter, G., Adam, R., Neubert, J., Claßen, M., van Gemmern, R., Wirth, S., 2008. Vitamin E treatment for children with chronic hepatitis B: randomized placebo controlled trial. World J. Gastroenterol. 14 (47), 7208–7213.

Grajeda-Cota, P., Ramirez-Mares, M.V., Gonzalez de Mejia, E., 2004. Vitamin C protects against *in vitro* cytotoxicity of cypermethrin in rat hepatocytes. Toxicol. In Vitro 18, 13–19.

Ha, H.-L., Shin, H.-J., Feitelson, M.A., Yu, D.-Y., 2010. Oxidative stress and antioxidants in hepatic pathogenesis. World J. Gastroenterol. 16 (48), 6035–6043.

Hadi, H.E., Vettor, R., Rossato, M., 2018. Vitamin E as a treatment for non-alcoholic fatty liver disease: reality or myth? Antioxidants 7 (1). https://doi.org/10.3390/antiox7010012.

Hamza, R.Z., Al-Harbi, M.S., El-Shenawy, N.S., 2017. Ameliorative effect of vitamin E and selenium against oxidative stress induced by sodium azide in liver, kidney, testis and heart of male mice. Biomed. Pharmacother. 91, 602–610.

Hardy, T., Anstee, Q.M., Day, C.P., 2015. Nonalcoholic fatty liver disease: new treatments. Curr. Opin. Gastroenterol. 31, 175–183.

Harrison, S.A., Torgerson, S., Hayashi, P., Ward, J., Schenker, S., 2003. Vitamin E and vitamin C treatment improves fibriosis in patients with nonalcoholic steatohepatitis. Am. J. Gastroenterol. 98 (11), 2485–2490.

Hashemian, Z., Hashemi, A., Fateminasab, M., 2012. The benefits of vitamin E on liver function and the homopoietic system in thalassemia patients. Iran. J. Pediatr. Hematol. Oncol. 2 (4), 153–158.

He, W., Xu, Y., Ren, X., Xiang, D., Lei, K., Zhang, C., Liu, D., 2019. Vitamin E ameliorates lipid metabolism in mice with nonalcoholic fatty liver disease via Nrf2/CES1 signalling pathway. Dig. Dis. Sci. https://doi.org/10.1007/s10620-019-05657-9.

Ipsen, D.H., Tveden-Nyborg, P., Lykkesfeldt, J., 2014. Does vitamin C deficiency promote fatty liver disease development? Nutrients 6, 5473–5499.

Khalaf, H.M., Ibrahim, M.A., Amin, E.F., Ibrahim, S.A., Abdel-Wahab, S., Fouad, Y.M., 2019. Allopurinol potentiates the hepatoprotective effect of metformin and vitamin E in fructose-induced fatty liver in rats. Clin. Exp. Hepatol. 5 (1), 65–74.

Kim, J.-H., Jeong, Y.-J., Hong, J.-M., Kim, H.-R., Kang, J.S., Lee, W.J., Hwang, Y., 2014. Chronic vitamin C insuffiency aggravated thioacetamide-induced liver fibrosis in gulo-knockout mice. Free Radic. Biol. Med. 67, 81–90.

Lavine, J.E., Schwimmer, J.B., van Natta, M.L., Molleston, J.P., Murray, K.F., Rosenthal, P., Abrams, S.H., Scheimann, A.O., Sanyal, A.J., Chalasani, N., Tonascia, J., Ünalp, A., Clark, J.M., Brunt, E.M., Kleiner, D.E., Hoofnagle, J.H., Robuck, P.R., Nonalcoholic Steatohepatitis Clinical Research Network, 2011. Effect of vitamin E or metformin for treatment of nonalcoholic fatty liver disease in children and adolescents: the TONIC randomized controlled trial. JAMA 305, 1659–1668.

Li, X., Millar, J.S., Brownell, N., Briand, F., Rader, D.J., 2010. Modulation of HDL metabolism by the niacin receptor GPR109A in mouse hepatocytes. Biochem. Pharmacol. 80, 1450–1457.

Liebler, D.C., 1993. The role of metabolism in the antioxidant function of vitamin E. Crit. Rev. Toxicol. 23, 147–169.

McCarty, M.F., 2000. Co-administration of equimolar doses of betaine may alleviate the hepatotoxic risk associated with niacin therapy. Med. Hypotheses 55 (3), 189–194.

Mondal, R., Biswas, S., Chatterjee, A., Mishra, R., Mukhopadhyay, A., Bhadra, R.K., Mukhopadhyay, P.K., 2016. Protection against arsenic-induced hematological and hepatic anomalies by supplementation of vitamin C and vitamin E in adult male rats. J. Basic Clin. Physiol. Pharmacol. 27 (6), 643–652.

Mostafavi-Pour, Z., Arianfar, F., Khademi, F., Zal, F., 2019. Altered antioxidant enzymes activity in Csa-treated HepG2 cells in the presence of vitamin E and in the combination with quercetin. Clin. Chim. Acta 493, S711–S729.

Mouzaki, M., Allard, J., 2012. Non-alcoholic steatohepatitis: the therapeutic challenge of a global epidemic. Ann. Gastroenterol. 25, 207–217.

Nagashimada, M., Ota, T., 2019. Role of vitamin E in nonalcoholic fatty liver disease. IUBMB 71 (4), 516–522.

Nan, Y.-M., Wu, W.-J., Fu, N., Liang, B.-L., Wang, R.-Q., Li, L.-X., Zhao, S.-X., Zhao, J.-M., Yu, J., 2009. Antioxidants vitamin E and 1-aminobenzotriazole prevent experimental non-alcoholic steatohepatitis in mice. Scand. J. Gastroenterol. 44 (9), 1121–1131.

Okamura, Y., Omori, A., Asada, N., Ono, A., 2018. Effects of vitamin C and E on toxic action of alcohol on partial hepatectomy-induced liver regeneration in rats. J. Clin. Biochem. Nutr. 63 (1), 50–57.

Oliveira, C.P.M.S., da Costa Gayotto, L.C., Tatai, C., Nina, B.I.D., Lima, E.S., Abdalla, D.S.P., Lopasso, F.P., Laurindo, F.R.M., Carrilho, F.J., 2003. Vitamin C and vitamin E in prevention of nonalcoholic fatty liver disease (NAFLD) in choline deficient diet fed rats. Nutr. J. 2 (9), 5.

Papandreou, D., Andreou, E., 2015. Role of diet on non-alcoholic fatty liver disease: an updated narrative review. World J. Hepatol. 7 (3), 575–582.

Perumpail, B.J., Li, A.A., John, N., Sallam, S., Shah, N.D., Kwong, W., Cholankeril, G., Kim, D., Ahmed, A., 2018. The role of vitamin E in the treatment of NAFLD. Disease 6 (86). https://doi.org/10.3390/diseases6040086.

Prathibha, P., Rejitha, S., Harikrishnan, R., Das, S.S., Abhilash, P.A., Indira, M., 2013. Additive effect of alpha-tocopherol and ascorbic acid in combating ethanol-induced hepatic fibrosis. Redox Rep. 18, 36–46.

Presa, N., Clugston, R.D., Lingrell, S., Kelly, S.E., Merrill Jr., A.H., Jana, S., Kassiri, Z., Gomez-Munoz, A., Vance, D.E., Jacobs, R.L., van der Veen, J.N., 2019. Vitamin E alleviates non-alcoholic fatty liver disease in phosphaditylethanolamine N-methyltransferase deficient mice. Biochim. Biophys. Acta (BBA) – Mol. Basis Dis. 1865, 14–25.

Roth, C.L., Elfers, C.T., Figlewicz, D.P., Melhorn, S.J., Morton, G.J., Hoofnagle, A., Yeh, M.M., Nelson, J.E., Kowdley, K.V., 2012. Vitamin D deficiency in obese rats exacerbates nonalcoholic fatty liver disease and increases hepatic resistin and toll-like receptor activation. Hepatology 55, 1103–1111.

Sanyal, A.J., Chalasani, N., Kowdley, K.V., McCullough, A., Diehl, A.M., Bass, N.M., Neuschwander-Tetri, B.A., Lavine, J.E., Tonascia, J., Unalp, A., Natta, M.V., Clark, J., Brunt, E.M., Kleiner, D.E., Hoofnagle, J.H., Robuck, P.R., 2010. Pioglitazone, vitamin E, or placebo for nonalcoholic steatohepatitis. N. Engl. J. Med. 362, 1675–1685.

Shalan, M.G., Mostafa, M.S., Hassouna, M.M., El-Nabi, S.E.H., El-Refaie, A., 2005. Amelioration of lead toxicity on rat liver with vitamin C and silymarin supplements. Toxicology 206, 1–15.

Sharifi, N., Amani, R., Hajiani, E., Cheraghian, B., 2014. Does vitamin D improve liver enzymes, oxidative stress, and inflammatory biomarkers in adults with non-alcoholic fatty liver disease? A randomized clinical trial. Endocrine 47, 70–80.

Simon, V., Sreerag, K.V., Sasikumar, R., Kanthlal, S.K., 2019. *In vitro* protective effect of ascorbic acid against antibiotic induced hepatotoxicity. Curr. Drug Discov. Technol. 16, 1–8.

Singh, S., Rana, S.V.S., 2010. Ascorbic acid improves mitochondrial function in liver of arsenic-treated rat. Toxicol. Ind. Health 26 (5), 265–272.

Skaaby, T., Husemoen, L.L.N., Borglykke, A., Jorgensen, T., Thuesen, B.H., Pisinger, C., Schmidt, L.E., Linneberg, A., 2014. Vitamin D status, liver enzymes, and incident liver disease and mortality: a general population study. Endocrine 47, 213–220.

Sriram, P., Venkateswaran, A., Malar, V., Thinakar, M., 2018. Association between serum 25-hydroxyvitamin D deficiency and hepatic encephalopathy in chronic liver disease. J. Clin. Exp. Hepatol. 8 (S1), S71.

Stellavato, A., Pirozzi, A.V.A., de Novellis, F., Scognamiglio, I., Vassalo, V., Giori, A.M., De Rosa, M., Schiraldi, C., 2018. *In vitro* assessment of nutraceutical compounds and novel nutraceutical formulations in a liver-steatosis-based model. Lipids Health Dis. 17 (24), 11.

Su, M., Guo, C., Liu, M., Liang, X., Yang, B., 2019a. Therapeutics targets of vitamin C on liver injury and associated biological mechanisms: a study of network pharmacology. Int. Immunopharmacol. 66, 383–387.

Su, M., Liang, X., Xu, X., Wu, X., Yang, B., 2019b. Hepatoprotective benefits of vitamin C against perfluorooctanensulfonate-induced liver damage in mice through suppressing inflammatory reaction and ER stress. Environ. Toxicol. Pharmacol. 65, 60–65.

Talpur, M., Palli, A.Y., Qureshi, S.S., 2017. Drug induced liver injury; role of ascorbic acid in a laboratory animal. Professional Med. J. 24 (11), 1697–1701.

Tavakoli, H., Rostami, H., Avan, A., Bagheriya, M., Ferns, G.A., Khayyatzadeh, S.S., Ghayour-Mobarhan, M., 2019. High dose vitamin D supplementation is associated with an improvement in serum markers of liver function. IUBMB 45 (3), 335–342.

Uzunhisarcikli, M., Kalender, Y., 2011. Protective effects of vitamins C and E against hepatotoxicity induced by methyl parathion in rats. Ecotoxicol. Environ. Saf. 74, 2112–2118.

Wahlang, B., McClain, C., Barve, S., Gobejishvaili, L., 2018. Role of cAMP and phosphodiesterase signaling in liver health and disease. Cell. Signal. 49, 105–115.

Wei, J., Lei, G.-H., Fu, L., Zeng, C., Yang, T., Peng, S.-F., 2016. Association between dietary vitamin C intake and non-alcoholic fatty liver disease: a cross-sectional study among middle-aged and older adults. PLoS One 11 (1). https://doi.org/10.1371/journal.pone.0147985.

Wimalawansa, S.J., 2018. Associations of vitamin D with insulin resistance, obesity, type 2 diabetes, and metabolic syndrome. J. Steroid Biochem. Mol. Biol. 175, 177–189.

Xiaoqiang, G., Wenjie, L., Qiliang, X., Hui, D., Caiyun, Z., Yanzhong, C., Xianglin, D., 2010. Vitamin C protective role for alcoholic liver disease in mice through regulating iron metabolism. Toxicol. Ind. Health 27 (4), 341–348.

Xu, P., Li, Y., Yu, Z., Yang, L., Shang, R., Yan, Z., 2019. Protective effect of vitamin C on triptolide-induced acute hepatotoxicity in mice through mitigation of oxidative stress. An. Acad. Bras. Cienc. 91 (2), e20181257.

Zhang, A., Wang, Y., Xie, H., Zheng, S., 2007. Calcitriol inhibits hepatocyte apoptosis in rat allograft by regulating apoptosis-associated genes. Int. Immunopharmacol. 7, 1122–1128.

Zhang, J., Song, W., Sun, Y., Shan, A., 2017. Effects of phoxim-induced hepatotoxicity on SD rats and the protection of vitamin E. Environ. Sci. Pollut. Res. 24, 24916–24927.

Zhong, X., Zheng, M., Bian, H., Zhong, C., Xiao, F., 2017. An evaluation of the protective role of vitamin C in reactive oxygen species-induced hepatotoxicity due to hexavalent chromium *in vitro* and *in vivo*. J. Occup. Med. Toxicol. 12 (15). https://doi.org/10.1186/s12995-017-0161-x.

Influence of other nutrients (e.g., L-arginine, taurine, and choline) on liver diseases

Jaime López-Cervantes, Dalia I. Sánchez-Machado, Olga N. Campas-Baypoli, Ernesto U. Cantú-Soto, and Gabriela Servín de la Mora-López
Sonora Institute of Technology, Ciudad Obregon, Sonora, Mexico

11.1 Introduction

The liver is the central organ of metabolism with functions that include protein synthesis, nutrient metabolism, and detoxification (Miyazaki and Matsuzaki, 2014). It also regulates the production, storage, and release of sugar, fat, and cholesterol (Wu et al., 2013).

Nonalcoholic fatty liver disease is the most common liver disease, and its prevalence continues to increase in tandem with obesity (Vernon et al., 2011). It is characterized by the accumulation of triglycerides in hepatocytes (Murakami, 2015).

Liver cancer is the fourth-leading cause of cancer death worldwide. Risk factors include chronic hepatitis C virus or hepatitis B virus infection, excessive alcohol consumption, diabetes, and nonalcoholic fatty liver disease (El-Serag, 2020).

Taurine is considered a conditionally essential nutrient due to its physiological functions; however, it is maintained in abundance in the liver (Miyazaki and Matsuzaki, 2014). Likewise, choline is a conditionally essential nutrient because endogenous biosynthesis is not sufficient to protect the liver from fat accumulation, especially in postmenopausal women (Yu et al., 2014). Arginine is an amino acid that is involved in liver detoxification by neutralizing ammonia, so it can be included in the treatment of liver diseases such as liver cirrhosis and fatty liver (Al-Dalaen et al., 2016).

In liver diseases, a decrease in the taurine content of the liver has been found. Therefore, in the body, there is less protection against oxidative stress and toxins as well as the absence of conjugation of bile acids (Miyazaki and Matsuzaki, 2014). According to Zhang et al. (2014), taurine has a protective effect against hepatotoxicity induced by chemical agents. In addition, it stabilizes biological membranes by acting as an antioxidant and eliminating reactive oxygen species (ROS).

The liver is responsible for the metabolism of choline, where it is found as phosphatidylcholine. To date, the mechanisms that explain the effects of choline on the liver from the accumulation of fat in the liver to hepatocellular carcinomas have been identified (Corbin and Zeisel, 2012). It has also been found that the incidence of fatty liver is higher in people with diets deficient in choline.

Therefore, finding safe hepatoprotective nutrients with therapeutic potential could have great clinical value (Heidari et al., 2015). In this review, we summarize the recent scientific findings that examine the hepatic functions of arginine, taurine, and choline as conditionally essential nutrients, highlighting the clinical implications in animals and humans.

11.2 Liver diseases

Hepatocellular carcinoma occurs after liver diseases such as hepatitis B or C, toxic chemical agents, alcoholism, or metabolic dysregulation (Sen et al., 2015). Other risk factors for this carcinoma are alcoholic or nonalcoholic liver disease. In addition, active liver damage to myofibroblasts leads to fibrosis, inflammation, oxidative stress, and cirrhosis. Therefore, in this microenvironment, mutations that lead to tumorigenesis are favored.

Liver disease, known as alcoholic fatty liver disease (AFLD), is one of the most well-known consequences of alcohol abuse (Ventura-Cots et al., 2019). In addition, it is responsible for 60% of cirrhosis in North America and Europe. In the mid-20th century, alcohol was identified as a hepatotoxin, and the first response to alcohol consumption is the accumulation of fat (Goh and Morgan, 2017). After the accumulation of fat, inflammation and scars, called fibrosis, have been found in the liver. When the disease progresses, lesions are called cirrhosis, and the liver has the highest degree of fibrosis. Alcoholic liver disease treatment includes alcohol withdrawal and some specific pharmacological treatments (Rosato et al., 2016).

The most common liver disease in the Western world is nonalcoholic fatty liver disease (NAFLD). This is characterized by the accumulation of fat within the liver in individuals who do not have a significant consumption of alcohol (Bashiardes et al., 2016). Its clinical and pathological manifestations cannot be differentiated from those developed in alcoholic patients (Martín-Domínguez et al., 2013). Obesity and type II diabetes mellitus have been associated with nonalcoholic fatty liver disease. The latter two are related to insulin resistance, glucose intolerance, and hypertriglyceridemia. Patients with this disease, with and without being overweight, progress slowly from fatty liver and liver fibrosis to cirrhosis and hepatocellular carcinoma (Wieland et al., 2015). Insulin resistance and oxidative stress have been proposed as the mechanisms responsible for the accumulation of fat (Bugianesi et al., 2004). For Carbone et al. (2016), there are no proven pharmacological treatments for nonalcoholic fatty liver disease. Currently, evidence has been found that both macronutrients and micronutrients are linked to the development and treatment of this liver disease (Mouzaki and Allard, 2012). Specifically, among the components of the diet that are linked to the disease are carbohydrates, fat in general, fructose, polyunsaturated fatty acids, choline, vitamin E, vitamin C, and minerals.

For both alcoholic and nonalcoholic liver diseases, nutritional therapy and physical exercise can improve patient survival and reverse other specific pathologies.

Hepatic lesions caused by drugs are the main cause of acute or chronic hepatic insufficiency. The diagnosis of these lesions is by exclusion and is performed by eliminating the common causes of liver diseases such as alcoholic hepatitis, metabolic and genetic liver diseases, and hepatitis A, B, and C virus infections (Davern et al., 2011). In the pathogenesis of hepatic drug-induced diseases, the cellular biochemistry or the immune response is altered by the original drug or its metabolites. Drug metabolism occurs in the liver, which determines its susceptibility to lesions induced by chemical agents (Kaplowitz, 2004). In addition, this susceptibility can be modified by age, gender, environment, and genetic factors. In Asian countries, more than 50% of cases of hepatic insufficiency are caused by herbal or dietary supplements (Leise et al., 2014). Most of these liver disorders decrease when treatments with herbal drugs or supplements cease.

11.3 Arginine

11.3.1 Structural characteristics and metabolism

Structurally, arginine is a diamino monocarboxylic amino acid called 2-amino-5-guanidino-pentanoic acid. It has been classified as a conditionally essential amino acid in infants, growing children, and adults with dysfunctions of the small intestine and kidney. However, in healthy adults, it is a nonessential amino acid due to its endogenous synthesis, which is sufficient to maintain muscle mass and connective tissue. Arginine is available in meat, nuts, wheat germ, and dairy products. The maximum intake of arginine with a typical diet is 5 g/day. Lüneburg et al. (2011) reported the plasma levels of L-arginine and the L-arginine:dimethylarginine (ADMA) ratio and pointed out that these reference limits allow us to know the nutritional status of people at risk of cardiovascular disease.

Arginine can be synthesized in the liver by the ornithine cycle and in the kidney from citrulline (Correa et al., 2014). The metabolic pathways of arginine produce polyamines, glutamate, proline, nitric oxide (NO), creatine phosphate, and other molecules with pharmacological actions in various body systems (Stechmiller et al., 2005).

11.3.2 Functional links with the liver

According to Wu et al. (2013), in the healthy liver, approximately 80% of the amino acids required by the body, including arginine, are produced. However, during the stages of growth or tissue repair, the dietary contribution of arginine is insufficient, and endogenous synthesis in the liver is essential. In patients with a liver transplant or liver injuries, there is arginine deficiency due to its hydrolysis caused by plasma arginase (Buijs et al., 2012).

This amino acid is a dietary alternative for improving the metabolic syndrome and hepatic and cardiovascular changes (Alam et al., 2013). It has been suggested that arginine reduces multiorgan damage caused by metabolic syndrome because endothelial NO limits inflammation stimulated by insulin resistance (Alam et al., 2013).

Arginine influences wound healing, endothelial and immune function, hormone secretion, and insulin sensitivity (Tong and Barbul, 2004). In addition, because it stimulates several hormones, arginine participates in the regulation of the metabolism of fatty acids, amino acids, proteins, and glucose (Buijs et al., 2012).

11.3.3 Evidence of hepatoprotective functions

Recently, there has been an increase in studies that relate dietary supplementation with arginine and liver lesions in experimental animals. Rishi et al. (2011) found that *Lactobacillus plantarum* directs the metabolism of arginine to the production of polyamines, with a synergistic effect against hepatic lesions in rats. Wu et al. (2013) reported that treatment with arginine improves liver health in piglets.

Arginine supplementation and exercise training improve hepatic and renal lesions in rats with myocardial infarction due to reduced oxidative stress (Ranjbar et al., 2018). In this trial, male rats were divided into groups combining exercise and drinking water supplemented with 4% arginine. In all groups, tissue oxidative stress and functional indices of the liver were measured.

Abdelhalim et al. (2018) confirmed that arginine and quercetin antioxidants protect hepatocytes from damage by oxidative stress caused by gold nanoparticles. Elbassuoni et al. (2018) demonstrated in experimental animals that sodium monoglutamate causes oxidative damage in the liver and kidneys as well as alterations in body weight. These authors also found that arginine and vitamin D restore lesions in the liver and suppress the increase in food intake that increases body weight. This was confirmed through histological exams and the analysis of markers of oxidative stress. Al-Dalaen et al. (2016) reported that in rats, arginine has protective and curative effects against lipid peroxidation induced by CCl_4, oxidative stress, and liver damage. Methotrexate is a drug for the treatment of cancer with possible side effects. Ashour et al. (2016), in a trial with albino rats, concluded that arginine protects the liver from methotrexate hepatotoxicity due to its antioxidant activity.

Li et al. (2012) indicate that arginine supplementation decreases morphological and functional lesions of the liver of weaned pigs. Hepatic lesions were induced by the injection of lipopolysaccharides of *Escherichia coli,* and the effects of arginine were evaluated for their antiinflammatory activity.

Alam et al. (2013), in a study with rats, found that oral supplementation with arginine decreases the changes associated with obesity in the liver because it reduces oxidative stress and inflammation when feeding is rich in fats and carbohydrates. In rats, the accumulation of lipids in the liver and the lipid profile in plasma decreased.

Reports of clinical trials with arginine supplementation in humans are limited with reference to those with various experimental animals. At the same time, there are many animal trials that report the benefits of arginine to reduce obesity. McKnight et al. (2010) noted that arginine supplementation can reduce obesity in humans by promoting fat loss and reducing the increase in white adipose tissue. They also indicate that this supplementation favors the development of brown adipose tissue due to the production of molecular signaling molecules such as nitric oxide and polyamides, among others. This is complemented by an increase in the expression of genes that contribute to the oxidation of glucose and fatty acids.

Niu et al. (2012), through a clinical study, found that the metabolism of histidine and arginine is abnormal in obese women, and both amino acids are closely related to oxidative stress and inflammation. This is attributed to the fact that arginine increases antioxidant capacity in obese humans, as was previously reported in a human study by Lucotti et al. (2006).

According to Bi'e Tan et al. (2012), there are currently molecular and biochemical mechanisms that explain the relationship of arginine with the metabolism of energy substrates; however, more clinical evidence is needed to support its benefits.

11.4 Taurine

11.4.1 Chemical structure and biological functions

Structurally, taurine is 2-aminoethane sulfonic acid and it is a nonprotein amino acid with many vital functions in physiological processes. It is synthesized endogenously from cysteine and methionine in the kidney, liver, and white adipose tissue (Craig, 2004). In the liver, taurine is synthesized because it is required for the conjugation of bile acids (Murakami, 2015).

Taurine is the most abundant amino acid with approximately 0.1% of body weight in humans (Murakami, 2015). Fish and shellfish are the main sources of taurine. Therefore, in some epidemiological studies, it has been found that there is a lower incidence of hypertension, obesity, and other metabolic diseases when people include large amounts of seafood in their diet.

For humans, it is considered a conditionally essential nutrient. Therefore, cells lacking taurine present certain pathologies (Schaffer and Kim, 2018). Thus, nutritional supplements with taurine prevent metabolic disorders such as obesity, insulin resistance, and atherosclerosis (Gentile et al., 2011). For its therapeutic actions, taurine is being added to energy drinks and infant milk as a nutritional supplement.

According to Heidari et al. (2015), many physiological and pharmacological properties can be attributed to taurine. Recently, it has been reported that taurine has cytoprotective action due to its antioxidant activity, regulation of energy metabolism, attenuation of endoplasmic reticulum stress, neuromodulator activity, and calcium modulation (Schaffer and Kim, 2018).

Its antioxidant function is due to its ability to stabilize membranes, eliminate ROS, and reduce the production of final products of lipid peroxidation (Başaran-Küçükgergin et al., 2016). Taurine decreases the damage caused by oxygen free radicals, so it is recognized as a free radical scavenger (Zhang et al., 2014).

Likewise, it has been shown that taurine attenuates steatosis and hepatotoxicity in model animals (Abdel-Moneim et al., 2015). In addition, in liver cirrhosis due to nonalcoholic fatty liver, it has been reported that taurine levels decrease.

In relation to its hepatic functions, taurine improves the flow of bile, increases the production of bile acid, and prevents cholestasis (Lourenco and Camilo, 2002).

11.4.2 Potential effects as a therapeutic agent

Batista et al. (2013) demonstrated that taurine supplementation prevents obesity and improves glucose levels in adult mice fed high-fat diets. In a trial with rats fed a diet rich in sucrose and mice injected with tunicamycin as a stress inducer, Gentile et al. (2011) found that dietary supplementation with taurine offers significant potential in the preventive treatment of nonalcoholic fatty liver disease. Fukuda et al. (2011) reported that taurine reduces the hepatic and serum concentrations of cholesterol esters, which improves hypercholesterolemia and the development of fatty liver caused by the consumption of diets rich in cholesterol in rats.

Wu et al. (2015) concluded that taurine accelerates lipid metabolism in the liver of rats, so it acts as a preventive and curative agent of liver damage caused by alcohol consumption. In another study, Wu et al. (2017) found that taurine inhibits the activation of Kupffer cells induced by lipopolysaccharides in rats with alcoholic liver disease. Because taurine maintains its structure and intestinal osmotic pressure, it reduces the release of lipopolysaccharides from the intestine. Additionally, taurine decreases the synthesis and release of inflammatory cytokines that damage the liver. In another study with rats, Wu et al. (2018) reported that taurine decreases the apoptosis of hepatocytes exposed to alcohol via mitochondrial pathways. In addition, it improves the antioxidant capacity of hepatocytes by protecting them from alcohol damage.

Liu et al. (2017) investigated the effect of taurine on liver damage caused by lipopolysaccharides in rats. Initially, the animals were pretreated with taurine by intravenous injection. They were then administered a solution with lipopolysaccharides by intraperitoneal injection. In the plasma, indicators of liver damage were quantified, such as proinflammatory cytokines and superoxide dismutase activity. Finally, the authors found that taurine increases antioxidant and antiinflammatory capacity, thus preventing liver damage caused by lipopolysaccharides.

At present, it is known that the hepatic taurine concentration decreases in hepatic lesions induced by xenobiotics and in some liver diseases. Başaran-Küçükgergin et al. (2016) reported that taurine improves hepatic lesions in rats due to the reduction of oxidative stress caused by chemical agents such as *N*-diethylnitrosamine.

Heidari et al. (2015) studied hepatic lesions induced by sulfasalazine and taurine as hepatoprotective agents in rats. The results of the trial revealed the therapeutic properties of taurine. In addition, oxidative stress was proposed as a mechanism for these hepatic lesions because they found significant quantities of reactive oxygen species and lipid peroxidation.

Heidari et al. (2016) designed a trial to evaluate the effect of taurine in models of liver damage and hyperammonemia. Thioacetamine and acetaminophen were used to induce liver damage in rats, in which a high level of ammonia was found in the brain and blood. These authors confirmed that taurine is effective in preserving liver function and preventing hyperammonemia. Jamshidzadeh et al. (2017) presented taurine as a therapeutic drug against ammonia toxicity in hepatic encephalopathy.

Zhang et al. (2014) reported that taurine supplementation improves liver function and inhibits hepatocyte apoptosis in mice overloaded with iron. In the trial, it was found that taurine reduces hepatic oxidative stress, decreases lipid peroxidation, increases the activity of antioxidant enzymes, and reduces glutathione levels. Thus, taurine decreases the toxicity of iron in the liver.

11.4.3 Clinical studies linked to liver diseases

Compared to studies with experimental animals, there are few clinical studies with humans on the effects of taurine in liver disease (Table 11.1).

In the liver, taurine is produced in response to paracetamol poisoning. To test this hypothesis, Ghandforoush-Sattari and Mashayekhi (2008) investigated the correlation between the concentration of taurine and biomarkers of liver damage in plasma in three groups of patients. Hu et al. (2008) studied the benefits of dietary taurine in liver function in patients with chronic hepatitis. Rosa et al. (2014) evaluated the inflammatory response and modulation of oxidative stress in obese women supplemented with taurine because chronic inflammation in adipose tissue and the liver has been linked to obesity. Taurine is safe and effective for the treatment of muscle cramps in people with cirrhosis (Vidot et al., 2018).

Table 11.1: Human clinical studies of the influence of taurine in liver diseases.

Reference/study	Subjects/study design	Conclusions
Ghandforoush-Sattari and Mashayekhi (2008) Evaluation of taurine as a biomarker of liver damage in paracetamol poisoning	217 Patients poisoned with paracetamol (mean 26.4 ± 1.6 mg/L). 100 Patients not poisoned with paracetamol (mean 18.1 ± 1.1 mg/L). 90 Healthy subjects (mean 5.6 ± 0.2 mg/L).	The plasma taurine concentration may be a marker of hepatic damage from paracetamol overdose. In addition, taurine is stable, easy to measure, and does not rise transiently.
Hu et al. (2008) Dietary amino acid taurine ameliorates liver injury in chronic hepatitis patients	Men and women with chronic hepatitis and with high levels of ALT or AST. Treatment group (mean age 58 years and mean weight of 63 kg): the patients took 2 g of taurine three times a day for 3 months, and the fourth month without taurine. Control group treatment (58 years of average age and average weight of 59 kg): patients took placebo without taurine for 4 months.	Taurine can improve liver injury caused by viruses in patients with chronic hepatitis because plasma ALT and AST activity decreased significantly at the end of treatment.
Rosa et al. (2014) Oxidative stress and inflammation in obesity after taurine supplementation: a double-blind, placebo-controlled study	16 Obese women (47 kg/m^2) and 8 women in the normal weight range (21 kg/m^2). Obese patients formed two groups of 8 people, one group received 3 g of taurine/day and the other 3 g of starch/day for 8 weeks. Nutritional assessment and quantification of sulfur amino acids, insulin, adiponectin, markers of inflammatory response, and oxidative stress in plasma were performed.	Supplementation with taurine decreases inflammation and lipid peroxidation markers in obese women.
Vidot et al. (2018) Randomized clinical trial: oral taurine supplementation versus placebo reduces muscle cramps in patients with chronic liver disease	Patients with cirrhosis and at least three cramps per week. They were given stepwise oral supplementation to prevent gastrointestinal effects.	In patients with chronic liver disease, supplementation with taurine reduces the frequency, duration, and intensity of muscle cramps.

Alanine aminotransferase (ALT) or aspartate aminotransferase (AST).

11.5 Choline

11.5.1 Its metabolites and dietary sources

Choline is classified as a B complex vitamin and has been referred to as vitamin J. This vitamin is a very stable molecule during food preparation or storage (Fennema, 2008).

Structurally, choline is a quaternary amine with a positive charge. It can be found free, phosphorylated, oxidized, and acetylated. It is essential for the synthesis of acetylcholine, which acts as a neurotransmitter, of the phospholipids of cellular membranes, and of lipid transporters as plasma lipoproteins (Al Rajabi et al., 2014). The oxidized form of choline is known as betaine and is a trimethylglycine that acts as a donor of methyl groups in the methionine cycle (Zeisel and da Costa, 2009).

There are many foods that are sources of choline. According to the USDA database (2008), the highest content of choline belongs to whole eggs, followed in descending order by meat-fish, whole grains, breakfast cereals, vegetables-fruits, milk, and fats-oils (Table 11.2). Eggs

Table 11.2: Main dietary sources of choline.

Description	mg choline/100 g of food	
	Free choline	Total choline
Whole eggs		
Egg, whole, cooked, fried	0.7	270
Egg, whole, cooked, hard boiled	0.7	230
Meat and fish		
Chicken, liver, all classes, cooked, pan-fried	69	330
Turkey, liver, all classes, cooked, simmered	9.7	220
Pork, cured, bacon, cooked, baked	12	120
Beef, choice, cooked, grilled	0.7	100
Fish, salmon, Atlantic, farmed, cooked, dry heat	7.8	91
Fish, tilapia, cooked, dry heat	21	83
Turkey, gizzard, all classes, cooked, simmered	9.5	82
Chicken, broilers and fryers, meat only, roasted	5.7	79
Pork sausage, fresh, cooked	7.1	67
Whole grains		
Quinoa	38	70
Amaranth	37	70
Breakfast cereal		
Cereals ready-to-eat, Kellogg's All-Bran Original	26	49
Cereals ready-to-eat, Kellogg's Special K	12	31
Cereals ready-to-eat, General Mills, Cheerios	4.4	26
Vegetables and fruits		
Broccoli, cooked, boiled, drained, without salt	8.5	40
Potatoes, red, flesh and skin, baked	8.5	19
Bananas, raw	3.2	9.8
Carrots, raw	6.8	8.8
Oranges, raw, navel	4.7	8.4
Melons, cantaloupe, raw	4.1	7.6
Tomatoes, red, ripe, raw, year-round average	4.4	6.7
Milk		
Milk, fluid, 1% milkfat, with added vitamin A	4	18
Yogurt, fruit variety, nonfat	3.3	16
Milk, whole, 3.25% milkfat	3.7	14

are the main source of phospholipids in the Western diet, including phosphatidylcholine, phosphatidylethanolamine, sphingomyelin, and phosphatidylinositol (Blesso, 2015). However, foods rich in choline contain a large amount of cholesterol or fats and are avoided by many people, which can lead to choline deficiencies.

The liver is the central organ responsible for the metabolism of choline, and choline influences liver function. The accumulation of fat in the liver and damage to liver cells occur when humans consume diets with low choline content (Fan and Cao, 2013). The adequate intake of choline is a function of the age and gender of individuals, for example, for children (250 mg/d), men (550 mg/d), female adolescents (400 mg/d), and adult women (425 mg) (IOM, 1998). Some researchers have reported that choline requirements vary among people according to their genetic characteristics, gender, and the composition of the intestinal microbiota (Corbin and Zeisel, 2012).

Bacteria can obtain phosphatidylcholine for their cell walls from endogenous or exogenous choline-based synthesis (Spencer et al., 2011). In addition, da Costa et al. (2006) reported that certain common genetic polymorphisms influence the susceptibility of some people to develop liver disease by eating diets deficient in choline.

It has been concluded that the dietary requirement of choline is modulated by estrogens and by single nucleotide polymorphisms in specific genes of choline and folate metabolism (Corbin and Zeisel, 2012). Therefore, the decrease in choline consumption is significantly associated with increased fibrosis in postmenopausal women with nonalcoholic fatty liver disease (NAFLD) (Fan and Cao, 2013). When the contribution of choline decreases, choline is recycled in the liver and redistributed from the kidney, lung, and intestine to return to the liver and brain (Li and Vance, 2008).

11.5.2 Aspects of its metabolism

Choline is synthesized in the bodies of humans and mammals, but some evidence suggests that it should be provided by the diet. Dietary choline is absorbed in the intestine, and uptake is carried out by choline transporters. In cells, choline is phosphorylated to become phosphatidylcholine, which is the most abundant phospholipid in cell membranes (Al Rajabi et al., 2014). Likewise, choline can be oxidized to betaine in some cells, such as hepatocytes. Both choline and betaine participate in the donation of methyl groups to form methionine. Additionally, betaine participates in the synthesis of methionine from homocysteine and restores the levels of S-adenosyl methionine, which plays essential roles in the metabolism of phospholipids and the structure of the membrane (Başaran-Küçükgergin et al., 2016). Phosphatidylcholine is necessary for the packaging and secretion of triglycerides in very low-density lipoproteins and for the solubilization of bile salts (Corbin and Zeisel, 2012).

The intestinal microbiota can metabolize choline to trimethylamine (TMA), which in the liver is oxidized by the action of monooxygenases and forms trimethylamine N-oxide (TMAO). TMAO influences lipid absorption, cholesterol homeostasis, glucose modulation, and lipid metabolism by decreasing the size of bile acids (Chen et al., 2016).

High-fat diets lead to the formation of intestinal microbiota that convert choline from the diet into methylamines, reducing circulating levels of phosphatidylcholine in the plasma to produce similar effects of diets deficient in choline and causing nonalcoholic fatty liver disease. This deficiency of choline induced by the microbiota results in an accumulation of triglycerides in hepatocytes (Schnabl and Brenner, 2014).

11.5.3 Clinical evidence of the effect on liver health

The effects of choline on the liver vary from fatty liver to hepatocellular carcinoma. It has been reported that the mechanisms involved in these liver diseases involve the abnormal synthesis of phospholipids, failures in the secretion of lipoproteins, oxidative damage caused by alterations in the mitochondria, and stress in the endoplasmic reticulum (Corbin and Zeisel, 2012).

There are few clinical studies with humans that associate choline-deficient diets with liver and fatty liver damage (Chen et al., 2016). Spencer et al. (2011) associated the composition of microbial communities in the human gastrointestinal tract with choline levels. The group of adult and healthy women who participated in the study received controlled diets while the levels of choline supplementation varied. These authors found that the bacterial levels of *Gammaproteobacteria* and *Erysipelotrichia* are associated with changes in the amount of liver fat in patients with choline deficiency.

Chen et al. (2016) related the presence and severity of nonalcoholic fatty liver disease (NAFLD) with the content of trimethylamine N-oxide, choline, and betaine in the blood. The study included Chinese adults with NAFLD and a control group in a hospital. In another group, adults from the community were included. The authors found adverse associations between the level of trimethylamine and the presence and severity of NAFLD in Chinese hospitals and communities, and for betaine with NAFLD, the association was favorable.

For children, men, and premenopausal women, choline intake does not contribute to the severity of NAFLD. However, in postmenopausal women with NAFLD, decreasing choline intake increases fibrosis. All the above was demonstrated by Guerrerio et al. (2012), who proposed the hypothesis that the limited intake of choline is associated with histological changes in the liver. To do this, they performed a cross-sectional analysis with 664 people, including children, adult men, women 19 years of age, and postmenopausal women. They included data on diet composition and liver biopsies. Premenopausal women and men showed the same trend. They suggest that men have additional mechanisms of genetic regulation for the synthesis of choline that compensate for moderate but not severe deficiencies.

Sha et al. (2010) found that through a directed metabolic profile, it is possible to predict the risk of developing hepatic dysfunction when diets are deficient in choline. To this end, they conducted a clinical study with healthy men and women with body mass indices from 19 to 33 who initially received a reference control diet and then a diet deficient in choline. In addition, the participants were evaluated for liver fat by magnetic resonance spectroscopy. Metabolites that decreased with choline deficiency were betaine, dimethylglycine, sarcosine, methionine, and choline in blood plasma.

Yu et al. (2014) studied the association between nonalcoholic fatty liver and dietary choline ingestion in the general population. The study included nonalcoholic Chinese adult men and women (40–75 years). Dietary frequency questionnaires were administered to determine dietary intake. It was discovered that the main sources of choline were eggs, soy derivatives, red meat, fish, and vegetables. They concluded that when the diet is high in choline, the risk of NAFLD decreases in normal-weight Chinese women.

Based on their research with mice, Al Rajabi et al. (2014) reported that the dietary supply of choline or one of its metabolites improves liver health because the cholesterol metabolism is regulated. Haubert et al. (2015) designed an experiment with rats to study the efficacy of choline and fructo-oligosaccharides in the treatment of NAFLD caused by a diet rich in carbohydrates. All groups of animals received a standard diet, but the diet of one group was supplemented with choline and the diet of another group was supplemented with fructo-oligosaccharides. It was found that both supplements are effective in reducing NAFLD. According to the biochemical analysis, choline increases the vitamin E content, and fructo-oligosaccharides decrease the cholesterol content in blood serum. The measurement of thiobarbituric acid indicates that the treatments had no protection against free radicals.

11.6 Conclusions

According to the evidence consulted, arginine, taurine, and choline have shown protective effects against liver damage due to their antioxidant activity, among other functions attributed to them. This has been shown through various tests with experimental animals and with humans, where it has been sought to understand the mechanisms that relate these nutrients to liver diseases, including obesity, fatty liver, and liver cancer. Dietary supplementation with arginine, taurine, or choline has also been recommended to keep the liver healthy due to its therapeutic effects. However, the therapeutic efficacy of these three nutrients requires more clinical studies with different groups of the population before reaching definitive conclusions.

References

Abdelhalim, M.A.K., Moussa, S.A.A., Qaid, H.A.Y., 2018. The protective role of quercetin and arginine on gold nanoparticles induced hepatotoxicity in rats. Int. J. Nanomedicine 13, 2821–2825.

Abdel-Moneim, A.M., Al-Kahtani, M.A., El-Kersh, M.A., Al-Omair, M.A., 2015. Free radical-scavenging, anti-inflammatory/anti-fibrotic and hepatoprotective actions of taurine and silymarin against CCl_4 induced rat liver damage. PLoS One 10, 1–16.

Al Rajabi, A., Castro, G.S., da Silva, R.P., Nelson, R.C., Thiesen, A., Vannucchi, H., Vine, D.F., Proctor, S.D., Field, C.J., Curtis, J.M., Jacobs, R.L., 2014. Choline supplementation protects against liver damage by normalizing cholesterol metabolism in Pemt/Ldlr knockout mice fed a high-fat diet. J. Nutr. 144, 252–257.

Alam, M.A., Kauter, K., Withers, K., Sernia, C., Brown, L., 2013. Chronic L-arginine treatment improves metabolic, cardiovascular and liver complications in diet-induced obesity in rats. Food Funct. 4, 83–91.

Al-Dalaen, S., Alzyoud, J., Al-Qtaitat, A., 2016. The effects of L-arginine in modulating liver antioxidant biomarkers within carbon tetrachloride induced hepatotoxicity: experimental study in rats. Biomed. Pharmacol. J. 9, 293–298.

Ashour, A., Abdel-Mawla, S., Hassan, S.M., Abd Al-Haleem, E.N., El-Hangoor, S.Z., 2016. Effect of L-arginine on methotrexate induced hepatotoxicity in albino rats. J. Biosci. Appl. Res. 2 (2), 88–99.

Başaran-Küçükgergin, C., Bingül, I., Tekkeşin, M.S., Olgaç, V., Doğru-Abbasoğlu, S., Uysal, M., 2016. Effects of carnosine, taurine, and betaine pretreatments on diethylnitrosamine-induced oxidative stress and tissue injury in rat liver. Toxicol. Ind. Health 32, 1405–1413.

Bashiardes, S., Shapiro, H., Rozin, S., Shibolet, O., Elinav, E., 2016. Non-alcoholic fatty liver and the gut microbiota. Mol. Metab. 5, 782–794.

Batista, T.M., Ribeiro, R.A., da Silva, P.M., Camargo, R.L., Lollo, P.C., Boschero, A.C., Carneiro, E.M., 2013. Taurine supplementation improves liver glucose control in normal protein and malnourished mice fed a high-fat diet. Mol. Nutr. Food Res. 57, 423–434.

Bi'e Tan, X.L., Yin, Y., Wu, Z., Liu, C., Tekwe, C.D., Wu, G., 2012. Regulatory roles for L-arginine in reducing white adipose tissue. Front. Biosci. 17, 2237.

Blesso, C.N., 2015. Egg phospholipids and cardiovascular health. Nutrients 7, 2731–2747.

Bugianesi, E., Marzocchi, R., Villanova, N., Marchesini, G., 2004. Non-alcoholic fatty liver disease/non-alcoholic steatohepatitis (NAFLD/NASH): treatment. Best Pract. Res. Clin. Gastroenterol. 18, 1105–1116.

Buijs, N., Marges, E., Visser, M., van Leeuwen, P.A.M., 2012. Arginina en nutrición especializada. In: Nutrición enteral y parenteral, second ed. McGraw-Hill Interamericana, México, p. 584.

Carbone, L.J., Angus, P.W., Yeomans, N.D., 2016. Incretin-based therapies for the treatment of non-alcoholic fatty liver disease: a systematic review and meta-analysis. J. Gastroenterol. Hepatol. 31, 23–31.

Chen, Y.M., Liu, Y., Zhou, R.F., Chen, X.L., Wang, C., Tan, X.Y., Wang, L.J., Zheng, R.D., Zhang, H.W., Ling, W.H., Zhu, H.L., 2016. Associations of gut-flora-dependent metabolite trimethylamine-N-oxide, betaine and choline with non-alcoholic fatty liver disease in adults. Sci. Rep. 6, 1–9.

Corbin, K.D., Zeisel, S.H., 2012. Choline metabolism provides novel insights into non-alcoholic fatty liver disease and its progression. Curr. Opin. Gastroenterol. 28, 159–165.

Correa, J.M.I., Gutiérrez, C.M.V., Lopera, M.M.V., 2014. Arginine and cancer: implications in the regulation of antitumoral respons. Iatreia 27, 63–72.

Craig, S.A., 2004. Betaine in human nutrition. Am. J. Clin. Nutr. 80 (3), 539–549.

da Costa, K.A., Kozyreva, O.G., Song, J., Galanko, J.A., Fischer, L.M., Zeisel, S.H., 2006. Common genetic polymorphisms affect the human requirement for the nutrient choline. FASEB J. 20, 1336–1344.

Davern, T.J., Chalasani, N., Fontana, R.J., Hayashi, P.H., Protiva, P., Kleiner, D.E., Engle, R.R., Emerson, S.U., Purcell, R.H., Tillmann, H.L., 2011. Acute hepatitis E infection accounts for some cases of suspected drug-induced liver injury. Gastroenterology 141 (5), 1665–1672.

Elbassuoni, E.A., Ragy, M.M., Ahmed, S.M., 2018. Evidence of the protective effect of L-arginine and vitamin D against monosodium glutamate-induced liver and kidney dysfunction in rats. Biomed. Pharmacother. 108, 799–808.

El-Serag, H.B., 2020. Epidemiology of hepatocellular carcinoma. In: The Liver: Biology and Pathobiology. Wiley, pp. 758–772.

Fan, J.G., Cao, H.X., 2013. Role of diet and nutritional management in non-alcoholic fatty liver disease. J. Gastroenterol. Hepatol. 28, 81–87.

Fennema, 2008. Fennema's Food Chemistry, fourth ed. Taylor & Francis Group, Florida.

Fukuda, N., Yoshitama, A., Sugita, S., Fujita, M., Murakami, S., 2011. Dietary taurine reduces hepatic secretion of cholesteryl ester and enhances fatty acid oxidation in rats fed a high-cholesterol diet. J. Nutr. Sci. Vitaminol. 57, 144–149.

Gentile, C.L., Nivala, A.M., Gonzales, J.C., Pfaffenbach, K.T., Wang, D., Wei, Y., Jiang, H., Orlicky, D.J., Petersen, D.R., Pagliassotti, M.J., Maclean, K.N., 2011. Experimental evidence for therapeutic potential of taurine in the treatment of nonalcoholic fatty liver disease. Am. J. Physiol. Regul. Integr. Comp. Physiol. 301, R1710–R1722.

Ghandforoush-Sattari, M., Mashayekhi, S., 2008. Evaluation of taurine as a biomarker of liver damage in paracetamol poisoning. Eur. J. Pharmacol. 581, 171–176.

Goh, E.T., Morgan, M.Y., 2017. Pharmacotherapy for alcohol dependence—the why, the what and the wherefore. Aliment. Pharmacol. Ther. 45 (7), 865–882.

Guerrerio, A.L., Colvin, R.M., Schwartz, A.K., Molleston, J.P., Murray, K.F., Diehl, A., Mohan, P., Schwimmer, J.B., Lavine, J.E., Torbenson, M.S., Scheimann, A.O., 2012. Choline intake in a large cohort of patients with nonalcoholic fatty liver disease. Am. J. Clin. Nutr. 95, 892–900.

Haubert, N.J.B.G.B., Marchini, J.S., Cunha, S.F.C., Suen, V.M.M., Padovan, G.J., Junior, A.A.J., Alves, C.M.M.M., Marchini, J.F.M., Vannucchi, H., 2015. Choline and fructooligosaccharide: non-alcoholic fatty liver disease, cardiac fat deposition, and oxidative stress markers. Nutr. Metab. Insights 8, 1–6.

Heidari, R., Sadeghi, N., Azarpira, N., Niknahad, H., 2015. Sulfasalazine-induced hepatic injury in an ex vivo model of isolated perfused rat liver and the protective role of taurine. Pharm. Sci. 21, 211–219.

Heidari, R., Jamshidzadeh, A., Niknahad, H., Mardani, E., Ommati, M.M., Azarpira, N., Khodaei, F., Zarei, A., Ayarzadeh, M., Mousavi, S., Abdoli, N., Yeganeh, B.S., Saeedi, A., Abdoli, N., 2016. Effect of taurine on chronic and acute liver injury: focus on blood and brain ammonia. Toxicol. Rep. 3, 870–879.

Hu, Y.H., Lin, C.L., Huang, Y.W., Liu, P.E., Hwang, D.F., 2008. Dietary amino acid taurine ameliorates liver injury in chronic hepatitis patients. Amino Acids 35, 469–473.

Institute of Medicine (US) Standing Committee on the Scientific Evaluation of Dietary Reference Intakes, 1998. Dietary Reference Intakes for Thiamin, Riboflavin, Niacin, Vitamin B6, Folate, Vitamin B12, Pantothenic acid, Biotin, and Choline. National Academies Press, US.

Jamshidzadeh, A., Heidari, R., Abasvali, M., Zarei, M., Ommati, M.M., Abdoli, N., Khodaei, F., Yeganeh, Y., Jafari, F., Zarei, A., Latifpour, Z., Mardani, E., Azarpira, N., Asadi, B., Najibi, A., 2017. Taurine treatment preserves brain and liver mitochondrial function in a rat model of fulminant hepatic failure and hyperammonemia. Biomed. Pharmacother. 86, 514–520.

Kaplowitz, N., 2004. Drug-induced liver injury. Clin. Infect. Dis. 38 (2), S44–S48.

Leise, M.D., Poterucha, J.J., Talwalkar, J.A., 2014. Drug-induced liver injury. Mayo Clin. Proc. 89 (1), 95–106.

Li, Z., Vance, D.E., 2008. Thematic review series: glycerolipids. Phosphatidylcholine and choline homeostasis. J. Lipid Res. 49 (6), 1187–1194.

Li, Q., Liu, Y., Che, Z., Zhu, H., Meng, G., Hou, Y., Ding, B., Yin, Y., Chen, F., 2012. Dietary L-arginine supplementation alleviates liver injury caused by *Escherichia coli* LPS in weaned pigs. J. Innate Immun. 18, 804–814.

Liu, Y., Li, F., Zhang, L., Wu, J., Wang, Y., Yu, H., 2017. Taurine alleviates lipopolysaccharide-induced liver injury by anti-inflammation and antioxidants in rats. Mol. Med. Rep. 16, 6512–6517.

Lourenco, R., Camilo, M.E., 2002. Taurine: a conditionally essential amino acid in humans? An overview in health and disease. Nutr. Hosp. 17, 262–270.

Lucotti, P., Setola, E., Monti, L.D., Galluccio, E., Costa, S., Sandoli, E.P., Fermo, I., Rabaiotti, G., Gatti, R., Piatti, P., 2006. Beneficial effects of a long-term oral L-arginine treatment added to a hypocaloric diet and exercise training program in obese, insulin-resistant type 2 diabetic patients. Am. J. Physiol. Endocrinol. Metab. 291 (5), E906–E912.

Lüneburg, N., Xanthakis, V., Schwedhelm, E., Sullivan, L.M., Maas, R., Anderssohn, M., Riederer, U., Glazer, N.L., Vasan, R.S., Böger, R.H., 2011. Reference intervals for plasma L-arginine and the L-arginine: asymmetric dimethylarginine ratio in the Framingham Offspring Cohort. J. Nutr. 141 (12), 2186–2190.

Martín-Domínguez, V., Gonzalez-Casas, R., Mendoza-Jimenez-Ridruejo, J., García-Buey, L., Moreno-Otero, R., 2013. Pathogenesis, diagnosis and treatment of non-alcoholic fatty liver disease. Rev. Esp. Enferm. Dig. 105, 409–420.

McKnight, J.R., Satterfield, M.C., Jobgen, W.S., Smith, S.B., Spencer, T.E., Meininger, C.J., McNeal, C.J., Wu, G., 2010. Beneficial effects of L-arginine on reducing obesity: potential mechanisms and important implications for human health. Amino Acids 39 (2), 349–357.

Miyazaki, T., Matsuzaki, Y., 2014. Taurine and liver diseases: a focus on the heterogeneous protective properties of taurine. Amino Acids 46, 101–110.

Mouzaki, M., Allard, J.P., 2012. The role of nutrients in the development, progression, and treatment of nonalcoholic fatty liver disease. J. Clin. Gastroenterol. 46, 457–467.

Murakami, S., 2015. Role of taurine in the pathogenesis of obesity. Mol. Nutr. Food Res. 59, 1353–1363.

Niu, Y.C., Feng, R.N., Hou, Y., Li, K., Kang, Z., Wang, J., Sun, C.-H., Li, Y., 2012. Histidine and arginine are associated with inflammation and oxidative stress in obese women. Br. J. Nutr. 108 (1), 57–61.

Ranjbar, K., Nazem, F., Sabrinezhad, R., Nazari, A., 2018. Aerobic training and L-arginine supplement attenuates myocardial infarction-induced kidney and liver injury in rats via reduced oxidative stress. Indian Heart J. 70, 538–543.

Rishi, P., Bharrhan, S., Singh, G., Kaur, I.P., 2011. Effect of *Lactobacillus plantarum* and L-arginine against endotoxin-induced liver injury in a rat model. Life Sci. J. 89, 847–853.

Rosa, F.T., Freitas, E.C., Deminice, R., Jordao, A.A., Marchini, J.S., 2014. Oxidative stress and inflammation in obesity after taurine supplementation: a double-blind, placebo-controlled study. Eur. J. Nutr. 53, 823–830.

Rosato, V., Abenavoli, L., Federico, A., Masarone, M., Persico, M., 2016. Pharmacotherapy of alcoholic liver disease in clinical practice. Int. J. Clin. Pract. 70, 119–131.

Schaffer, S., Kim, H.W., 2018. Effects and mechanisms of taurine as a therapeutic agent. Biomol. Ther. 26, 225–241.

Schnabl, B., Brenner, D.A., 2014. Interactions between the intestinal microbiome and liver diseases. Gastroenterology 146, 1513–1524.

Sen, S., Langiewicz, M., Jumaa, H., Webster, N.J., 2015. Deletion of serine/arginine-rich splicing factor 3 in hepatocytes predisposes to hepatocellular carcinoma in mice. Hepatology 61 (1), 171–183.

Sha, W., da Costa, K.A., Fischer, L.M., Milburn, M.V., Lawton, K.A., Berger, A., Jia, W., Zeisel, S.H., 2010. Metabolomic profiling can predict which humans will develop liver dysfunction when deprived of dietary choline. FASEB J. 24, 2962–2975.

Spencer, M.D., Hamp, T.J., Reid, R.W., Fischer, L.M., Zeisel, S.H., Fodor, A.A., 2011. Association between composition of the human gastrointestinal microbiome and development of fatty liver with choline deficiency. Gastroenterology 140, 976–986.

Stechmiller, J.K., Childress, B., Cowan, L., 2005. Arginine supplementation and wound healing. Nutr. Clin. Pract. 20, 52–61.

Tong, B.C., Barbul, A., 2004. Cellular and physiological effects of arginine. Mini-Rev. Med. Chem. 4, 823–832.

United States Department of Agriculture, Agricultural Research Services USDA, 2008. National Nutrient Database for Standard Reference, Release Two. Nutrient Data Laboratory. Web Site: http://www.ars.usda.gov/nutrientdata.

Ventura-Cots, M., Ballester-Ferré, M.P., Ravi, S., Bataller, R., 2019. Public health policies and alcohol-related liver disease. JHEP Rep. 1 (5), 403–413.

Vernon, G., Baranova, A., Younossi, Z.M., 2011. Systematic review: the epidemiology and natural history of non-alcoholic fatty liver disease and non-alcoholic steatohepatitis in adults. Aliment. Pharmacol. Ther. 34, 274–285.

Vidot, H., Cvejic, E., Carey, S., Strasser, S.I., McCaughan, G.W., Allman-Farinelli, M., Shackel, N.A., 2018. Randomised clinical trial: oral taurine supplementation versus placebo reduces muscle cramps in patients with chronic liver disease. Aliment. Pharmacol. Ther. 48, 704–712.

Wieland, A., Frank, D.N., Harnke, B., Bambha, K., 2015. Systematic review: microbial dysbiosis and nonalcoholic fatty liver disease. Aliment. Pharmacol. Ther. 42, 1051–1063.

Wu, X., Xie, C., Yin, Y., Li, F., Li, T., Huang, R., Ruan, Z., Deng, Z., 2013. Effect of L-arginine on HSP70 expression in liver in weanling piglets. BMC Vet. Res. 9, 63.

Wu, G., Tang, R., Yang, J., Tao, Y., Liu, Z., Feng, Y., Lin, S., Yang, Q., Lv, Q., Hu, J., 2015. Taurine accelerates alcohol and fat metabolism of rats with alcoholic fatty liver disease. In: Taurine 9. Springer, Cham, pp. 793–805.

Wu, G., Yang, Q., Yu, Y., Lin, S., Feng, Y., Lv, Q., Yang, J., Hu, J., 2017. Taurine inhibits Kupffer cells activation induced by lipopolysaccharide in alcoholic liver damaged rats. In: Taurine 10. Springer, Dordrecht, pp. 789–800.

Wu, G., Yang, J., Lv, H., Jing, W., Zhou, J., Feng, Y., Lin, S., Yang, Q., Hu, J., 2018. Taurine prevents ethanol-induced apoptosis mediated by mitochondrial or death receptor pathways in liver cells. Amino Acids 50, 863–875.

Yu, D., Shu, X.O., Xiang, Y.B., Li, H., Yang, G., Gao, Y.T., Zheng, W., Zhang, X., 2014. Higher dietary choline intake is associated with lower risk of nonalcoholic fatty liver in normal-weight Chinese women. J. Nutr. 144, 2034–2040.

Zeisel, S.H., Da Costa, K.A., 2009. Choline: an essential nutrient for public health. Nutr. Rev. 67, 615–623.

Zhang, Z., Liu, D., Yi, B., Liao, Z., Tang, L., Yin, D., He, M., 2014. Taurine supplementation reduces oxidative stress and protects the liver in an iron-overload murine model. Mol. Med. 10, 2255–2262.

CHAPTER 12

Antioxidants with hepatoprotective activity

Gökçe Şeker Karatoprak

Department of Pharmacognosy, Faculty of Pharmacy, Erciyes University, Kayseri, Turkey

12.1 Introduction

The liver is a frequent target for many toxic substances as an organ that has an important role in many metabolic functions (Meyer and Kulkarni, 2001). Reactive oxygen metabolites are mainly caused by the peroxidation of lipids, the induction of cytokines and the Fas ligand, and steatohepatitis. Prooxidants in the liver include CYP2E-1 from the cytochrome P450 enzyme system, reactive oxygen metabolites from mitochondria, hydrogen peroxide, mitochondrial or peroxisome-induced hydrogen peroxide, nitroradicals, some Kupffer cell-derived substances, activated neutrophils, and macrophages (Li et al., 2015). However, the main event leading to liver damage is the reduction of the amount of defect-dependent glutathione sulfate (GS) in the mitochondrial uptake system. Free oxygen radicals activate lipid peroxidation by affecting unsaturated fats. Oxidative stress not only causes liver damage, but also has a role in the continuation of the inflammatory event in the liver with various chemokines and cytokines, particularly tumor necrosis factor-alpha (TNF-α) (Cichoz-Lach and Michalak, 2014). Lipid peroxidation and free reactive oxygen species (ROS) decrease the amounts of antioxidants such as beta-carotene, vitamin C, vitamin E, and glutathione (GSH), thus causing the liver to become susceptible to oxidative damage. However, other factors, such as the formation of large amounts of ROS by mitochondria and hepatic iron accumulation, may have roles in increasing oxidative damage in the fatty liver (Meyer and Kulkarni, 2001). Oxidative stress, also known as excessive free radicals and oxidants, is an important parameter in liver ailments. Various antioxidant treatments and antioxidants have been suggested for the prevention and treatment of liver diseases. A number of studies have tested some antioxidants such as vitamin E and C, mitoquinone, *N*-acetylcysteine, polaprezinc, silymarin, and silibinin in the treatment of patients with different liver ailments such as chronic hepatitis C infection, cirrhosis, and nonalcoholic fatty liver disease. In addition, many natural plants have recently been tried in animal models to eliminate hepatic damage, and polyphenols and flavonoids have been reported to be bioactive compounds that eliminate oxidative stress (Li et al., 2015).

Influence of Nutrients, Bioactive Compounds, and Plant Extracts in Liver Diseases. https://doi.org/10.1016/B978-0-12-816488-4.00008-5

12.2 Natural hepatoprotective agents

12.2.1 Ursodeoxycholic acid

Ursodeoxycholic acid (UDCA), which is about 3% of the bile acid pool in humans, is extracted from the gallbladders of bears. Hepatoprotective effects have also been studied because of its worldwide use in the treatment of primary biliary cirrhosis. In a study of children with acute lymphoblastic leukemia, the hepatoprotection efficacy and safety of UDCA in combination with chemotherapy were investigated. The beneficial effect of UDCA has been associated with its cytoprotective, antiapoptotic, membrane stabilizing, antioxidant, and immunomodulatory activity. Also, UDCA has been shown to inhibit hepatic lipid peroxidation in experimental cholestatic liver disease featured by increased OH^- formation. It has been reported that the antioxidant effect of UDCA is associated with the hepatoprotective effects surveyed in this study (Mohammed Saif et al., 2012). The chemical structure of ursodeoxycholic acid is given Fig. 12.1.

12.2.2 Choline

Hepatosteatosis, liver cell damage, and death occur when there is a lack of the essential nutrient choline in humans. A low choline diet results in fatty liver and liver damage. Estrogen and single nucleotide polymorphisms in certain genes of choline and folate metabolism regulate the dietary requirement for choline (Corbin and Steven, 2012). The antioxidant properties of choline with a lipotropic role have been demonstrated in research using C3A cells (human hepatic cells). According to the results of the study, it was determined that choline increased the GSH-Px levels in LOP (lactate, octanoate, and pyruvate-supplemented medium)-treated C3A cells (human hepatocellular carcinoma cells). Choline also showed radical scavenging activity and lipid catabolism-promoting activity under LOP perturbation, which reduced the amount of hepatocellular triglycerides (Zhu et al., 2014). The chemical structure of choline is given in Fig. 12.2.

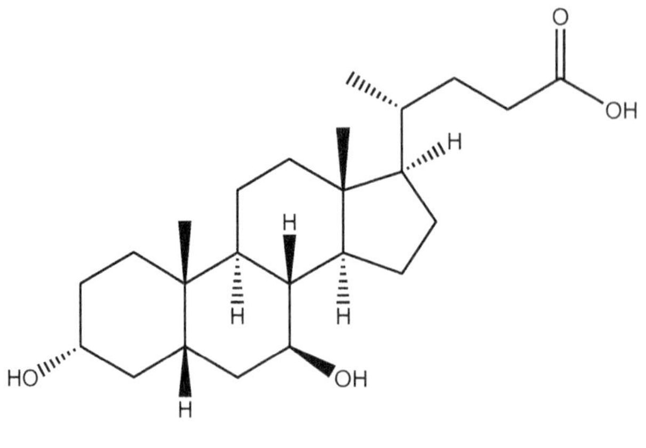

Fig. 12.1
Chemical structure of ursodeoxycholic acid.

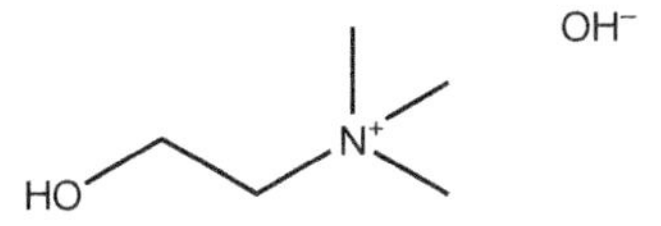

Fig. 12.2
Chemical structure of choline.

12.2.3 Betaine

Betaine, a methyl group donor, that affects lipid partitioning, but its metabolism is also associated with various metabolites, including choline, homocysteine,and methionine, which has an important place in the health of humans and other mammals. Also, it has protective effects on different types of liver cells.

In research by Hasanzadeh-Moghadam et al. (2018), the effects of betaine on a liver injury after a heart attack were evaluated. Rats with myocardial infarction with isoprenaline were treated with betaine (50, 150, and 250 mg kg^{-1} body weight) via gastric gavage for 60 days. The research outcomes showed that the antioxidant capacity in the betain-applied group resulted in a statistically significant increase compared to the control group. It has also been reported that the degenerative changes in the liver tissue in the betaine group significantly decreased. The chemical structure of betaine is given in Fig. 12.3.

12.2.4 S-Adenosyl-ʟ-methionine

S-Adenosyl-ʟ-methionine (SAM) is a metabolite that is involved in glutathione synthesis and functions as a methyl donor for methylation reactions. SAM also regulates hepatocyte growth, specialization, and death (Cederbaum, 2010).

In a study comparing melatonin with *S*-adenosyl-ʟ-methionine, protection against oxidative stress and hepatic cholestasis in adult male Wistar rats was investigated in vivo. Hepatic oxidative stress was assessed by differences in the amount of lipid peroxides and reduced GSH content in erythrocytes and hepatic tissue. SAM was found to be efficient in prohibiting GSH loss; the findings confirmed the function of SAM as an antioxidant and hepatoprotector (López et al., 2000). The chemical structure of *S*-adenosyl-ʟ-methionine is given in Fig. 12.4.

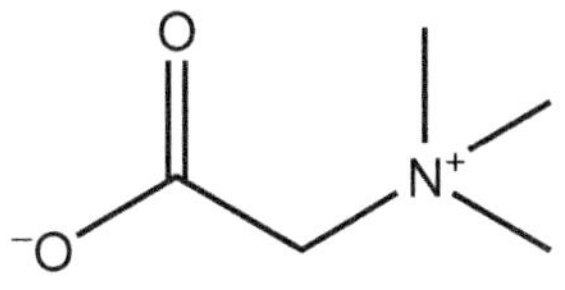

Fig. 12.3
Chemical structure of betaine.

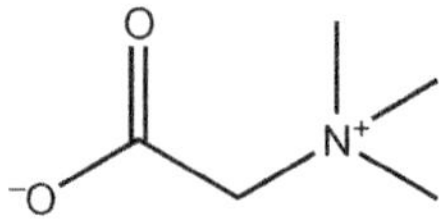

Fig. 12.4
Chemical structure of S-adenosyl-L-methionine.

12.2.5 Melatonin

Melatonin, which is known to directly and indirectly show strong antioxidant properties, is the hormone of darkness and a messenger of the photoperiod. The fact that melatonin is a strong organ preservative has been linked to the intense radical scavenging capacity of the hormone by working on many injury models (Mathes, 2010).

The effects of melatonin on liver function and lipid peroxidation were investigated in Sprague-Dawley rats with hepatic ischemia-reperfusion injury. Changes in alanine aminotransferase (ALT), aspartate aminotransferase (AST), lactate dehydrogenase (LDH), malondialdehyde (MDA), superoxide dismutase (SOD), and GSH levels were investigated. In the melatonin-treated group, a significant decrease in MDA levels as well as enhanced SOD activity and GSH levels were detected (Deng et al., 2016). The chemical structure of melatonin is given in Fig. 12.5.

12.2.6 Glutathione

Glutathione is a low molecular weight water-soluble tripeptide with a reduced thiol group that binds electrophilic molecules while modulating intracellular redox balance; it is present in a large amount in hepatocytes. It is an important compound for antioxidant activity involved in the detoxification of xenobiotic compounds (pollutants, heavy metals, and drugs) and endogenous metabolic products. GSH preserves the normal cell metabolism and cell

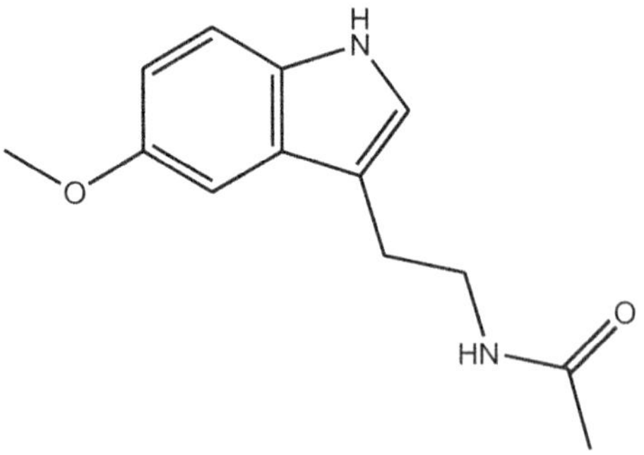

Fig. 12.5
Chemical structure of melatonin.

membrane integrity, and promotes the metabolism of sugars, fats, and proteins (Kantah et al., 2016; Lin et al., 2018). GSH is widely used today in the treatment of certain liver diseases such as viral-induced hepatitis, liver cirrhosis, and liver damage caused by drugs.

The effect of reduced glutathione treatment was studied in oxaliplatin (OXA)-initiated liver injury model-induced mice. The mice were administered OXA (10 mg/kg, i.p.) and GSH (400 mg/kg, i.p.) for 4 days. The ALT, AST, hepatic pathology, and oxidative stress parameters were analyzed in the hepatic tissues. According to the test results, it was found that GSH, used to treat the OXA-induced liver-damaged mouse model, alleviates pathological damage in liver tissues and significantly reduces serum ALT and AST amounts. In addition, GSH treatment caused a decrease in MDA levels caused by OXA (Lin et al., 2018).

In research conducted by Kantah et al. (2016), an orally bioavailable glutathione-based hepatoprotective compound (GLU-9599) was evaluated in experimental acute liver injury.

In this study, rats were treated with GLU-9599 for 5 days, then exposed to CCl_4.

Liver enzymes and hepatic histology criteria have been used to evaluate the effectiveness of the treatments. The lowest histological damage was scored in the group treated with GLU-9599, and treatment with GLU-9599 significantly decreased the elevation levels of AST and ALT. The chemical structure of glutathione is given in Fig. 12.6.

12.2.7 N-Acetylcysteine

N-Acetylcysteine (NAC) is the initiator of the L-cysteine amino acid and is found in the structure of the GSH, an endogenous antioxidant. NAC has a direct and indirect antioxidant effect.

The indirect antioxidant effect is exemplified by the formation of GSH while the direct antioxidant effect is exemplified by the interaction of the free thiol group with the ROS electrophilic groups (Saleem et al., 2018). The hepatoprotective effect of NAC, which has beneficial effects in situations characterized by GSH reduction or oxidative stress, has been shown with many studies (Saleem et al., 2018; Saito et al., 2010; Penumathsa et al., 2006; Galicia-Moreno et al., 2012).

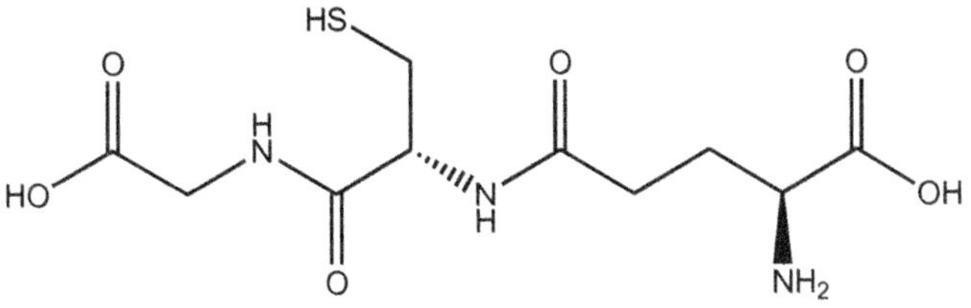

Fig. 12.6
Chemical structure of glutathione.

In a study evaluating the hepatoprotective activity of *N*-acetyl cysteine against hepatotoxicity due to carbamazepine (CBZ), it was observed that NAC increased glutathione content, decreased lipid peroxidation, and reversed histopathological abnormalities caused by CBZ. (Maheswari et al., 2014). The chemical structure of *N*-acetylcysteine is given Fig. 12.7.

12.2.8 Minerals in antioxidant enzymes

Steatosis can enhance oxidative stress by cellular enzymatic [Cu/Zn-SOD, Mn-SOD, glutathione peroxidase (GPx), and catalase] and nonenzymatic systems. These antioxidant enzymes effectively detoxify ROS (Perlemuter et al., 2005). Mitochondrial manganese superoxide dismutase (MnSOD), cytosolic Cu-Zn dismutase (Cu-ZnSOD), and extracellular dismutase (EcSOD) are the different forms of superoxide dismutase. Of these, MnSOD is believed to be the most important enzyme in ROT detoxification in cells (Tiebosch et al., 2013)

Copper plays a key role in the antioxidant defense in biological systems, preventing lipid peroxidation and mitochondrial function. In one study, the effect of copper on the hepatic histology in individuals with chronic hepatitis C, hemochromatosis, alcoholic liver lubrication, autoimmune hepatitis, and other liver insufficiencies was investigated in 124 subjects with nonalcoholic fatty liver disease (NAFLD). Liver copper amounts were lower in NAFLD and other liver patients against the control group (Aigner et al., 2010).

MnSOD expression significantly reduced the effectiveness of hepatic stellate cells, which are efficient in the development of hepatic fibrosis. Chronic liver diseases are most often caused by damage to the liver by extreme ROS production (Tiebosch et al., 2013).

Serum ALT, AST, ALP, GGT, and SOD levels were investigated in a study evaluating the preventive efficacy of manganese chloride ($MnCl_2$) against liver damage caused by carbon tetrachloride (CCl_4) in rats. Treatment with $MnCl_2$ reduced these changes to almost normal levels. The outcomes of this study support the antioxidant features of $MnCl_2$ against CCl_4-caused oxidative liver injury (Eidi et al., 2013).

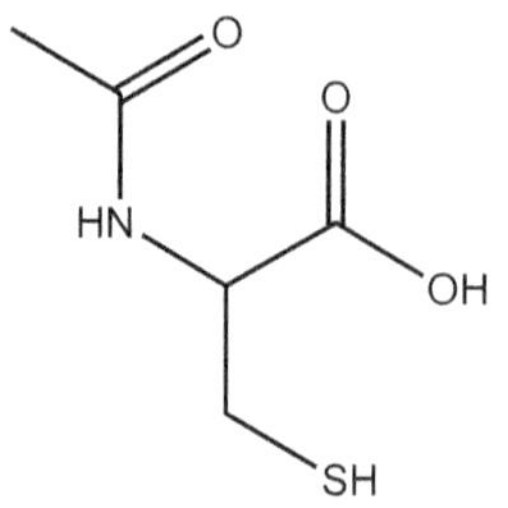

Fig. 12.7
Chemical structure of *N*-acetylcysteine.

Selenium (Se) is a well-known essential micronutrient with detoxifying effects in heavy metal poisoning. Many diseases such as chronic degenerative diseases, cognitive dysfunctions, and neurological disorders are correlated with Se deficiency. It can also restore glutathione peroxidase (GSH-Px) and Trx reductase (Ansar et al., 2017). In an in vivo study investigating the antioxidant and hepatoprotective efficiency of selenium nanoparticles against acetaminophen-induced (APAP) hepatic damage, 24 male rats were divided into three groups: a control group receiving 0.9% NaCl, an oral-administered APAP group, and a nano-Se (10–20 nm, intraperitoneal (ip) injection) and APAP (oral administration) applied group. The nano-Se treatment strengthened the hepatic antioxidant preservation mechanism and reduced cellular susceptibility to DNA fragmentation. Nano-Se showed a preventive effect against APAP-mediated hepatotoxicity by increasing the catalase, SOD, and GSH levels and reducing hepatic DNA degradation, a hepatic biological marker of cell death (Amin et al., 2017).

12.2.9 Vitamins E and C

Antioxidant vitamins have advantageous effects, especially on the pathogenesis of steatohepatitis and fibrosis, due to their ability to prevent oxidative stress and inflammation. Supporting this hypothesis, obese patients with nonalcoholic steatohepatitis (NASH) have less consumption of vitamins E and C compared to obese controls. Vitamin E supplementation improves fibrosis and inflammation in patients with NASH while also suppressing oxidative stress and lipid peroxidation (Stefan et al., 2008). Sanyal and colleagues assessed the efficacy of vitamin E in 247 patients with nonalcoholic steatohepatitis. An improved liver histology compared with the placebo was found 96 weeks after treatment with vitamin E (800 IU/day) (Sanyal et al., 2010). Harrison et al. gave vitamin C (1000 mg) and vitamin E (1000 IU) daily during 6 months to 45 patients with nonalcoholic steatohepatitis. Treatment with vitamins E and C significantly improved the degree of fibrosis in these individuals (Harrison et al., 2003). The chemical structures of vitamins E and C are given in Figs. 12.8 and 12.9.

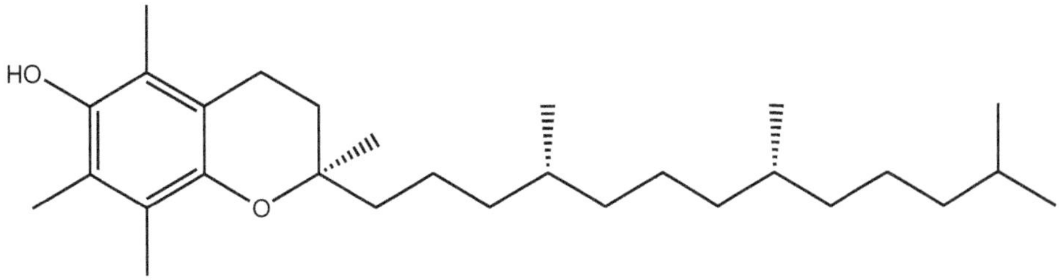

Fig. 12.8
Chemical structure of vitamin E.

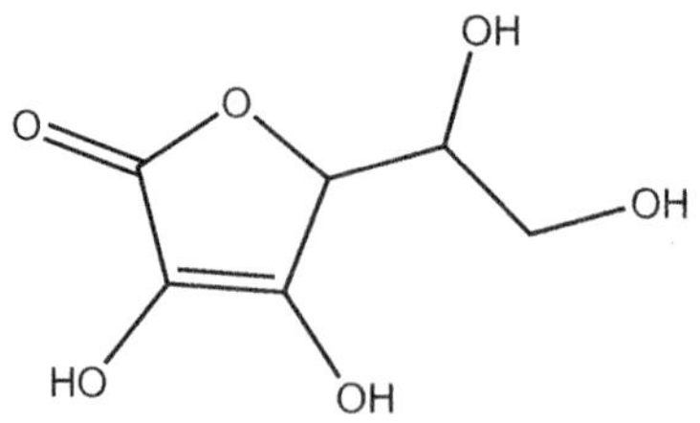

Fig. 12.9
Chemical structure of vitamin C.

12.2.10 Lycopene

Lycopene is a nonprovitamin A carotenoid. It is also the basic pigment that gives the tomato and its products a characteristic dark red color; that color is also given to some fruits and vegetables. The preventive efficacy of lycopene on oxidative stress and inflammation-related disorders in humans due to its antioxidant and antiinflammatory properties is remarkable. Studies have shown that the use of tomatoes and tomato products as food prevents lipid peroxidation in humans and strengthens the antioxidant system. A relationship has recently been discovered between liver cancer and lycopene. NASH patients had significantly lower plasma lycopene, which is important evidence of possible interactions between lycopene and liver disease development (Ip and Wang, 2014). In a study conducted to analyze the effect of lycopene on NASH with a high-fat diet, rats were divided into four groups. Rats with a standard diet, a high-fat diet, a high-fat diet + 2 mg/lycopene per kg, and a high-fat diet + 4 mg/kg of lycopene per 6 weeks were fed separately. The expressions of inflammation, steatosis, α-smooth muscle actin (α-SMA), and cytochrome P450 2E1 (CYP 2E1) decreased in rats fed with lycopene and increased in rats fed with a high-fat diet. Lycopene supplementation decreased the amount of malondialdehyde and TNF-α and increased the level of glutathione. These data show that lycopene addition can decrease oxidative stress in cells derived from a high-fat diet (Bahcecioglu et al., 2010). The chemical structure of lycopene is given in Fig. 12.10.

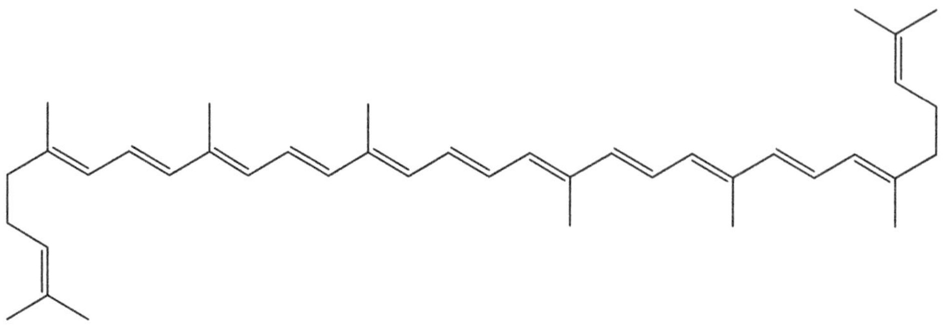

Fig. 12.10
Chemical structure of lycopene.

12.2.11 Beta-carotene

Beta-carotene, the main precursor of vitamin A, is an abundant compound in plants and has many immune and antioxidant properties. Beta-carotene shows its antioxidant activity by scavenging singlet oxygen, cleansing peroxide radicals, and reacting directly with peroxy radicals, thereby protecting membrane lipids from free radical damage. The role of oxidative stress on acetaminophen (APAP)-induced hepatic damage and the possible protective effects of beta-carotene supplementation against this damage were investigated by Morakinyo et al. (2012). In the study, rats were randomly divided into four groups: control, APAP, beta-carotene, and APAP + beta-carotene. According to the results of the study, it was stated that beta-carotene showed a hepatoprotective effect in rats against APAP-induced hepatotoxicity. A significant reversal of oxidative stress by beta-carotene treatment with an effective control of the level of liver enzymes showed that beta-carotene has a strong antioxidant effect on hepatotoxicity (Morakinyo et al., 2012). The chemical structure of beta-carotene is given in Fig. 12.11.

12.2.12 Silymarin

Silymarin is a natural compound found in *Silybum marianum*, known as the milk thistle. Seven flavanolignans—silibin A, silibin B, isosilibin A, isosilibin B, silichristin, isosilichristin, silidianin, and taxifolin—form silymarin (Hellerbrand et al., 2016). It has been used as a complementary medicine for many years because of its useful effects on the treatment of liver diseases. The natural hepatoprotective and antioxidant activities of silymarin have been shown to be due to its ability to remove ROS generated by the hepatic metabolism of toxic agents such as Et-OH, paracetamol, or CCL_4. The ability to donate electrons for scavenging free radicals is due to the phenolic structure of silymarin; it also affects cellular glutathione, which inhibits the lipid peroxidation of membranes (Vargas-Mendoza et al., 2014).

Clinical studies of silymarin administration in toxic hepatological disorders have shown a reduction in AST and ALT serum levels (Feher et al., 1989; Di Mario et al., 1981; Salmi

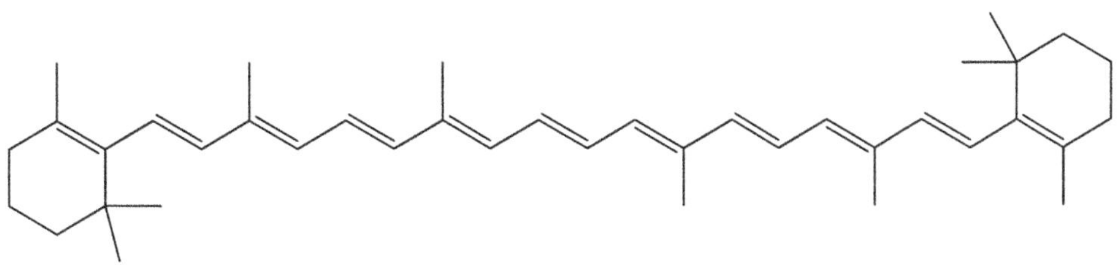

Fig. 12.11
Chemical structure of beta-carotene.

and Sarna, 1982). In a different study involving 12 patients treated with milk thistle extract (420 mg) per day for 6 months, concentrated on the activity of silymarin on superoxide dismutase expression in macrophages and erythrocytes, the silymarin treatment significantly developed the SOD activity of erythrocytes and lymphocytes and also repaired the SOD expression in lymphocytes. In addition, silymarin treatment significantly enhanced the serum levels of free −SH groups and glutathione peroxidase activity while decreasing serum MDA levels (Muzes et al., 1990). The chemical structure of silymarin is given in Fig. 12.12.

12.2.13 Alpha-lipoic acid

Alpha-lipoic acid, also called thioctic acid, has two different forms: oxidized (disulfide, LA) and reduced (di-thiol: dihydro-lipoic acid, DHLA). LA is available in two enantiomers: biologically active R-isomer and S-isomer. Low amounts of R-(+)-LA are found as lipoyllysine in plant and animal tissues. Herbal sources rich in R-LA are spinach, broccoli, and tomatoes. LA is distributed in the membrane and cytosol of plant and animal cells due to its hydrophilic and hydrophobic structure. Numerous studies have shown that LA and DHLA may have potent antioxidant potential with chemical reduction and oxidation (redox) properties (Rochette et al., 2015). Significant in vitro studies to date have shown the hepatoprotective activity of alpha-lipoic acid as an antioxidant agent by inhibiting lipid peroxidation, decreasing ROS levels, and increasing the amounts of SOD, GSH, and catalase (Khalaf et al., 2017; Sudheesh et al., 2013; Maheswari et al., 2014).

In a clinical trial, the effect of alpha-lipoic acid (ALA) versus vitamin E in 40 obese patients with nonalcoholic fatty liver disease (NAFLD) was investigated. ALA (200 mg) and vitamin E (700 IU) once a day were given to patients for 24 weeks. Orally given ALA was found more successful versus vitamin E in normalizing ALT, increasing the HDL and homeostasis model evaluation-insulin resistance (HOMA-IR) score, leptin, LDL, triglycerides, TNF-α and diastolic blood pressure reduced efficiency. Researchers have reported that ALA may be a medical choice for NAFLD (Basu et al., 2009). The chemical structure of alpha-lipoic acid is given in Fig. 12.13.

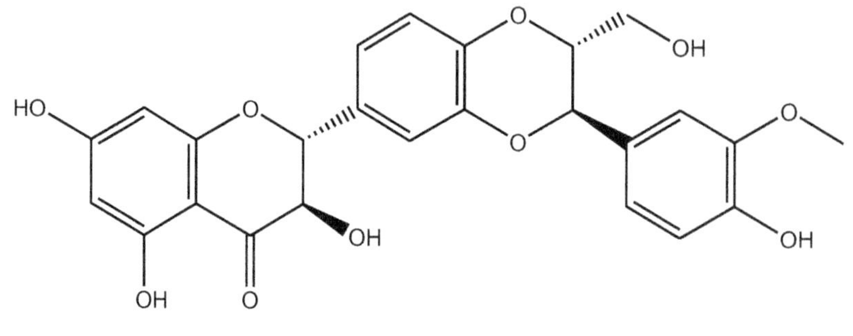

Fig. 12.12
Chemical structure of silymarin.

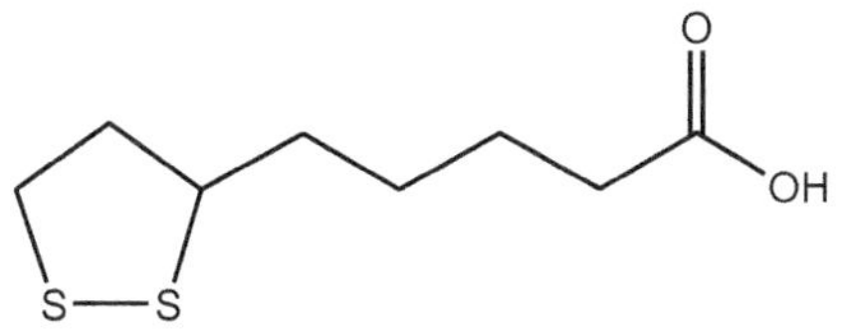

Fig. 12.13
Chemical structure of alpha-lipoic acid.

12.2.14 Coenzyme Q10

Coenzyme Q10 (2-methyl-5,6-dimethoxy-1,4-benzoquinone, ubiquinone, UQ) is a molecule that is found in all cells and cellular membranes that plays a crucial role in the mitochondrial respiratory chain and cellular metabolism. Coenzyme Q10 has the potential to protect lipoproteins and cellular membranes due to its strong lipophilic antioxidant properties (Sayiner and Kismali, 2016). In many studies carried out with animal models exposed to medicinal drugs, toxic chemicals, and lipopolysaccharides, CoQ10 showed the ability to decrease or avoid the formation of liver cirrhosis (Fouad and Jresat, 2012; Baskaran and Sabina, 2015; Song et al., 2017). In a study by Song et al. (2017), the ability of CoQ10 on blood biochemical compounds and the hepatic antioxidant system against LPS-induced oxidative damage was demonstrated. The addition of CoQ10 (100 and 300 mg of CoQ_{10}/kg BW) to the LPS-treated rat groups improved the SOD amounts to a level analogous to that of the control group. Also, the mRNA expression and activity of GPx in both CoQ10 groups were distinctly higher than the LPS group.

Although the activity of CoQ10 on liver function is mostly studied in animal models, there are a restricted number of clinical studies. In a clinical study, the systemic markers of oxidative stress and antioxidants were investigated in NAFLD patients and the depletion of the coenzyme Q10 was observed (Yesilova et al., 2005). In a randomized controlled clinical study, oxidative stress parameters, including total antioxidant capacity (TAC) and MDA, were observed in the blood samples of NAFLD participants supplemented with 100 mg/day of CoQ10. The researchers reported that unlike many previous animal experiments, the addition of CoQ10 caused a decrease in serum TAC levels in NAFLD patients. However, the limitations of this clinical trial to assess oxidative stress were reported as a small number of participants and no measurements of the activity of glutathione peroxidase and superoxide dismutase antioxidant enzymes (Farhangi et al., 2014). The chemical structure of coenzyme Q10 is given in Fig. 12.14.

12.2.15 Curcumin

Curcumin is the most important major bioactive compound of the plant *Curcuma longa* from the Zingiberaceae family. In traditional medicine, curcumin is used to treat various diseases such as dyspepsia, ureter infections, liver diseases, and rheumatoid arthritis (Cooper et al., 1994).

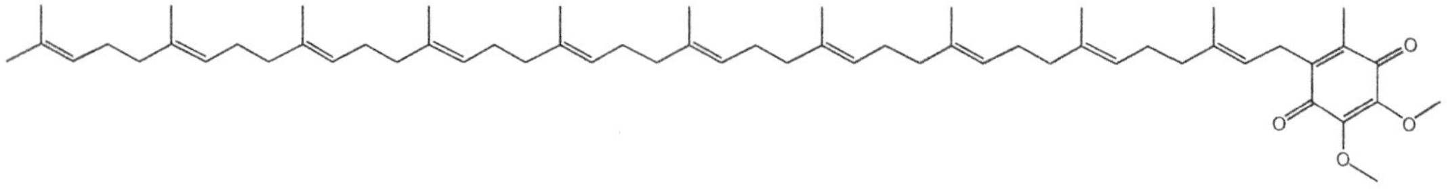

Fig. 12.14
Chemical structure of coenzyme Q10.

Curcumin, an effective scavenging agent for ROS, has a role in the prevention of pathogenesis. Experimental animal models have been used in many curcumin studies on different liver damage such as alcoholic liver disease, nonalcoholic fatty liver disease, and drug-induced hepatotoxicity. The main protective mechanism of curcumin and its derivatives against drug-caused liver damage is its antioxidant ability. The curative effect is shown in experimental models using some drugs such as paracetamol, chloroquine, methotrexate, erythromycin estolate, isoniazid, rifampicin, and pyrazinamide (Nabavi et al., 2013). In a murine model of nonalcoholic steatohepatitis, curcumin inhibited the generation of hepatic oxidative stress. Moreover, it inhibited ROS generation in myofibroblastic hepatic stellate cells and modified the excretion of the tissue inhibitor of metalloprotease-1 (Vizzutti et al., 2009). Curcumin has also been shown to reduce malondialdehyde caused by ethanol and increased GSH levels in empirical examples of alcoholic liver diseases (Nanji et al., 1999). The chemical structure of curcumin is given in Fig. 12.15.

12.2.16 Other natural antioxidants with hepatoprotective effects

Many natural plants have been tested in animal models in recent years to eliminate liver damage, and polyphenols and flavonoids have been reported to be bioactive compounds that eliminate oxidative stress. The studied effects of some antioxidants from natural sources on hepatic damage are summarized in Table 12.1.

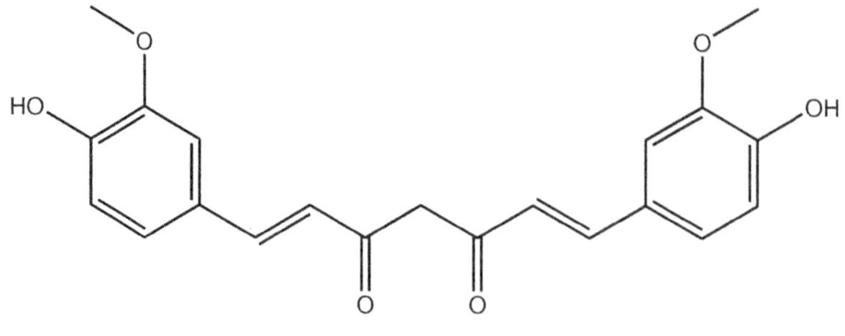

Fig. 12.15
Chemical structure of curcumin.

Table 12.1: Effects of antioxidant compounds obtained from natural sources in in vitro models with different liver injuries.

Model	Compound	Effect	Dose	Reference
Paracetamol-stimulated hepatic toxicity in mice	Gallic acid	Antioxidant and hepatoprotective	100 mg/kg	Rasool et al. (2010)
Paracetamol-stimulated hepatic toxicity in mice	Genistein	Antioxidant and hepatoprotective	50, 100, and 200 mg/kg (dose-effect)	Fan et al. (2013)
Lipopolysaccharide-stimulated hepatic damage in rats	Carnosic acid	Antioxidant and hepatoprotective	15, 30, and 60 mg/kg (dose-effect)	Xiang et al. (2013)
Lipopolysaccharide/D-galactosamine-stimulated hepatic damage in rats	Betulinic acid	Antioxidant and hepatoprotective	20 and 50 mg/kg (no dose-effect)	Zheng et al. (2011)
Tert-butyl hydroperoxide-stimulated hepatic damage in rats	Propolis	Antioxidant and hepatoprotective	50 and 100 mg/kg (no dose-effect)	Wang et al. (2006)
Tamoxifen-stimulated hepatic damage in mice	Catechin	Antioxidation	40 mg/kg	Tabassum et al. (2007)
Nonalcoholic Steatohepatitis rats (high-fat liquid diet)	Silibinin	Antioxidation	200 mg/kg	Haddad et al. (2011)
Thioacetamide-stimulated hepatic damage in rats	Eugenol	Lipid peroxidation; antioxidation	10.7 mg/kg b.w.	Yogalakshmi et al. (2010)
Bile-duct ligated rats	Thymoquinone	Antioxidation	50 mg/kg b.w.	Oguz et al. (2012)
Streptozotocin-stimulated diabetic rats	Berberine	Antioxidation	75, 150, and 300 mg/kg	Zhou and Zhou (2011)
Streptozotocin-stimulated diabetic rats	Resveratrol	Antioxidation	20 mg/kg	Sadi et al. (2014)

12.3 Synthetic hepatoprotectors with antioxidant activity

12.3.1 Pentoxiyfylline

The mechanism of action of pentoxifylline, a peripheral vasodilator that is widely used in vascular perfusion disorders, has been studied in rats with acute hepatic damage caused by galactosamine (Mohamed et al., 2015; Taye et al., 2009). Rats were treated with 100 mg/kg pentoxifylline during 3 weeks. Pretreatment with pentoxifylline has been reported to inhibit galactosamine-induced antioxidant enzyme activities, to reduce SOD and CAT, and to attenuate increased levels of malondialdehyde in hepatic tissue. The results of the study showed that pentoxifylline is a potential hepatoprotective agent and this effect may be related to its antioxidant features (Taye et al., 2009).

12.3.2 Angiotensin-converting enzyme inhibitors

It is stated that some angiotensin-converting enzyme inhibitors may exhibit antioxidant and radical clearing activities due to their structural thiol groups (Mikrut et al., 2016; Mashhoody et al., 2013).

The hepatoprotective efficacy of captopril and enalapril against oxidative stress cytotoxicity in isolated rat hepatocytes stimulated with paraquat on oxidative stress cytotoxicity markers such as cell lysis, ROS formation, lipid peroxidation, glutathione depletion, mitochondrial membrane potential reduction, lysosomal membrane oxidative damage, and cellular proteolysis was investigated (Pourahmad et al., 2011). The results of the research reported that enalapril, which does not have a thiol group, is as effective as thiol-containing captopril in inhibiting oxidative stress cytotoxicity parameters. As a hypothesis, it has been shown that the antioxidant activity of ACE inhibitors is not due to the presence of the thiol group, but an increase in nitric oxide synthesis (Pourahmad et al., 2011).

12.4 Conclusion

Although the concept of antioxidant therapy in liver disease has been studied in many studies and extensive efforts have been made, there remains a long process for these treatments to be applicable in liver diseases. The parameters of proven and safe antioxidants such as dosage, duration of treatment, absorption, and bioavailability require extensive research. Large-scale clinical trials and appropriate antioxidative treatment should be applied for several liver diseases.

References

Aigner, E., Strasser, M., Haufe, H.A., 2010. Role for low hepatic copper concentrations in nonalcoholic fatty liver disease. Am. J. Gastroenterol. 105, 1978–1985.

Amin, K.A., Hashem, K.S., Alshehri, F.S., Awad, S.T., Hassan, M.S., 2017. Antioxidant and hepatoprotective efficiency of selenium nanoparticles against acetaminophen-induced hepatic damage. Biol. Trace Elem. Res. 175, 136–145.

Ansar, S., Alshehri, S.M., Abudawood, M., Hamed, S.S., Ahamad, T., 2017. Antioxidant and hepatoprotective role of selenium against silver nanoparticles. Int. J. Nanomedicine 12, 7789–7797.

Bahcecioglu, I.H., Kuzu, N., Metin, K., Ozercan, I.H., Ustündag, B., Sahin, K., Kucuk, O., 2010. Lycopene prevents development of steatohepatitis in experimental nonalcoholic steatohepatitis model induced by high-fat diet. Vet. Med. Int. 2010. https://doi.org/10.4061/2010/262179. pii: 262179.

Baskaran, U.L., Sabina, E.P., 2015. The food supplement coenzyme Q10 and suppression of antitubercular drug-induced hepatic injury in rats: the role of antioxidant defence system, anti-inflammatory cytokine IL-10. Cell Biol. Toxicol. 31, 211–219.

Basu, P.P., Rayapudi, K., Pacana, T., Ramamurthy, S., Brown, R.S., 2009. M1733 A randomised open label clinical trial with oral alpha lipoic acid and vitamin E in non alcoholic fatty liver disease. Gastroenterology 136 (5), A-420. https://doi.org/10.1016/s0016-5085(09)61933-8.

Cederbaum, A.I., 2010. Hepatoprotective effects of *S*-adenosyl-L-methionine against alcohol- and cytochrome P450 2E1-induced liver injury. World J. Gastroenterol. 16 (11), 1366–1376.

Cichoz-Lach, H., Michalak, A., 2014. Oxidative stress as a crucial factor in liver diseases. World J. Gastroenterol. 20, 8082–8091.

Cooper, T.H., Clark, J.G., Guzınski, J.A., 1994. Analysis of curcuminoids by high-performance liquid chromatography. In: Ho, C.T., Osawa, T., Huang, M.T., Rosen, R.T. (Eds.), Food Phytochemicals for Cancer Prevention II. ACS Publications, New York, pp. 231–236.

Corbin, K.D., Steven, H., 2012. Zeisel choline metabolism provides novel insights into non-alcoholic fatty liver disease and its progression. Curr. Opin. Gastroenterol. 28 (2), 159–165.

Deng, W., Xu, Q., Liu, Y., Jiang, C., Zhou, H., Gu, L., 2016. Effects of melatonin on liver function and lipid peroxidation in a rat model of hepatic ischemia/reperfusion injury. Exp. Ther. Med. 11, 1955–1960.

Di Mario, F.R., Melzer, J., Meier, R., 1981. Die Wirkung von Silymarin auf Leberfunktionsproben bei Patienten mit alkoholbedingter Leberererkrankung. Doppelblindstudie. In: Di Ritis, F., Csomos, G., Braatz, R. (Eds.), Der toxisch-metabolische Leberschaden. Hansisches Verlagskontor, Lübeck, pp. 54–58.

Eidi, A., Mortazavi, P., Behzadi, K., Rohani, A.H., Safi, S., 2013. Hepatoprotective effect of manganese chloride against CCl$_4$-induced liver injury in rats. Biol. Trace Elem. Res. 155 (2), 267–275.

Fan, Y.J., Rong, Y., Li, P.F., Dong, W.L., Zhang, D.Y., Zhang, L., Cui, M.J., 2013. Genistein protection against acetaminophen-induced liver injury via its potential impact on the activation of UDP-glucuronosyltransferase and antioxidant enzymes. Food Chem. Toxicol. 55, 172–181.

Farhangi, M.A., Alipour, B., Jafarvand, E., Khoshbaten, M., 2014. Oral CoQ10 supplementation in patients with NAFLD: effects on serum vaspin, chemerin, pentraxin, insulin resistance and oxidative stress. Arch. Med. Res. 45, 589–595.

Feher, J.D.G., Muzes, G., Lang, I., Niederland, V., Nekam, K., Karteszi, M., 1989. Liver-protective action of silymarin therapy in chronic alcoholic liver diseases. Orv. Hetil. 130, 2723–2727.

Fouad, A.A., Jresat, I., 2012. Hepatoprotective effect of coenzyme Q10 in rats with acetaminophen toxicity. Environ. Toxicol. Pharmacol. 33 (2), 158–167.

Galicia-Moreno, M., Favari, L., Muriel, P., 2012. Antifibrotic and antioxidant effects of *N*-acetylcysteine in an experimental cholestatic model. Eur. J. Gastroenterol. Hepatol. 24, 179–185.

Haddad, Y., Vallerand, D., Brault, A., Haddad, P.S., 2011. Antioxidant and hepatoprotective effects of silibinin in a rat model of nonalcoholic steatohepatitis. Evid. Based Complement. Alternat. Med. 2011, nep164. https://doi.org/10.1093/ecam/nep164.

Harrison, S.A., Torgerson, S., Hayashi, P., 2003. Vitamin E and vitamin C treatment improves fibrosis in patients with nonalcoholic steatohepatitis. Am. J. Gastroenterol. 98 (11), 2485–2490.

Hasanzadeh-Moghadam, M., Khadem-Ansari, M.H., Farjah, G.H., Rasmi, Y., 2018. Hepatoprotective effects of betaine on liver damages followed by myocardial infarction. Vet. Res. Forum 9 (2), 129–135.

Hellerbrand, C., Schattenberg, J.M., Peterburs, P., Lechnerr, A., Brignoli, R., 2016. The potential of silymarin for the treatment of hepatic disorders. Clin. Phytosci. 2, 7. https://doi.org/10.1186/s40816-016-0019-2.

Ip, B.C., Wang, X.D., 2014. Non-alcoholic steatohepatitis and hepatocellular carcinoma: implications for lycopene intervention. Nutrients 6, 124–162.

Kantah, M.K., Kumari, A., He, F., Sollano, J., Alagozlu, H., Min, C.H., Lorenzetti, A., Morita, Y., Marotta, F., 2016. An orally-bioavailable glutathione-based hepatoprotective compound in experimental acute liver injury: more effective than silymarin and YHK. J. Gastrointest. Dig. Syst. 6, 462. https://doi.org/10.4172/2161-069X.1000462.

Khalaf, A.A., Zaki, A.R., Galal, M.K., Ogaly, H.A., Ibrahim, M.A., Hassan, A., 2017. The potential protective effect of α-lipoic acid against nanocopper particle-induced hepatotoxicity in male rats. Hum. Exp. Toxicol. 36 (9), 881–891.

Li, S., Tan, H.Y., Wang, N., Zhang, Z.J., Lao, L., Wong, C.W., Feng, Y., 2015. The role of oxidative stress and antioxidants in liver diseases. Int. J. Mol. Sci. 16, 26087–26124.

Lin, Y., Li, Y., Hu, X., Liu, Z., Chen, J., Lu, Y., Liu, J., Liao, S., Zhang, Y., Liang, R., Lin, Y., Li, Q., Liang, C., Yuan, C., Liao, X., 2018. The hepatoprotective role of reduced glutathione and its underlying mechanism in oxaliplatin-induced acute liver injury. Oncol. Lett. 15 (2), 2266–2272.

López, P.M., Fiñana, I.T., Muñoz De Agueda, M.C., Sánchez, E.C., Montilla Muñoz, M.C., Álvarez, J.P., 2000. Protective effect of melatonin against oxidative stress induced by ligature of extra-hepatic biliary duct in rats: comparison with the effect of *S*-adenosyl-L-methionine. J. Pineal Res. 28, 143–149.

Maheswari, E., Saraswathy, G.R., Santhranii, T., 2014. Hepatoprotective and antioxidant activity of *N*-acetyl cysteine in carbamazepine-administered rats. Indian J. Pharm. 46 (2), 211–215.

Mashhoody, T., Rastegar, K., Zal, F., 2013. Perindopril may improve the hippocampal reduced glutathione content in rats. Adv. Pharm. Bull. 4 (2), 155–159.

Mathes, A.M., 2010. Hepatoprotective actions of melatonin: possible mediation by melatonin receptors. World J. Gastroenterol. 16 (48), 6087–6097.

Meyer, S.A., Kulkarni, A.P., 2001. Hepatotoxicity. In: Hodgson, E., Smart, R.C. (Eds.), Introduction to Biochemical Toxicology, third ed. John Wiley and Sons, New York, p. 487.

Mikrut, K., Kupsz, J., Kozlik, J., Krauss, H., Pruszynska-Oszmałek, E., Gibas-Dorna, M., 2016. Angiotensin-converting enzyme inhibitors reduce oxidative stress intensity in hyperglicemic conditions in rats independently from bradykinin receptor inhibitors. Croat. Med. J. 57 (4), 371–380.

Mohamed, E.E., Husien, S., Osama, A.A., Fatma, A.M., Engy, R.F., 2015. Studies on hepatoprotective effect of pentoxifylline on CCL$_4$ induced liver fibrosis in guinea pigs. Int. Clin. Pathol. J. 1, 95–100.

Mohammed Saif, M., Farid, S.F., Khaleel, S.A., Sabry, N.A., El-Sayed, M.H., 2012. Hepatoprotective efficacy of ursodeoxycholic acid in pediatrics' acute lymphoblastic leukemia. Pediatr. Hematol. Oncol. 29, 627–632.

Morakinyo, A.O., Iranloye, B.O., Oyelowo, O.T., Nnaji, J., 2012. Anti-oxidative and hepatoprotective effect of beta-carotene on acetaminophen-induced liver damage in rats. Biol. Med. 4 (3), 134–140.

Muzes, G., Deak, G., Lang, I., Nekam, K., Niederland, V., Feher, J., 1990. Effect of silimarin (Legalon) therapy on the antioxidant defense mechanism and lipid peroxidation in alcoholic liver disease (double blind protocol). Orv. Hetil. 131 (16), 863–866.

Nabavi, S.F., Daglia, M., Moghaddam, A.H., Habtemariam, S., 2013. Curcumin and liver disease: from chemistry to medicine. Compr. Rev. Food Sci. Food Saf. 13, 62–77.

Nanji, A.A., Jokelainen, K., Rahemtulla, A., Miao, L., Fogt, F., Matsumoto, H., Tahan, S.R., Su, G.L., 1999. Activation of nuclear factor kappa B and cytokine imbalance in experimental alcoholic liver disease in the rat. Hepatology 30 (4), 934–943.

Oguz, S., Kanter, M., Erboga, M., Erenoglu, C., 2012. Protective effects of thymoquinone against cholestatic oxidative stress and hepatic damage after biliary obstruction in rats. J. Mol. Histol. 43, 151–159.

Penumathsa, S.V., Kode, A., Rajagopalan, R., Menon, V.P., 2006. Changes in activities of MMP in alcohol and thermally oxidized sunflower oil-induced liver damage: NAC antioxidant therapy. Toxicol. Mech. Methods 16, 267–274.

Perlemuter, G., Davit-Spraul, A., Cosson, C., 2005. Increase in liver antioxidant enzyme activities in non-alcoholic fatty liver disease. Liver Int. 25 (5), 946–953.

Pourahmad, J., Hosseini, M.-J., Bakan, S., Ghazi-Khansari, M., 2011. Hepatoprotective activity of angiotensin-converting enzyme (ACE) inhibitors, captopril and enalapril, against paraquat toxicity. Pestic. Biochem. Physiol. 99 (1), 105–110.

Rasool, M.K., Sabina, E.P., Ramya, S.R., Preety, P., Patel, S., Mandal, N., Mishra, P.P., Samuel, J., 2010. Hepatoprotective and antioxidant effects of gallic acid in paracetamol-induced liver damage in mice. J. Pharm. Pharmacol. 62, 638–643.

Rochette, L., Ghibu, S., Muresan, A., Vergely, C., 2015. Alpha-lipoic acid: molecular mechanisms and therapeutic potential in diabetes. Can. J. Physiol. Pharmacol. 93, 1021–1027.

Sadi, G., Bozan, D., Yildiz, H.B., 2014. Redox regulation of antioxidant enzymes: post-translational modulation of catalase and glutathione peroxidase activity by resveratrol in diabetic rat liver. Mol. Cell. Biochem. 393, 111–122.

Saito, C., Zwingmann, C., Jaeschke, H., 2010. Novel mechanisms of protection against acetaminophen hepatotoxicity in mice by glutathione and N-acetylcysteine. Hepatology 51 (1), 246–254.

Saleem, T.H., Abo El-Maali, N., Hassan, M.H., Mohamed, N.A., Mostafa, N., Abdel-Kahaar, E., Tammam, A.S., 2018. Comparative protective effects of N-acetylcysteine, N-acetyl methionine, and N-acetyl glucosamine against paracetamol and phenacetin therapeutic doses-induced hepatotoxicity in rats. Int. J. Hepatol. 2018. https://doi.org/10.1155/2018/7603437.

Salmi, H.A., Sarna, S., 1982. Effect of silymarin on chemical, functional, and morphological alterations of the liver. A double-blind controlled study. Scand. J. Gastroenterol. 17, 517–521.

Sanyal, A.J., Chalasani, N., Kowdley, K.V., 2010. Pioglitazone, vitamin E, or placebo for nonalcoholic steatohepatitis. N. Engl. J. Med. 362 (18), 1675–1685.

Sayiner, S., Kismali, G., 2016. Coenzyme Q and relation with diseases. Atatürk Üniversitesi Vet. Bil. Derg. 11 (2), 247–253.

Song, M.H., Kim, H.N., Lim, Y., Jang, I.S., 2017. Effects of coenzyme Q$_{10}$ on the antioxidant system in SD rats exposed to lipopolysaccharide-induced toxicity. Lab. Anim. Res. 33 (1), 24–31.

Stefan, N., Kantartzis, K., Häring, H.U., 2008. Causes and metabolic consequences of fatty liver. Endocr. Rev. 29 (7), 939–960.

Sudheesh, N.P., Ajith, T.A., Janardhanan, K.K., 2013. Hepatoprotective effects of DL-α-lipoic acid and α-tocopherol through amelioration of the mitochondrial oxidative stress in acetaminophen challenged rats. Toxicol. Mech. Methods 23 (5), 368–376.

Tabassum, H., Parvez, S., Rehman, H., Banerjee, B.D., Raisuddin, S., 2007. Catechin as an antioxidant in liver mitochondrial toxicity: inhibition of tamoxifen-induced protein oxidation and lipid peroxidation. J. Biochem. Mol. Toxicol. 21, 110–117.

Taye, A., El-Moselhy, M.A., Hassan, M.K., Ibrahim, H.M., Mohammed, A.F., 2009. Hepatoprotective effect of pentoxifylline against D-galactosamine-induced hepatotoxicity in rats. Ann. Hepatol. 8 (4), 364–370.

Tiebosch, M.H., Dunning, S., Rehman, A., 2013. Glutathione and antioxidant enzymes serve complementary roles in protecting activated hepatic stellate cells against hydrogen peroxide-induced cell death. Biochim. Biophys. Acta 1832 (12), 2027–2034.

Vargas-Mendoza, N., Madrigal-Santillán, E., Morales-González, A., Esquivel-Soto, J., Esquivel-Chirino, C., García-Luna, Y., González-Rubio, M., Gayosso-de-Lucio, J.A., Morales-González, J.A., 2014. Hepatoprotective effect of silymarin. World J. Hepatol. 6 (3), 144–149.

Vizzutti, F., Provenzano, A., Galastri, S., Milani, S., Delogu, W., Novo, E., Caligiuri, A., Zamara, E., Arena, U., Laffi, G., Parola, M., Pinzani, M., Marra, F., 2009. Curcumin limits the fibrogenic evolution of experimental steatohepatitis. Lab. Invest. 90 (1), 104–115.

Wang, B.J., Lien, Y.H., Su, C.L., Wu, C.P., Yu, Z.R., 2006. Fractionation using supercritical CO_2 influences the antioxidant and hepatoprotective activity of propolis against liver damage induced by tert-butyl hydroperoxide. Int. J. Food Sci. Technol. 41, 68–75.

Xiang, Q., Liu, Z., Wang, Y., Xiao, H., Wu, W., Xiao, C., Liu, X., 2013. Carnosic acid attenuates lipopolysaccharide-induced liver injury in rats via fortifying cellular antioxidant defense system. Food Chem. Toxicol. 53, 1–9.

Yesilova, Z., Yaman, H., Oktenli, C., Ozcan, A., Uygun, A., Cakir, E., Sanisoglu, S.Y., Erdil, A., Ates, Y., Aslan, M., Musabak, U., Erbil, M.K., Karaeren, N., Dagalp, K., 2005. Systemic markers of lipid peroxidation and antioxidants in patients with nonalcoholic fatty liver disease. Am. J. Gastroenterol. 100 (4), 850–855.

Yogalakshmi, B., Viswanathan, P., Anuradha, C.V., 2010. Investigation of antioxidant, anti-inflammatory and DNA-protective properties of eugenol in thioacetamide-induced liver injury in rats. Toxicology 268, 204–212.

Zheng, Z.W., Song, S.Z., Wu, Y.L., Lian, L.H., Wan, Y., Nan, J.X., 2011. Betulinic acid prevention of D-galactosamine/lipopolysaccharide liver toxicity is triggered by activation of Bcl-2 and antioxidant mechanisms. J. Pharm. Pharmacol. 63, 572–578.

Zhou, J.Y., Zhou, S.W., 2011. Protective effect of berberine on antioxidant enzymes and positive transcription elongation factor b expression in diabetic rat liver. Fitoterapia 82, 184–189.

Zhu, J., Wu, Y., Tang, Q., Leng, Y., Cai, W., 2014. The effects of choline on hepatic lipid metabolism, mitochondrial function and antioxidative status in human hepatic C3A cells exposed to excessive energy substrates. Nutrients 6 (7), 2552–2571.

CHAPTER 13

Plant extracts with putative hepatoprotective activity

Esra Köngül Şafak

Department of Pharmacognosy, Faculty of Pharmacy, Erciyes University, Kayseri, Turkey

13.1 Introduction

The liver is one of the most important organs and it has vital functions in physiological processes such as metabolism, secretion, storage, and detoxification (Abbaszadeh et al., 2018; Shirani et al., 2017). Therefore, liver diseases are considered among the most important health problems (Rabiul et al., 2011). Steatosis, viral hepatitis, cirrhosis, fibrosis, and liver cancer are among the most common liver diseases (Majee et al., 2019; Saral et al., 2016). Liver damage can be caused by fatty liver, bacterial and viral infections, alcohol abuse, various chemicals, heavy metals, and drugs (Kang and Koppula, 2014; Saral et al., 2016). Carbon tetrachloride, paracetamol, ethanol, antitubercular drugs (isoniazid and rifampicin), and galactosamine are some of the agents used to induce experimental hepatopathy in animal models (Saral et al., 2016). Cell necrosis, fibrosis, lipid peroxidation, and reduction of the levels of antioxidant enzymes such as glutathione are situations associated with liver injury (Abbaszadeh et al., 2018). Many chemicals lead to liver damage due to their oxidative properties or due to the impairment of the antioxidant defense system (Abbaszadeh et al., 2018). So, the use of antioxidants in liver disorders is an important approach (Li et al., 2015). Because of the possible side effects of existing drugs used in liver disorders, the discovery of more effective drugs with fewer side effects is needed (Yang et al., 2010). Therefore, natural products that are believed to be safer than conventional drugs have become popular in treatment (Lu et al., 2012). Most in vivo studies have shown that various plants and plant-derived products are promising to prevent hepatic damage, to reverse hepatic damage-related disorders, and to treat liver diseases (Saral et al., 2016). It has been reported that plants that are known as important natural antioxidant sources show their ameliorative effects by mainly scavenging free radicals, inhibiting lipid peroxidation, modulating the antioxidant-defense system, and being antiinflammatory agents (Yousuf et al., 2019). Plants with hepatoprotective effects and their possible mechanisms of action are summarized in Table 13.1.

Influence of Nutrients, Bioactive Compounds, and Plant Extracts in Liver Diseases. https://doi.org/10.1016/B978-0-12-816488-4.00006-1

Table 13.1: List of plants with hepatoprotective activity.

	Plants	Family	Part of used	Extract/extracts	Liver damage inducing agent	Possible mechanism of action	References
1	*Acacia catechu*	Mimosaceae	Heartwood powder	Aqueous slurry	CCl_4 (carbon tetrachloride)	Antioxidant, free radical scavenging, inhibiting lipid peroxidation	Pingale (2010)
2	*Acalypha racemosa*	Euphorbiaceae	Leaves	Aqueous	CCl_4	Antioxidant	Iniaghe et al. (2008)
3	*Acantholimon gilliati*	Plumbaginaceae	Aerial parts	Methanol	Formaldehyde	Antioxidant	Gazor et al. (2017)
4	*Achillea millefolium*	Asteraceae	Aerial parts	Hydroalcoholic	D-Galactosamine, lipopolysaccharide	Calcium-channel blocking	Yaeesh et al. (2006)
5	*Acrocarpus fraxinifolius*	Fabaceae	Leaves	*n*-Hexane	Paracetamol	Antioxidant	Abd El-Ghffar et al. (2017)
6	*Actinidia deliciosa*	Actinidiaceae	Pulp of the fruits	Hydroalcoholic	CCl_4	Antioxidant	Kang et al. (2012)
7	*Aegiceras corniculatum*	Aegicerataceae	Aerial parts	*n*-Hexane, ethyl acetate, and methanol	CCl_4	Antioxidant	Roome et al. (2008)
8	*Aegle marmelos*	Rutaceae	Leaves	Methanol	CCl_4	Antioxidant, free radical scavenging	Siddique et al. (2011)
9	*Aerva lanata*	Amaranthaceae	Whole plant	Petroleum ether	CCl_4	Antioxidant	Nevin and Vijayammal (2005)
10	*Ageratum conyzoides*	Asteraceae	Whole plant	*n*-Hexane	Paracetamol	Restoring the levels of total thiols, GSH and GST activity	Verma et al. (2013)
11	*Albizzia lebbeck*	Fabaceae	Bark of plant	70% Ethanol	CCl_4	Antioxidant	Patel et al. (2010)
12	*Alchornea cordifolia*	Euphorbiaceae	Leaves	Methanol	CCl_4	Antioxidant, free radical scavenging	Osadebe et al. (2012)
13	*Allium cepa*	Alliaceae	Bulbs	Aqueous	Ethanol	Antioxidant	Kumar et al. (2013a)
14	*Aloe vera*	Liliaceae	Whole plant	Aqueous	Alcohol	Antioxidant and membrane stabilizing	Saka et al. (2011)
15	*Alpinia oxyphylla*	Zingiberaceae	Fruits	Ethanol extract and its dichloromethane fraction	CCl_4	Free radical scavenging, inhibition of ROS generation and lipid peroxidation, activation of Nrf2 pathway	Zhang et al. (2017)
16	*Andrographis paniculata*	Acanthaceae	Leaves	Aqueous	Hexachlorocyclohexane	Activation of antioxidative enzymes	Trivedi and Rawal (2001)

No.	Plant	Family	Part	Extract	Inducer	Activity	Reference
17	*Anethum graveolens*	Apiaceae	Leaves	Ethanol	CCl_4	Restoring levels of antioxidant enzymes	Tamilarasi et al. (2012)
18	*Angelica keiskei*	Apiaceae	Aerial parts	Methanol	D-Galactosamine and CCl_4	Increase in aniline hydroxylase activity	Choi and Park (2011)
19	*Annona squamosa*	Annonaceae	Leaves	Methanolic extract	Isoniazid-rifampicin	Antioxidant, free radical scavenging	Uduman et al. (2011)
20	*Anoectochilus formosanus*	Orchidoideae	Whole plants	Standardized aqueous fraction	CCl_4	Free radical scavenging	Fang et al. (2008)
21	*Aquilaria agallocha*	Thymelaeaceae	Leaves	Ethanol	Paracetamol	Antioxidant	Alam et al. (2017)
22	*Arctium lappa*	Asteraceae	Root	Aqueous	CCl_4 and paracetamol	Antioxidant, free radical scavenging	Lin et al. (2000)
23	*Ardisia solanacea*	Myrsinaceae	Leaves	Alcoholic	CCl_4	Inhibition of cytochrome P-450 activity, inhibition of lipid peroxidation, membrane stabilizing, enhancing protein and glycoprotein biosynthesis	Samal (2013)
24	*Artemisia aucheri*	Asteraceae	Aerial parts	Hydroalcoholic	CCl_4	Free radical scavenging	Ghavamizadeh and Mirzaei (2015)
25	*Artemisia capillaris*	Asteraceae	Aerial parts	Aqueous	Alcohol-pyrazole	Antioxidant, modulation of proinflammatory cytokines	Choi et al. (2013)
26	*Artocarpus lakoocha*	Moraceae	Fruits	Methanolic	Paracetamol	Antioxidant	Saleem et al. (2018)
27	*Aspalathus linearis*	Theaceae	Aerial parts	Aqueous	CCl_4	Antioxidant, free radical scavenging	Bosek and Nakano (2003)
28	*Asparagus racemosus*	Liliaceae	Roots	Hydroalcoholic extract and its fractions (methanol, ethyl acetate, *n*-butanol, and precipitated aqueous)	CCl_4	Antioxidant, free radical scavenging	Acharya et al. (2012)
29	*Asteracantha longifolia*	Acanthaceae	Aerial parts	95% Ethanol	Isoniazid, rifampicin	Cell membrane stabilizing	Lina et al. (2012)
30	*Azadirachta indica*	Meliaceae	Leaves	70% Ethanol	Paracetamol	Antioxidant	Chattopadhyay (2003)

Continued

Table 13.1: List of plants with hepatoprotective activity—cont'd

	Plants	Family	Part of used	Extract/extracts	Liver damage inducing agent	Possible mechanism of action	References
31	Azima tetracantha	Salvadoraceae	Leaves	Chloroform, ethanol	CCl_4	Antioxidant	Ekbote et al. (2010)
32	Bacopa monnieri	Schrophulariaceae	Aerial parts	Ethanol	Paracetamol	Antioxidant	Ghosh et al. (2007)
33	Baliospermum montanum	Euphorbiaceae	Roots	Methanol subfraction	Paracetamol	Stimulation of hepatic cell regeneration, stabilization of plasma membrane, and activation of the reticuloendothelial system	Kumar and Mishra (2014)
34	Bauhinia purpurea	Fabaceae	Leaves	Methanolic	Paracetamol	Antioxidant	Yahya et al. (2013)
35	Berberis tinctoria	Berneridaceae	Leaves	Methanol	Paracetamol	Antioxidant	Murugesh et al. (2005)
36	Berberis vulgaris	Berberidaceae	Leaves	70% Ethanol	CCl_4	Antioxidant	Tahmasebi et al. (2018)
37	Bixa orellana	Bixaceae	Seeds	Seed oils	CCl_4	Inhibition of lipid peroxidation	Obidah et al. (2011)
38	Boerhaavia diffusa	Nyctaginaceae	Leaves	Ethanol	Paracetamol	Increasing of antioxidant defenses	Olaleye et al. (2010)
39	Boesenbergia rotunda	Zingiberaceae	Rhizome	Ethanol	Thioacetamide	Antioxidant, antiinflammatory	Salama et al. (2013a)
40	Boswellia dalzielii	Burseraceae	Stem bark	Aqueous	Paracetamol	Antioxidant	Said et al. (2017)
41	Boswellia ovalifoliolata	Burseraceae	Bark	Alcoholic	Paracetamol	Antioxidant, free radical scavenging	Mahesh et al. (2014)
42	Caesalpinia bonducella	Caesalpiniaceae	Leaves	Methanol	CCl_4	Antioxidant, free radical scavenging	Kumar et al. (2010)
43	Cajanus cajan	Papilionaceae	Leaves	Ethanol	D-Galactosamine	Antiperoxidative	Akinloye and Olaniyi (2011)
44	Calotropis procera	Asclepiadaceae	Flowers	70% Ethanol	CCl_4	Antioxidant	Qureshi et al. (2007)
45	Camellia sinensis	Theaceae	Aerial parts	Aqueous	CCl_4	Antioxidant	Sengottuvelu et al. (2008)
46	Capparis spinosa	Capparidaceae	Root Bark	Ethanol	CCl_4	Antioxidant	Aghel et al. (2010)
47	Careya arborea	Myrtaceae	Stem bark	Methanol	CCl_4	Antioxidant	Kumar et al. (2005)
48	Carica papaya	Caricaceae	Fruits	Aqueous and ethanol	CCl_4	Antioxidant	Sadeque and Begum (2010)
49	Carissa carandas	Apocyanaceae	Roots	Ethanol	CCl_4	Antioxidant, free radical scavenging, inhibition of lipid peroxidation	Hegde and Joshi (2009)

50	*Carissa opaca*	Apocyanaceae	Leaves	Methanol	CCl_4	Antioxidant, membrane stabilizing	Sahreen et al. (2011)
51	*Carissa spinarum*	Apocyanaceae	Roots	Ethanol	CCl_4 and paracetamol	Free radical scavenging	Hegde and Joshi (2010)
52	*Carthamus tinctorius*	Compositae	Flowers	Methanol	CCl_4	Antioxidant and antiinflammatory	Yar et al. (2012)
53	*Cassia fistula*	Fabaceae	Leaves	Ethanol	Isoniazid, rifampicin	Antioxidant	Jehangir et al. (2010)
54	*Celosia argentea*	Amaranthaceae	Seeds	70% Ethanol	CCl_4	Antioxidant	Jain (2005)
55	*Chenopodium album*	Chenopodiaceae	Seeds	Ethanol	CCl_4	Antioxidant	Baldi and Choudhary (2013)
56	*Chrozophora tinctoria*	Euphobiaceae	Leaves	Hydroalcoholic	CCl_4	Antioxidant	Maurya and Upadhyay (2019)
57	*Cichorium intybus*	Asteraceae	Aerial parts	Hydroalcholic	CCl_4	Antioxidant	Heibatollah et al. (2008)
58	*Cinnamomum zeylanicum*	Lauraceae	Bark	Ethanol	CCl_4	Increasing the activity of the antioxidant defense system, inhibition of lipid peroxidation	Eidi et al. (2012)
59	*Citrus maxima*	Rutaceae	Leaves	Water	Dietary-induced	Hypolipidemic, antiinflammatory, antioxidant	Feksa et al. (2018)
60	*Clerodendrum infortunatum*	Verbanaceae	Leaves	Methanol	CCl_4	Increase in the activity of the antioxidant defense system, inhibition of lipid peroxidation	Sannigrahi et al. (2009)
61	*Coccinia grandis*	Cucurbitaceae	Fruits	Alcohol	CCl_4	Antioxidant	Vadivu et al. (2008)
62	*Coldenia procumbens*	Boraginaceae	Whole plant	Chloroform	D-Galactosamine	Antioxidant	Venkatanarasimhan et al. (2014)
63	*Colocasia esculenta*	Araceae	Leaves	Water	Thioacetamide	Free radical scavenging	Chinonyelum et al. (2015)
64	*Commiphora berryi*	Burseraceae	Bark	Methanol	CCl_4	Antioxidant, free radical scavenging	Shankar et al. (2008)
65	*Coriandrum sativum*	Apiaceae	Leaves	Ethanol	CCl_4	Antioxidant	Pandey et al. (2011)
66	*Costus after*	Zingiberaceae	Stem	Methanol	Ethanol	Increase in the activity of the antioxidant defense system, inhibition of lipid peroxidation	Tonkiri et al. (2014)
67	*Crassocephalum crepidioides*	Asteraceae	Aerial parts	Water	CCl_4	Antioxidant, free radical scavenging	Aniya et al. (2005)

Continued

Table 13.1: List of plants with hepatoprotective activity—cont'd

	Plants	Family	Part of used	Extract/extracts	Liver damage inducing agent	Possible mechanism of action	References
68	Croton hypoleucus	Euphorbiaceae	Aerial parts	Ethanol	Thioacetamide	Antioxidant, modulation of the antioxidant defense system	Urrutia-Hernández et al. (2019)
69	Croton zehntneri	Euphorbiaceae	Leaves	Essential oil	Paracetamol	Free radical scavenging	Lima et al. (2008)
70	Curculigo orchioides	Amaryllidaceae	Rhizomes	Methanol	CCl_4	Antioxidant, antilipid peroxidative	Venukumar and Latha (2002)
71	Curcuma longa	Zingiberaceae	Rhizome	Ethanol	Thioacetamide	Antioxidan, antiinflammatory	Salama et al. (2013b)
72	Curcuma xanthorrhiza	Zingiberaceae	Rhizome	Ethanol	CCl_4	Antioxidant, free radical scavenging	Devaraj et al. (2010)
73	Cyathea gigantea	Cyatheaceae	Leaves	Methanol	Paracetamol	Antioxidant	Kiran et al. (2012)
74	Cymbopogon citratus	Poaceae	Leaves	Aqueous	Hydrogen peroxide	Increasing levels of antioxidative enzymes	Rahim et al. (2014)
75	Cynara scolymus	Asteraceae	Leaves	Aqueous	CCl_4	Restoring of antioxidant defense systems, reducing lipid peroxidation	Colak et al. (2016)
76	Cynodon dactylon	Poaceae	Leaves	Protein fraction	CCl_4	Antioxidant	Prabha and Annapoorani (2009)
77	Cyperus articulatus	Cyperaceae	Rhizome	Methanol	Paracetamol	Increasing activity of the antioxidant defense system, inhibition of lipid peroxidation	Datta et al. (2013)
78	Decalepis hamiltonii	Apocynaceae	Roots	Aqueous	CCl_4	Antioxidant	Srivastava and Shivanandappa (2010)
79	Delonix regia	Caesalpiniaceae	Leaves	Methanol	CCl_4	Antioxidant, free radical scavenging	Azab et al. (2013)
80	Dendrocnide sinuata	Urticaceae	Roots	Water	CCl_4	Antioxidant	Angom et al. (2018)
81	Dendrophthoe pentandra	Loranthaceae	Leaves	Aqueous, ethanol, chloroform and petroleum ether	CCl_4	Restoring the activities of antioxidant enzymes, scavenging of free radicals, preventing cytochrom P450 enzyme	Haque et al. (2018)
82	Dracocephalum rupestre	Lamiaceae	Whole plant	Ethyl acetate fraction	CCl_4	Antioxidant	Zhu et al. (2018)

#	Plant	Family	Part	Extract	Hepatotoxin	Mechanism	Reference
83	Eclipta alba	Asteraceae	Leaves	Aqueous	CCl_4	Restoring levels of antioxidant enzymes	Thirumalai et al. (2011)
84	Emblica officinalis	Euphorbiaceae	Fruits	Hydroalcoholic	Isoniazid, rifampicin	Antioxidant, membrane stabilizing, inhibition of CYP 2E1	Tasduq et al. (2005)
85	Enicostemma axillare	Gentianaceae	Aerial parts	Water	Paracetamol	Increasing in levels of antioxidative enzymes	Gite et al. (2010)
86	Epaltes divaricata	Asteraceae	Whole plant	Aqueous	CCl_4	Antioxidant	Hewawasam et al. (2004)
87	Euphorbia antiquorum	Euphorbiaceae	Aerial parts	Aqueous	CCl_4	Antioxidant	Jyothi et al. (2008)
88	Falcaria vulgaris	Apiaceae	Leaves	Aqueous	CCl_4	Antioxidant, antiinflammatory	Zangeneh et al. (2018)
89	Feronia elephantum	Rutaceae	Fruits	Methanolic	Paracetamol	Antioxidant	Kangralkar et al. (2010)
90	Feronia limonia	Rutaceae	Fruits	Petroleum ether, chloroform, and methanol	CCl_4	Cell membrane stabilization, hepatic cell regeneration, and activation of antioxidative enzymes	Upadhyay et al. (2010)
91	Ficus carica	Moraceae	Leaves	Ethanol	CCl_4	Antioxidant, inhibition of cytochrome P450	Mujeeb et al. (2011)
92	Flacourtia indica	Flacourtiaceae	Leaves	Aqueous	CCl_4	Alteration of cytochrome P-450	Gnanaprakash et al. (2010)
93	Foeniculum vulgare	Apiaceae	Seeds	Essential oil	CCl_4	Antioxidant	Rabeh et al. (2014)
94	Fraxinus rhynchophylla	Oleaceae	Seeds	Hydroalcholic	CCl_4	Increasing in levels of antioxidative enzymes	Guo et al. (2017)
95	Fumaria indica	Fumariaceae	Whole plant	50% Ethanol	N-nitrosodiethylamine and CCl_4	Restoring antioxidant defense systems, reducing lipid peroxidation, free radical scavenging	Hussain et al. (2012)
96	Funtumia africana	Apocynaceae	Leaves	Methanol	CCl_4	Restoring antioxidant defense systems, inhibition of lipid peroxidation	Uroko et al. (2019)
97	Garcinia kola	Clusiaceae	Seed	Seed flour	CCl_4	Antioxidant	Wegwu and Didia (2007)
98	Gardenia gummifera	Rubiaceae	Roots	Methanol	Thioacetamide	Antioxidant	Prabha et al. (2012)

Continued

Table 13.1: List of plants with hepatoprotective activity—cont'd

	Plants	Family	Part of used	Extract/extracts	Liver damage inducing agent	Possible mechanism of action	References
99	Ginkgo biloba	Ginkgoaceae	Leaves	Standardized dry extract	CCl_4	Antioxidant	Shenoy et al. (2001)
100	Glycyrrhiza glabra	Fabaceae	Roots	Powdered roots	CCl_4	Antioxidant, free radical scavenging, inhibition of lipid peroxidation	Rajesh and Latha (2004)
101	Gundelia tourenfortii	Asteraceae	Whole plant	Hydroalcholic	CCl_4	Antioxidant	Jamshidzadeh et al. (2005)
102	Hedera helix	Araliaceae	Leaves	Standardized extract	Paracetamol	Antioxidant, free radical scavenging	Moshaie-Nezhad et al. (2019)
103	Hedyotis corymbosa	Rubiaceae	Whole plant	Ethanol	Perchloroethylene	Increasing levels of antioxidative enzymes, reducing lipid peroxidation	Rathi et al. (2009)
104	Hemidesmus indicus	Asclepiadaceae	Roots	50% Ethanol	CCl_4	Free radical scavenging	Rao et al. (2005)
105	Hibiscus sabdariffa	Malvaceae	Flower	Aqueous	CCl_4	Antioxidant	Liu et al. (2006)
106	Hippophae rhamnoides	Elaegnaceae	Leaves	Phenolic-rich ethyl acetate fraction	CCl_4	Antioxidant	Maheshwari et al. (2011)
107	Homalium letestui	Flacourtiaceae	Stem	Ethanol	Paracetamol	Antioxidant	Okokon et al. (2017b)
108	Hygrophila spinosa	Acanthaceae	Roots	Aqueous	CCl_4	Antilipid peroxidative, free radical scavenging	Shanmugasundaram and Venkataraman (2006)
109	Hypericum perforatum	Hypericaceae	Leaves	Fat-free hydroalcoholic extract	Hepatic ischemia/ reperfusion injury	Antioxidant, free radical scavenging	Bayramoglu et al. (2014)
110	Ichnocarpus frutescens	Apocynaceae	Flowers	Chloroform, methanol	Paracetamol	Free radical scavenging	Dash et al. (2007)
111	Indigofera tinctoria	Fabaceae	Whole plant	Methanol	D-Galactosamine / endotoxin	Antioxidant	Sreepriya et al. (2001)
112	Indigofera aspalathoides	Fabaceae	Whole plant	Methanol	CCl_4	Antioxidant, antilipid peroxidative	Gupta et al. (2004)

#	Species	Family	Part	Extract	Inducer	Activity	Reference
113	Ipomoea aquatica	Convolvulaceae	Whole plant	Ethanol	Thioacetamide	Antioxidant, free radical scavenging, modulation of detoxification enzymes	Alkiyumi et al. (2012)
114	Juniperus phoenicea	Cupressaceae	Berries	Aqueous	CCl_4	Antioxidant	Laouar et al. (2017)
115	Kigelia africana	Bignoniaceae	Fruits	Aqueous and methanol	CCl_4	Antioxidant	Shama and Marwa (2013)
116	Launaea intybacea	Asteraceae	Aerial parts	Aqueous	CCl_4	Increasing levels of antioxidative enzymes	Takate et al. (2010)
117	Lawsonia inermis	Lythraceae	Leaves	Methanol	CCl_4	Antioxidant	Mohamed et al. (2016)
118	Luffa acutangula	Cucurbitaceae	Leaves	Ethanol	CCl_4	Antioxidant, free radical scavenging	Ulganathan et al. (2010)
119	Lygodium flexuosum	Lygodiaceae	Fruits	n-Hexane	D-Galactosamine	Inhibition of the UDP-sugar derivatives and the membrane stabilizing effect	Wills and Asha (2006)
120	Macrotyloma uniflorum	Fabaceae	Seeds	Hydroalcoholic	Ethanol	Increasing of endogenous antioxidants, inhibition of lipid peroxidation	Panda et al. (2015)
121	Mammea suriga	Calophyllaceae	Flower buds	Aqueous	CCl_4	Antioxidant	Shastri et al. (2017)
122	Marrubium vulgare	Lamiaceae	Whole plant	Methanol	Paracetamol	Antioxidant	Akther et al. (2013)
123	Marsilea minuta	Marsileaceae	Whole plant	Methanol	CCl_4	Antioxidant	Praneetha et al. (2011)
124	Maytenus robusta	Celastraceae	Leaves	Methanol	CCl_4	Antioxidant, antiinflammatory	Thiesen et al. (2017)
125	Mentha longifolia	Lamiaceae	Aerial parts	Ethanol extract and its fractions	CCl_4	Increasing in hepatic glutathione and superoxide dismutase activity, and decreasing of cytochrome P450	Mimica-Dukic et al. (1999)
126	Mimosa pudica	Mimosaceae	Roots	Methanol	CCl_4	Antioxidant	Suneetha et al. (2011)
127	Momordica dioica	Cucurbitaceae	Leaves	Ethanol and aqueous	CCl_4	Antioxidant, free radical scavenging	Jain et al. (2008)
128	Momordica tuberose	Cucurbitaceae	Tubers	Hydroalcoholic	CCl_4	Antioxidant	Kumar (2008)

Continued

Table 13.1: List of plants with hepatoprotective activity—cont'd

	Plants	Family	Part of used	Extract/extracts	Liver damage inducing agent	Possible mechanism of action	References
129	*Moringa oleifera*	Moringaceae	Leaves	Ethanolic extracts (defatting and chlorophyll free)	CCl_4	Antioxidant and free radical scavenging	Singh et al. (2014)
130	*Morus nigra*	Moraceae	Leaves	Hydroalcoholic	Paracetamol	Antioxidant and free radical scavenging	Mallhi et al. (2014)
131	*Muntingia calabura*	Muntingiaceae	Leaves	Methanol	Paracetamol	Antioxidant	Mahmood et al. (2014)
132	*Murraya koenigii*	Rutaceae	Leaves	Aqueous	Lead	Antioxidant	Ghosh et al. (2013)
133	*Musanga cecropioides*	Urticaceae	Stem bark	Aqueous	Paracetamol	Antioxidant	Omoruyi et al. (2015)
134	*Nelumbo nucifera*	Nymphaeaceae	Leaves	Ethanol	CCl_4	Antioxidant and free radical scavenging	Huang et al. (2010)
135	*Nigella sativa*	Ranunculaceae	Seeds	Hydroalcoholic	Paracetamol	Antioxidant activity, suppressing lipid peroxidation and ROS generation	Adam et al. (2016)
136	*Oldenlandia umbellata*	Rubiaceae	Aerial parts	Methanol	CCl_4	Antioxidant, free radical scavenging, inhibition of lipid peroxidation	Gupta et al. (2007)
137	*Operculina turpethum*	Convolvulaceae	Roots	Ethanol	N-nitrosodimethylamine	Increasing antioxidative enzymes in liver	Sharma and Singh (2014)
138	*Opuntia ficus indica*	Cactaceae	Fruits	Juice	CCl_4	Antioxidant	Galati et al. (2005)
139	*Orthosiphon stamineus*	Lamiaceae	Leaves	Methanol/water	CCl_4	Antioxidant, free radical scavenging	Yam et al. (2007)
140	*Orychophragmus violaceus*	Brassicaceae	Seeds	Water	CCl_4	Regulation of the Nrf2 and NFκB pathways	Huo et al. (2017)
141	*Panax ginseng*	Araliaceae	Roots (black ginseng)	Powder	Paracetamol	Antioxidant, antiapoptotic, antiinflammatory, antinitrative	Hu et al. (2017)
142	*Parkinsonia aculeata*	Fabaceae	Leaves	50% Ethanol	CCl_4	Antioxidant	Hassan et al. (2008)
143	*Pergularia daemia*	Asclepiadaceae	Aerial parts	Aqueous and ethanolic extract	CCl_4 and paracetamol	Improving antioxidative enzyme activities	Bhaskar and Balakrishnan (2010)

144	*Phoenix dactylifera*	Palmae	Seeds (raw or roasted)	Aqueous suspensions	CCl_4	Antioxidant, free radical scavenging	Abdelaziz and Ali (2014)
145	*Phyllanthus fraternus*	Euphorbiaceae	Aerial parts	Aqueous extract	Cyclophosphamide	Antioxidant, free radical scavenging	Lata et al. (2014)
146	*Phyllanthus niruri*	Euphorbiacae	Leaves	Methanol and aqueous	CCl_4	Free radical scavenging, inhibition of ROS and lipid peroxidation	Harish and Shivanandappa (2006)
147	*Phyllanthus polyphyllus*	Euphorbiaceae	Leaves	Methanol	Paracetamol	Antioxidant, free radical scavenging activity, inhibition of lipid peroxidation	Rajkapoor et al. (2008)
148	*Physalis peruviana*	Solanaceae	Whole plants	Aqueous	Paracetamol	Cell membrane stabilization, hepatic cell regeneration, and increasing of antioxidative enzymes	Chang et al. (2008)
149	*Picrorhiza kurroa*	Scrofulariaceae	Rhizomes and roots	Ethanol	Isoniazid and rifampicin	Antioxidant, membrane-stabilizing	Jeyakumar et al. (2008)
150	*Pimpinella anisum*	Apiaceae	Seeds	Essential oil	CCl_4	Antioxidant	Jamshidzadeh et al. (2015)
151	*Pisonia aculeata*	Nyctaginaceae	Leaves	Ethanol	CCl_4	Free radical scavenging, inhibition of lipid peroxidation, increasing of antioxidative enzymes	Palanivel et al. (2008)
152	*Pistacia lentiscus*	Anacardiaceae	Leaves	Aqueous	CCl_4	Reducing in the activity of ALP, ALT, AST enzymes, and the level of bilirubin	Janakat and Al-Merie (2002)
153	*Pittosporum neelgherrense*	Pittosporaceae	Stem bark	Methanol	CCl_4, D-galactosamine, Paracetamol	Inhibition of cytochrome P-450 activity, prevention of lipid peroxidation, stabilizing of the hepatocellular membrane, and enhancing protein and glycoprotein biosynthesis	Shyamal et al. (2006)
154	*Plantago major*	Plantaginaceae	Seeds	Methanol	CCl_4	Antioxidant	Türel et al. (2009)
155	*Plumbago zeylanica*	Plumbaginaceae	Aerial parts	Methanol	CCl_4	Reducing the serum total bilirubin, SGPT, SGOT, and ALP levels	Kumar et al. (2009)
156	*Polygonum multiflorum*	Polygonaceae	Roots	Water	CCl_4	Reducing of lipid peroxidation and antiinflammation	Lee et al. (2012)

Continued

Table 13.1: List of plants with hepatoprotective activity—cont'd

	Plants	Family	Part of used	Extract/extracts	Liver damage inducing agent	Possible mechanism of action	References
157	*Polygonum orientale*	Polygonaceae	Fruits	Ethanol	CCl_4	Antioxidative, antiproinflammatory	Chiu et al. (2018)
158	*Portulaca oleracea*	Portulacaceae	Aerial parts	Fresh juice	Paracetamol	Antioxidant	Ahmida (2010)
159	*Prunus amygdalus*	Rosaceae	Seeds	Oil	CCl_4	Inhibition of lipid peroxidation, increasing antioxidant enzyme activity	Jia et al. (2011)
160	*Psidium guajava*	Myrtaceae	Leaves	Aqueous	CCl_4	Antioxidant	Roy et al. (2006)
161	*Pterocarpus marsupium*	Papilionaceae	Stem bark	Methanol and aqueous	CCl_4	Restoration of the levels of serum bilirubin, protein, and enzymes	Mankani et al. (2005)
162	*Punica granatum*	Punicaceae	Flowers	Ethanol	Fe-NTA	Antioxidant, free radical scavenging	Kaur et al. (2006)
163	*Pyrus pashia*	Rosaceae	Aerial parts	Aqueous	CCl_4	Antioxidant, free radical scavenging	Athokpam et al. (2017)
164	*Raphanus sativus*	Brassicaceae	Leaves	Aqueous and ethanol	CCl_4	Antioxidant	Syed et al. (2014)
165	*Rhododendron arboreum*	Ericaceae	Leaves	Ethanol	CCl_4	Antioxidant	Prakash et al. (2008)
166	*Rhus oxyacantha*	Anacardiaceae	Root cortex	Ethyl acetate	DDT	Antioxidant and free radical scavenging	Miled et al. (2017)
167	*Ricinus communis*	Euphorbiaceae	Leaves	Hydroalcoholic	CCl_4	Membrane stabilizing, antiperoxidative	Prince et al. (2011)
168	*Rosmarinus officinalis*	Lamiaceae	Aerial parts	Essential oil	CCl_4	Free radical scavenging	Rašković et al. (2014)
169	*Roylea elegans*	Lamiaceae	Aerial parts	Hydroalcoholic	CCl_4 and paracetamol	Antioxidant	Upadhyay et al. (2017)
170	*Rubia cordifolia*	Rubiaceae	Roots	Hydroalcoholic	CCl_4 and paracetamol	Ca ++ channel blocking	Gilani and Janbaz (1995)
171	*Salvia cryptantha*	Lamiaceae	Aerial parts	Ethanol	CCl_4	Improving levels of SOD, GPx, and catalase, reducing the serum levels of MDA	Yalcin et al. (2017)
172	*Salvia officinalis*	Lamiaceae	Aerial parts	Hydroalcoholic	Isoniazid	Antioxidant, free radical scavenging	Shahrzad et al. (2014)

No.	Species	Family	Part	Extract	Model	Activity/Mechanism	Reference
173	*Saponaria officinalis*	Caryophyllaceae	Roots	Ethyl acetate, chloroform, and methanol	Paracetamol	Free radical scavenging	Talluri et al. (2018)
174	*Schisandra chinensis*	Schizandraceae	Pollen	Hydroalcoholic	CCl_4	Antioxidant, free radical scavenging, inhibition of lipid peroxidation	Cheng et al. (2013)
175	*Schisandra sphenanthera*	Schisandraceae	–	Ethanolic extract (in a commercial tablet form)	Lithocholic acid	Activation of the PXR pathway and promotion of liver regeneration	Zeng et al. (2016)
176	*Schrebera swietenioides*	Oleaceae	Stem bark	Aqueous	CCl_4	Reducing of AST, ALT levels and total bilirubin levels, increasing catalase, SOD, and GSH levels	Kumar et al. (2017)
177	*Scoparia dulcis*	Scrophulariaceae	Whole plant	Ethanolic	CCl_4	Decreasing the level of MDA and increasing the level of GSH	Tsai et al. (2010)
178	*Sida rhombifolia*	Malvaceae	Roots	Ethanolic extract	Alcohol	Downregulation of the expression of transcription factors	Rejitha et al. (2012)
179	*Silene villosa*	Caryophyllaceae	Aerial parts	Methanol	CCl_4	Antioxidant, antiinflammatory activities	Yusufoglu et al. (2018)
180	*Silybum marianum*	Asteraceae	Aerial parts	Ethanol	CCl_4	Antioxidant	Ramadan et al. (2011)
181	*Smilax chinensis*	Liliaceae	Roots	Ethyl acetate fraction	Paracetamol	Antioxidant	Mandal et al. (2008)
182	*Solanum fastigiatum*	Solanaceae	Leaves	Aqueous	Paracetamol	Free radical scavenging, antilipid peroxidative	Sabir and Rocha (2008)
183	*Solanum nigrum*	Solanaceae	Whole plant	Water	CCl_4	Antioxidant, free radical scavenging, modulation of detoxification enzymes	Lin et al. (2008)
184	*Solanum pubescens*	Solanaceae	Whole plant	Ethanol	CCl_4	Antioxidant, free radical scavenging	Pushpalatha and Ananthi (2012)
185	*Solanum trilobatum*	Solanaceae	Whole plant	Methanol	CCl_4	Antioxidant	Shahjahan et al. (2004)
186	*Solanum xanthocarpum*	Solanaceae	Fruits	50% Ethanol	CCl_4	Antioxidant	Gupta et al. (2011)
187	*Solenostemon monostachyus*	Lamiaceae	Leaves	Ethanol	Paracetamol	Antioxidant	Okokon et al. (2017a)

Continued

Table 13.1: List of plants with hepatoprotective activity—cont'd

	Plants	Family	Part of used	Extract/extracts	Liver damage inducing agent	Possible mechanism of action	References
188	*Solidago microglossa*	Compositae	Leaves	Ethanol	Paracetamol	Free radical scavenging, antilipid peroxidative	Sabir et al. (2012)
189	*Sphaeranthus indicus*	Asteraceae	Flower heads	Aqueous and methanolic	Paracetamol	Increasing levels of antioxidative enzymes and reducing lipid peroxidation	Tiwari and Khosa (2009)
190	*Stachys pilifera*	Lamiaceae	Leaves	Ethanol	CCl_4	Antioxidant	Panahi Kokhdan et al. (2017)
191	*Stevia rebaudiana*	Asteraceae	Leaves	Aqueous	CCl_4	Antioxidant	Mohan and Robert (2009)
192	*Strychnos potatorum*	Loganiaceae	Seeds	Seed powder and aqueous extract	CCl_4	Antioxidant	Sanmugapriya and Venkataraman (2006)
193	*Syzygium aromaticum*	Myrtaceae	Flower	Essential oil	CCl_4	Antioxidant	El-Hadary and Ramadan Hassanien (2016)
194	*Tagetes lucida*	Asteraceae	Leaves	70% Ethanol	Paracetamol	Increasing antioxidative enzymes and antilipid peroxidative	El-Newary et al. (2016)
195	*Tamarindus indica*	Caesalpiniaceae	Fruits	Aqueous	Isoniazid and rifampicin	Free radical scavenging	Amir et al. (2016)
196	*Tanacetum parthenium*	Asteraceae	Aerial parts	Methanol	CCl_4	Antioxidant	Mahmoodzadeh et al. (2017)
197	*Tecomella undulata*	Bignoneaceae	Leaves	Methanol	Alcohol and paracetamol	Antioxidant	Singh and Gupta (2011)
198	*Telfairia occidentalis*	Cucurbitaceae	leaves	Aqueous, ethanol	Garlic	Antioxidant	Oboh (2005)
199	*Terminalia catappa*	Combretaceae	Leaves	Ethanol	D-Galactosamine	Mitochondrion protection, free radical scavenging	Tang et al. (2004)
200	*Thespesia lampas*	Malvaceae	Stems	Methanol	CCl_4	Antioxidant	Chumbhale and Upasani (2012)
201	*Thonningia sanguinea*	Balanophoraceae	Roots	Water	D-Galactosamine and CCl_4	Antioxidant, free radical scavenging	Gyamfi et al. (1999)
202	*Thymus capitatus*	Lamiaceae	Aerial parts	Essential oils	Paracetamol	Antioxidant	El-Banna et al. (2013)

#	Plant	Family	Part	Extract	Inducer	Activity	Reference
203	*Tinospora cordifolia*	Menispermaceae	Aerial parts	Water	CCl_4	Antioxidant, free radical scavenging	Kumar et al. (2013b)
204	*Trianthema portulacastrum*	Aizoaceae	Whole plant	Ethanol	CCl_4	Modulation of antioxidant defense enzymes, inhibition of lipid peroxidation	Mandal et al. (1997)
205	*Trigonella foenum graecum*	Fabaceae	Seed	50% Ethanol	Thioacetamide	Inhibiting the activity of enzymes, mainly xanthine oxidase, free radical scavenging	Zargar (2014)
206	*Urtica dioica*	Urticaceae	Whole plant	Hydroalcoholic	CCl_4	Antioxidant and free radical scavenging activities	Joshi et al. (2015)
207	*Vetiveria zizanioides*	Poaceae	Roots	Methanol	CCl_4	Accelerating liver regeneration by regulating the TNF-α and IL-6 mediated pathways	Parmar et al. (2013)
208	*Vicia calcarata*	Fabaceae	Aerial parts	Flavonol glycoside-rich fraction, prepared from 70% alcohol extract	CCl_4	Antioxidant	Singab et al. (2005)
209	*Vitex negundo*	Lamiaceae	Leaves	Ethanolic	Thioacetamide	Antioxidant	Kadir et al. (2013)
210	*Vitex trifolia*	Verbenaceae	Leaves	Aqueous and ethanol	CCl_4	Antioxidant	Manjunatha and Vidya (2008)
211	*Zanthoxylum armatum*	Rutaceae	Leaves	Ethanol	CCl_4	Antioxidant, free radical scavenging	Ranawat et al. (2010)
212	*Zataria multiflora*	Lamiaceae	Aerial parts	Ethanol	Cyclophosphamide	Increasing the activity of the antioxidant defense system, free radical scavenging	Shokrzadeh et al. (2015)
213	*Zingiber officinale*	Zingiberaceae	Rhizome	50% Ethanol	Paracetamol	Antioxidant, free radical scavenging	Ajith et al. (2007)
214	*Zizyphus jujube*	Rhamnaceae	Fruits	70% Ethanol	CCl_4	Free radical scavenging, antiinflammatory	Shen et al. (2009)

Although the hepatoprotective effects of plants are mostly investigated by in vitro and in vivo experimental models, some clinical studies are also available. Alanine transaminase (ALT), aspartate transaminase (AST), alkaline phosphatase (ALP), gammaglutamyl transferase (GGT), serum bilirubin, prothrombin time, or international normalized ratio and serum albumin are common liver function tests (Limdi and Hyde, 2003). In most liver diseases, the disorder of these tests coexists, but ALT and AST are associated with hepatocellular damage, GGT and ALP are associated with cholestasis, and bilirubin increases both liver damage and cholestasis. Also, total protein, albumin, and PTZ reflect liver synthesis capacity (Savaş, 2014). Clinical studies have shown that *Berberis vulgaris*, *Camellia sinensis*, *Cynara scolymus*, *Glycyrrhiza glabra,* and *Panax ginseng* reduce serum ALT and AST levels (Kashkooli et al., 2015; Hussain et al., 2017; Panahi et al., 2018; Hajiaghamohammadi et al., 2012; Abdel-Wahhab et al., 2011). It has also been reported that *Angelica keiskei* caused a significant decrease in GGT levels and *Picrorhiza kurroa* in bilurubin levels (Noh et al., 2015; Vaidya et al., 1996). Nonalcoholic fatty liver disease (NAFLD) is a disease that is characterized by the excessive accumulation of fat in the liver; it embraces a broad spectrum including simple steatosis, steatohepatitis, fibrosis, and ultimately cirrhosis (Anstee and Day, 2013; Hashimoto et al., 2013). An impaired pro- or antiinflammatory adipokine balance secreted from adipose tissue, cytokines that mediate hepatic inflammation, cell necrosis, apoptosis, and fibrosis can play an active role in the formation and progression of NAFDL (Göktaş and Erdem, 2017). *Panax ginseng* has been reported to reduce proinflammatory cytokine levels and increase adiponectin serum levels in patients with NAFLD (Hong et al., 2016). Also, *Camellia sinensis*, *Cynara scolymus*, and *Glycyrrhiza glabra* have been shown to have healing effects on the serum parameters of NAFLD with clinical trials (Hussain et al., 2017; Panahi et al., 2018; Hajiaghamohammadi et al., 2012). Details of the clinical trials on hepatoprotective plants are summarized in Table 13.2.

13.2 Conclusion

Plants and herbal products have been used frequently in the treatment or prevention of many diseases from the past to the present. Nowadays, exposure to many chemicals as well as changing lifestyles and dietary habits have led to increases in liver disorders. The disadvantages of conventional medicine have led to searches for new therapeutic strategies. Therefore, herbal medicine use against hepatic diseases has increased. Plants can affect many different pathways in hepatocytes with their rich phytochemical content, so they show hepatoprotective effects through diverse mechanisms. The potential hepatoprotective effects of plants have been mostly associated with their antioxidant activities. However, more detailed research is needed to understand the mechanisms of action. Although the obtained results from various in vivo and in vitro studies are promising, numerous clinical studies are required to accept the use of these plants in treatment.

Table 13.2: Clinical trials on hepatoprotective plants.

Plants	Study design	Subjects	Extract/dose	Outcomes/results	References
Angelica keiskei	Multicenter, randomized, double-blind, placebo-controlled two parallel groups trial	82 Habitual alcohol drinkers with abnormal livers.	**Treatment group:** *Angelica keiskei* extract capsules (500 mg extract). **Control group:** Placebo capsules. One capsule two times a day between meals over 12 weeks.	Significant decrease in GGT levels. AST and ALT levels were not significantly different from the placebo group.	Noh et al. (2015)
Berberis vulgaris	Randomized, placebo-controlled trial	80 Patients with lipid accumulation in the liver and increased liver enzymes.	**Treatment group:** *Berberis vulgaris* capsules (750 mg aqueous extract). **Control group** Placebo capsules. One capsule two times a day for 3 months.	A significant reduction in serum levels of ALT (49–27.48 μ/L), AST (48.22–29.8 μ/L) ($P < 0.001$), weight, triglycerides, and cholesterol. There was no significant change in fasting blood sugar, high-density lipoprotein cholesterol (HDL-C), or low-density lipoprotein cholesterol (LDL).	Kashkooli et al. (2015)
Camellia sinensis (green tea)	Randomized, placebo-controlled, two parallel groups trial	80 Overweight, nondiabetic, and dyslipidemic patients with NAFLD.	**Treatment group:** Green tea leaf extract capsules (500 mg). **Control group** Placebo capsules. One capsule two times a day for 12 weeks.	A significant improvement in body weight, body mass index, homeostasis model assessment-insulin resistance index, lipid profile (total cholesterol, triglycerides, low-density lipoprotein cholesterol, high-density lipoprotein cholesterol), aminotransferases (ALT, AST), and inflammatory markers (high sensitivity C-reactive protein, adiponectin). 67.5% regression of fatty liver changes in treatment group.	Hussain et al. (2017)
Cynara scolymus	Randomized, double-blind, placebo-controlled parallel-group trial	100 Patients with NAFLD.	**Treatment group:** Standardized artichoke leaf extract tablet (200 mg dried extract including 2 mg cynarine). **Control group:** Placebo tablet. One tablet three times a day for 2 months.	Reduction in serum cholesterol (total cholesterol, low-density lipoprotein cholesterol, high-density lipoprotein cholesterol, non-high-density lipoprotein cholesterol, and triglyceride) concentrations. Improvement in ultrasound liver parameters and liver serum parameters (ALT, AST, APRI ratio, and total bilirubin).	Panahi et al. (2018)

Continued

Table 13.2: Clinical trials on hepatoprotective plants—cont'd

Plants	Study design	Subjects	Extract/dose	Outcomes/results	References
Glycyrrhiza glabra	Randomized, double-blind, placebo-controlled trial	66 Patients with NAFLD.	**Treatment group:** Licorice root extract capsule (2 g aqueous extract including 20% glycyrrhizin). **Control group** Placebo capsules. One capsule per day for 2 months.	A significant reduction in levels of ALT (64.09–51.27 IU/mL, $P < 0.001$) and AST (58.18–49.45 IU/mL, $P < 0.001$). There was no significant change in BMI.	Hajiaghamohammadi et al. (2012)
Hibiscus sabdariffa	Randomized, double-blind, placebo-controlled trial	36 Patients with BMI ≥ 27 and fatty liver.	**Treatment group:** *Hibiscus sabdariffa* extract capsule (450 mg aqueous extract of dried flowers). **Control group:** Placebo capsule. Two capsules three times (after meal) a day for 12 weeks.	Decrease in body weight, BMI, body fat, waist-hip ratio, and free fatty acid in serum.	Chang et al. (2014)
Panax ginseng **(Korean red ginseng)**	Placebo-controlled trial	30 Patients with hepatocellular carcinoma (HCC) and 30 patients with liver cirrhosis related to hepatitis C virus (HCV).	**Treatment group:** Medical therapy+Korean red ginseng extract capsule. (HCC group; 900 mg capsules/day, HCV group; 600 mg capsules/day for 11 weeks). **Control group:** Medical therapy only.	Significant improvement in liver function tests, reduction in the tumor marker (AFP) levels and the viral titers in HCV patients.	Abdel-Wahhab et al. (2011)
Panax ginseng **(Korean red ginseng)**	Randomized, single-blind, placebo-controlled trial	80 Patients with NAFLD.	**Treatment group:** Korean red ginseng capsule (ginsenosides Rg1+Rb1 6.0 mg/g; 3000 mg/d). **Control group:** Placebo capsule. One capsule three times a day for 3 weeks.	Reduction in TNF-α serum levels, improvement in adiponectin serum levels, significant decrease in the fatigue score in overweight patients with NAFLD.	Hong et al. (2016)
Phyllanthus amarus	Randomized, comparative, interferon-controlled trial.	55 Patients with chronic viral hepatitis B.	**Treatment group:** *Phyllanthus amarus* capsule (275 mg *Phyllanthus amarus*). Four capsules three times a day for 3 months (orally). **Control group:** IFN-α 1b was given to control group intramuscularly at 3×10^6 U dose on alternate days for 3 months.	There is no significant difference ($P > 0.05$) between treatment and control group about the negative conversion rates of HBeAg (42.3%) and HBV-DNA (47.8%) but the beneficial effect on liver function was better than IFN ($P < 0.05$).	Xin-Hua et al. (2001)

Plant	Study design	Participants	Intervention	Results	Reference
Picrorhiza kurroa	Randomized, double-blind, placebo-controlled trial	33 Patients with acute viral hepatitis (HBsAg negative).	**Treatment group:** *Picrorhiza kurroa* root powder capsule (375 mg). **Control group** Placebo capsules. One capsule three times a day for 2 weeks.	There was significant difference in values of bilirubin, SGOT, and SGPT between placebo and treatment groups.	Vaidya et al. (1996)
Silybum marianum	Randomized, double-blind, placebo-controlled, crossover trial	24 Patients with chronic hepatitis C.	**Treatment group:** *Silybum marianum* extract containing 80% silymarin (either 600 mg or 1200 mg/day). **Control group:** Placebo. Once a day, randomly *S. marianum* and placebo by a 4-week washout interval for 12 weeks.	There was no significant difference in HCV RNA titers, serum ALT levels, and Short Form-36 scores between placebo and treatment groups.	Gordon et al. (2006)
Silybum marianum	Randomized, double-blind placebo-controlled trial	29 Healthy men.	**Treatment group:** *Silybum marianum* seed extract tablet (286 mg extract including 177 mg silymarin complex). **Control group:** Placebo tablet. One tablet three times a day (with meals) for 60 days.	Decrease in serum cholesterol and increase in HDL cholesterol. Significantly higher serum antioxidant capacity in treatment group.	Šimánek et al. (2001)

References

Abbaszadeh, S., Andevari, A.N., Koohpayeh, A., Naghdi, N., Alizadeh, M., Beyranvand, F., Harsej, Z., 2018. Folklore medicinal plants used in liver disease: a review. Int. J. Green Pharm. 12, S463–S472.

Abd El-Ghffar, E.A., El-Nashar, H.A., Eldahshan, O.A., Singab, A.N.B., 2017. GC-MS analysis and hepatoprotective activity of the *n*-hexane extract of *Acrocarpus fraxinifolius* leaves against paracetamol-induced hepatotoxicity in male albino rats. Pharm. Biol. 55, 441–449.

Abdelaziz, D.H., Ali, S.A., 2014. The protective effect of *Phoenix dactylifera* L. seeds against CCl_4-induced hepatotoxicity in rats. J. Ethnopharmacol. 155, 736–743.

Abdel-Wahhab, M.A., Gamil, K., El-Kady, A.A., El-Nekeety, A.A., Naguib, K.M., 2011. Therapeutic effects of Korean red ginseng extract in Egyptian patients with chronic liver diseases. J. Ginseng Res. 35, 69–79.

Acharya, S., Acharya, N., Bhangale, J., Shah, S., Pandya, S., 2012. Antioxidant and hepatoprotective action of *Asparagus racemosus* Willd. root extracts. Indian J. Exp. Biol. 50, 795–801.

Adam, G.O., Rahman, M.M., Lee, S.-J., Kim, G.-B., Kang, H.-S., Kim, J.-S., Kim, S.-J., 2016. Hepatoprotective effects of *Nigella sativa* seed extract against acetaminophen-induced oxidative stress. Asian Pac. J. Trop. Biomed. 9, 221–227.

Aghel, N., Rashidi, I., Mombeini, A., 2010. Hepatoprotective activity of *Capparis spinosa* root bark against CCl_4 induced hepatic damage in mice. Iran J. Pharm. Res. 6, 285–290.

Ahmida, M., 2010. Evaluation of *in vivo* antioxidant and hepatoprotective activity of *Portulaca oleracea* L. against paracetamol-induced. Am. J. Pharmacol. Toxicol. 5, 167–176.

Ajith, T., Hema, U., Aswathy, M., 2007. *Zingiber officinale* Roscoe prevents acetaminophen-induced acute hepatotoxicity by enhancing hepatic antioxidant status. Food Chem. Toxicol. 45, 2267–2272.

Akinloye, O.A., Olaniyi, M.O., 2011. Hepatoprotective effect of *Cajanus cajan* on tissue defense system in D-galactosamine-induced hepatitis in rats. Turk. J. Biochem. 36, 237–241.

Akther, N., Shawl, A., Sultana, S., Chandan, B., Akhter, M., 2013. Hepatoprotective activity of *Marrubium vulgare* against paracetamol induced toxicity. J. Pharm. Res. 7, 565–570.

Alam, J., Mujahid, M., Jahan, Y., Bagga, P., Rahman, M.A., 2017. Hepatoprotective potential of ethanolic extract of *Aquilaria agallocha* leaves against paracetamol induced hepatotoxicity in SD rats. J. Tradit. Complement. Med. 7, 9–13.

Alkiyumi, S.S., Abdullah, M.A., Alrashdi, A.S., Salama, S.M., Abdelwahab, S.I., Hadi, A.H.A., 2012. *Ipomoea aquatica* extract shows protective action against thioacetamide-induced hepatotoxicity. Molecules 17, 6146–6155.

Amir, M., Khan, M.A., Ahmad, S., Akhtar, M., Mujeeb, M., Ahmad, A., Khan, S.A., Al-Abbasi, F.A., 2016. Ameliorating effects of *Tamarindus indica* fruit extract on anti-tubercular drugs induced liver toxicity in rats. Nat. Prod. Res. 30, 715–719.

Angom, B., Mohan, P., Lalmuanthanga, C., Maurya, P., Chanu, K.V., 2018. Hepatoprotective activity of aqueous extract of *Dendrocnide sinuata* (Blume) Chew. J. Pharmacogn. Phytochem. 7, 1072–1077.

Aniya, Y., Koyama, T., Miyagi, C., Miyahira, M., Inomata, C., Kinoshita, S., Ichiba, T., 2005. Free radical scavenging and hepatoprotective actions of the medicinal herb, *Crassocephalum crepidioides* from the Okinawa Islands. Biol. Pharm. Bull. 28, 19–23.

Anstee, Q.M., Day, C.P., 2013. The genetics of NAFLD. Nat. Rev. Gastroenterol. Hepatol. 10, 645.

Athokpam, R., Bawari, M., Choudhury, M.D., 2017. Hepatoprotective activity of aqueous extract of *Pyrus pashia* Buch.-Ham. Ex D. Don against CCl_4 induced liver damage. Int. J. Pharm. Sci. Res. 8, 4195–4200.

Azab, S.S., Abdel-Daim, M., Eldahshan, O.A., 2013. Phytochemical, cytotoxic, hepatoprotective and antioxidant properties of *Delonix regia* leaves extract. Med. Chem. Res. 22, 4269–4277.

Baldi, A., Choudhary, N.K., 2013. *In vitro* antioxidant and hepatoprotective potential of *Chenopodium album* extract. Int. J. Green Pharm. 7, 50–56.

Bayramoglu, G., Bayramoglu, A., Engur, S., Senturk, H., Ozturk, N., Colak, S., 2014. The hepatoprotective effects of *Hypericum perforatum* L. on hepatic ischemia/reperfusion injury in rats. Cytotechnology 66, 443–448.

Bhaskar, V., Balakrishnan, N., 2010. Protective effects of *Pergularia daemia* roots against paracetamol and carbon tetrachloride-induced hepatotoxicity in rats. Pharm. Biol. 48, 1265–1272.

Bosek, P., Nakano, M., 2003. Hepatoprotective effect of rooibos tea (*Aspalathus linearis*) on CCl$_4$-induced liver damage in rats. Physiol. Res. 52, 461–466.

Chang, J., Lin, C., Wu, S., Lin, D., Wang, S., Miaw, C., Ng, L., 2008. Antioxidative and hepatoprotective effects of *Physalis peruviana* extract against acetaminophen-induced liver injury in rats. Pharm. Biol. 46, 724–731.

Chang, H.C., Peng, C.H., Yeh, D.M., Kao, E.S., Wang, C.J., 2014. *Hibiscus sabdariffa* extract inhibits obesity and fat accumulation, and improves liver steatosis in humans. Food Funct. 5, 734–739.

Chattopadhyay, R.R., 2003. Possible mechanism of hepatoprotective activity of *Azadirachta indica* leaf extract: part II. J. Ethnopharmacol. 89, 217–219.

Cheng, N., Ren, N., Gao, H., Lei, X., Zheng, J., Cao, W., 2013. Antioxidant and hepatoprotective effects of *Schisandra chinensis* pollen extract on CCl$_4$-induced acute liver damage in mice. Food Chem. Toxicol. 55, 234–240.

Chinonyelum, A.N., Uwadiegwu, A.P., Nwachukwu, O.C., Emmanuel, O., 2015. Evaluation of hepatoprotective activity of *Colocasia esculenta* (L. Schott) leaves on thioacetamide-induced hepatotoxicity in rats. Pak. J. Pharm. Sci. 28, 2237–2241.

Chiu, Y.-J., Chou, S.-C., Chiu, C.-S., Kao, C.-P., Wu, K.-C., Chen, C.-J., Tsai, J.-C., Peng, W.-H., 2018. Hepatoprotective effect of the ethanol extract of *Polygonum orientale* on carbon tetrachloride-induced acute liver injury in mice. J. Food Drug Anal. 26, 369–379.

Choi, M.-K., Han, J.-M., Kim, H.-G., Lee, J.-S., Lee, J.-S., Wang, J.-H., Son, S.-W., Park, H.-J., Son, C.-G., 2013. Aqueous extract of *Artemisia capillaris* exerts hepatoprotective action in alcohol-pyrazole-fed rat model. J. Ethnopharmacol. 147, 662–670.

Choi, S.-H., Park, K.-H., 2011. Protective effects of *Angelica keiskei* extracts against *D*-galactosamine (GalN)-induced hepatotoxicity in rats. J. Food Hyg. Saf. 26, 235–241.

Chumbhale, D.S., Upasani, C.D., 2012. Hepatoprotective and antioxidant activity of *Thespesia lampas* (Cav.) Dalz & Gibs. Phytopharmacology 2, 114–122.

Colak, E., Ustuner, M.C., Tekin, N., Colak, E., Burukoglu, D., Degirmenci, I., Gunes, H.V., 2016. The hepatocurative effects of *Cynara scolymus* L. leaf extract on carbon tetrachloride-induced oxidative stress and hepatic injury in rats. SpringerPlus 5, 216.

Dash, D.K., Yeligar, V.C., Nayak, S.S., Ghosh, T., Rajalingam, R., Sengupta, P., Maiti, B.C., Maity, T.K., 2007. Evaluation of hepatoprotective and antioxidant activity of *Ichnocarpus frutescens* (Linn.) R. Br. on paracetamol-induced hepatotoxicity in rats. Trop. J. Pharm. Res. 6, 755–765.

Datta, S., Dhar, S., Nayak, S., Dinda, S.C., 2013. Hepatoprotective activity of *Cyperus articulatus* Linn. against paracetamol induced hepatotoxicity in rats. J. Chem. Pharm. Res. 5, 314–319.

Devaraj, S., Ismail, S., Ramanathan, S., Marimuthu, S., Fei, Y.M., 2010. Evaluation of the hepatoprotective activity of standardized ethanolic extract of *Curcuma xanthorrhiza* Roxb. J. Med. Plant Res. 4, 2512–2517.

Eidi, A., Mortazavi, P., Bazargan, M., Zaringhalam, J., 2012. Hepatoprotective activity of cinnamon ethanolic extract against CCl$_4$-induced liver injury in rats. EXCLI J. 11, 495.

Ekbote, M.T., Ramesh, C., Mahmood, R., Thippeswamy, B., Verapur, V., 2010. Hepatoprotective and antioxidant effect of *Azima tetracantha* Lam. leaves extracts against CCl$_4$-induced liver injury in rats. Indian J. Nat. Prod. Resour. 1, 493–499.

El-Banna, H., Soliman, M., Al-Wabel, N., 2013. Hepatoprotective effects of *Thymus* and *Salvia* essential oils on paracetamol-induced toxicity in rats. J. Physiol. Pharmacol. Adv. 3, 41.

El-Hadary, A.E., Ramadan Hassanien, M.F., 2016. Hepatoprotective effect of cold-pressed *Syzygium aromaticum* oil against carbon tetrachloride (CCl$_4$)-induced hepatotoxicity in rats. Pharm. Biol. 54, 1364–1372.

El-Newary, S.A., Ismail, R.F., Shaffie, N.M., Hendawy, S., Omer, E., 2016. Hepatoprotective, therapeutic and *in vivo* anti-oxidant activities of *Tagetes lucida* leaves alcoholic extract against paracetamol-induced hepatotoxicity rats. Int. J. PharmTech Res. 9, 327–341.

Fang, H.L., Wu, J.B., Lin, W.L., Ho, H.Y., Lin, W.C., 2008. Further studies on the hepatoprotective effects of *Anoectochilus formosanus*. Phytother. Res. 22, 291–296.

Feksa, D.L., Coelho, R.P., da Costa Güllich, A.A., Dal Ponte, E.S., Piccoli, J.d.C.E., Manfredini, V., 2018. Extract of *Citrus maxima* (pummelo) leaves improve hepatoprotective activity in Wistar rats submitted to the induction of non-alcoholic hepatic steatosis. Biomed. Pharmacother. 98, 338–346.

Galati, E., Mondello, M., Lauriano, E., Taviano, M., Galluzzo, M., Miceli, N., 2005. *Opuntia ficus indica* (L.) Mill. fruit juice protects liver from carbon tetrachloride-induced injury. Phytother. Res. 19, 796–800.

Gazor, R., Asgari, M., Pasdaran, A., Mohammadghasemi, F., Nasiri, E., Roushan, Z.A., 2017. Evaluation of hepatoprotective effect of *Acantholimon gilliati* aerial part methanolic extract. Iran J. Pharm. Res. 16, 135.

Ghavamizadeh, M., Mirzaei, A., 2015. Antioxidant activity and hepatoprotective potential of *Artemisia aucheri* in rat. Indian J. Sci. Technol. 8, 1–8.

Ghosh, T., Kumar Maity, T., Das, M., Bose, A., Kumar Dash, D., 2007. In vitro antioxidant and hepatoprotective activity of ethanolic extract of *Bacopa monnieri* Linn. aerial parts. Iran. J. Pharmacol. Ther. 6, 77–85.

Ghosh, D., Firdaus, S.B., Mitra, E., Dey, M., Chattopadhyay, A., Pattari, S.K., Dutta, S., Jana, K., Bandyopadhyay, D., 2013. Hepatoprotective activity of aqueous leaf extract of *Murraya koenigii* against lead-induced hepatotoxicity in male Wistar rat. Int. J. Pharm. Pharm. Sci. 5, 285–295.

Gilani, A.U.H., Janbaz, K.H., 1995. Effect of *Rubia cordifolia* extract on acetaminophen and CCl$_4$-induced hepatotoxicity. Phytother. Res. 9, 372–375.

Gite, V., Pokharkar, R., Chopade, V., Takate, S., 2010. Hepato-protective activity of *Enicostemma axillare* in paracetamol induced hepato-toxicity in albino rats. Int. J. Pharm. Life Sci. 1, 50–53.

Gnanaprakash, K., Chetty, M., Ramkanth, S., Alagusundaram, M., Vs, T., Angala Parameswari, S., Ts, M.S., 2010. Aqueous extract of *Flacourtia indica* prevents carbon tetrachloride induced hepatotoxicity in rat. World Acad. Sci. Eng. Technol. 37, 1117–1121.

Göktaş, Z., Erdem, N.B., 2017. Non-alkolik yağlı karaciğer hastalığında inflamatuvar proteinler. Beslenme ve Diyet Dergisi 45, 83–90.

Gordon, A., Hobbs, D.A., Bowden, D.S., Bailey, M.J., Mitchell, J., Francis, A.J., Roberts, S.K., 2006. Effects of *Silybum marianum* on serum hepatitis C virus RNA, alanine aminotransferase levels and well-being in patients with chronic hepatitis C. J. Gastroenterol. Hepatol. 21, 275–280.

Guo, S., Guo, T., Cheng, N., Liu, Q., Zhang, Y., Bai, L., Zhang, L., Cao, W., Ho, C.-T., Bai, N., 2017. Hepatoprotective standardized EtOH–water extract from the seeds of *Fraxinus rhynchophylla* Hance. J. Tradit. Complement. Med. 7, 158–164.

Gupta, M., Mazumder, U., Haldar, P., Manikandan, L., Senthilkumar, G., Kander, C., 2004. Hepatoprotective activity of *Indigofera aspalathoides* extract against CCl$_4$-induced liver damage. Orient. Pharm. Exp. Med. 4, 100–103.

Gupta, M., Mazumder, U., Thamilselvan, V., Manikandan, L., Senthilkumar, G., Suresh, R., Kakotti, B., 2007. Potential hepatoprotective effect and antioxidant role of methanol extract of *Oldenlandia umbellata* in carbon tetrachloride induced hepatotoxicity in Wistar rats. Iran. J. Pharmacol. Ther. 6, 5. 0.

Gupta, R.K., Hussain, T., Panigrahi, G., Das, A., Singh, G.N., Sweety, K., Faiyazuddin, M., Rao, C.V., 2011. Hepatoprotective effect of *Solanum xanthocarpum* fruit extract against CCl$_4$ induced acute liver toxicity in experimental animals. Asian Pac. J. Trop. Biomed. 4, 964–968.

Gyamfi, M.A., Yonamine, M., Aniya, Y., 1999. Free-radical scavenging action of medicinal herbs from Ghana: *Thonningia sanguinea* on experimentally-induced liver injuries. Gen. Pharmacol. 32, 661–667.

Hajiaghamohammadi, A.A., Ziaee, A., Samimi, R., 2012. The efficacy of licorice root extract in decreasing transaminase activities in non-alcoholic fatty liver disease: a randomized controlled clinical trial. Phytother. Res. 26, 1381–1384.

Haque, M.A., Haque, M.U., Islam, M.A.U., 2018. Evaluation of antioxidant and hepatoprotective effects of *Dendrophthoe pentranda* leaves on CCl$_4$-induced hepatotoxic rat. Bangladesh Pharm. J. 21, 71–79.

Harish, R., Shivanandappa, T., 2006. Antioxidant activity and hepatoprotective potential of *Phyllanthus niruri*. Food Chem. 95, 180–185.

Hashimoto, E., Taniai, M., Tokushige, K., 2013. Characteristics and diagnosis of NAFLD/NASH. J. Gastroenterol. Hepatol. 28, 64–70.

Hassan, S., Umar, R., Ebbo, A., Akpeji, A., Matazu, I., 2008. Hepatoprotective effect of leaf extracts of *Parkinsonia aculeata* L. against CCl$_4$ intoxication in albino rats. Int. J. Biol. Chem. 2, 42–48.

Hegde, K., Joshi, A.B., 2009. Hepatoprotective effect of *Carissa carandas* Linn root extract against CCl$_4$ and paracetamol induced hepatic oxidative stress. Indian J. Exp. Biol. 47, 660–667.

Hegde, K., Joshi, A.B., 2010. Hepatoprotective and anti-oxidant effect of *Carissa spinarum* root extract against CCl₄ and paracetamol-induced hepatic damage in rats. Bangladesh J. Pharmacol. 5, 73–76.

Heibatollah, S., Reza, N.M., Izadpanah, G., Sohailla, S., 2008. Hepatoprotective effect of *Cichorium intybus* on CCl₄-induced liver damage in rats. Afr. J. Biochem. Res. 2, 141–144.

Hewawasam, R., Jayatilaka, K., Pathirana, C., Mudduwa, L., 2004. Hepatoprotective effect of *Epaltes divaricata* extract on carbon tetrachloride induced hepatotoxicity in mice. Indian J. Med. Res. 120, 30–34.

Hong, M., Lee, Y.H., Kim, S., Suk, K.T., Bang, C.S., Yoon, J.H., Baik, G.H., Kim, D.J., Kim, M.J., 2016. Anti-inflammatory and antifatigue effect of Korean Red Ginseng in patients with nonalcoholic fatty liver disease. J. Ginseng Res. 40, 203–210.

Hu, J.-N., Liu, Z., Wang, Z., Li, X.-D., Zhang, L.-X., Li, W., Wang, Y.-P., 2017. Ameliorative effects and possible molecular mechanism of action of black ginseng (*Panax ginseng*) on acetaminophen-mediated liver injury. Molecules 22, 664.

Huang, B., Ban, X., He, J., Tong, J., Tian, J., Wang, Y., 2010. Hepatoprotective and antioxidant activity of ethanolic extracts of edible lotus (*Nelumbo nucifera* Gaertn.) leaves. Food Chem. 120, 873–878.

Huo, X., Liu, C., Gao, L., Xu, X., Zhu, N., Cao, L., 2017. Hepatoprotective effect of aqueous extract from the seeds of *Orychophragmus violaceus* against liver injury in mice and HepG2 cells. Int. J. Mol. Sci. 18, 1197.

Hussain, T., Siddiqui, H.H., Fareed, S., Sweety, K., Vijayakumar, M., Rao, C.V., 2012. Chemopreventive effect of *Fumaria indica* that modulates the oxidant-antioxidant imbalance during *N*-nitrosodiethylamine and CCl₄-induced hepatocarcinogenesis in Wistar rats. Asian Pac. J. Trop. Biomed. 2, S995–S1001.

Hussain, M., Habib-Ur-Rehman, Akhtar, L., 2017. Therapeutic benefits of green tea extract on various parameters in non-alcoholic fatty liver disease patients. Pak. J. Med. Sci. 33, 931–936.

Iniaghe, O., Malomo, S., Adebayo, J., 2008. Hepatoprotective effect of the aqueous extract of leaves of *Acalypha racemosa* in carbon tetrachloride treated rats. J. Med. Plant Res. 2, 301–305.

Jain, G., 2005. Hepatoprotective activity of ethanolic extract of *Celosia argentea* Linn. seeds in rats. J. Phytol. Res. 18, 87–90.

Jain, A., Soni, M., Deb, L., Jain, A., Rout, S., Gupta, V., Krishna, K., 2008. Antioxidant and hepatoprotective activity of ethanolic and aqueous extracts of *Momordica dioica* Roxb. leaves. J. Ethnopharmacol. 115, 61–66.

Jamshidzadeh, A., Fereidooni, F., Salehi, Z., Niknahad, H., 2005. Hepatoprotective activity of *Gundelia tourenfortii*. J. Ethnopharmacol. 101, 233–237.

Jamshidzadeh, A., Heidari, R., Razmjou, M., Karimi, F., Moein, M.R., Farshad, O., Akbarizadeh, A.R., Shayesteh, M.R.H., 2015. An *in vivo* and *in vitro* investigation on hepatoprotective effects of *Pimpinella anisum* seed essential oil and extracts against carbon tetrachloride-induced toxicity. Iran. J. Basic Med. Sci. 18, 205.

Janakat, S., Al-Merie, H., 2002. Evaluation of hepatoprotective effect of *Pistacia lentiscus*, *Phillyrea latifolia* and *Nicotiana glauca*. J. Ethnopharmacol. 83, 135–138.

Jehangir, A., Nagi, A., Shahzad, M., Zia, A., 2010. The hepatoprotective effect of *Cassia fistula* (amaltas) leaves in isoniazid and rifampicin induced hepatotoxicity in rodents. Biomedica 26, 25–29.

Jeyakumar, R., Rajesh, R., Meena, B., Rajaprabhu, D., Ganesan, B., Buddhan, S., An, R., 2008. Antihepatotoxic effect of *Picrorhiza kurroa* on mitochondrial defense system in antitubercular drugs (isoniazid and rifampicin)-induced hepatitis in rats. J. Med. Plant Res. 2, 017–019.

Jia, X.-Y., Zhang, Q.-A., Zhang, Z.-Q., Wang, Y., Yuan, J.-F., Wang, H.-Y., Zhao, D., 2011. Hepatoprotective effects of almond oil against carbon tetrachloride induced liver injury in rats. Food Chem. 125, 673–678.

Joshi, B.C., Prakash, A., Kalia, A.N., 2015. Hepatoprotective potential of antioxidant potent fraction from *Urtica dioica* Linn. (whole plant) in CCl₄ challenged rats. Toxicol. Rep. 2, 1101–1110.

Jyothi, T., Prabhu, K., Jayachandran, E., Lakshminarasu, S., Setty, R., 2008. Hepatoprotective and antioxidant activity of *Euphorbia antiquorum*. Pharmacogn. Mag. 4, 127.

Kadir, F.A., Kassim, N.M., Abdulla, M.A., Yehye, W.A., 2013. Hepatoprotective role of ethanolic extract of *Vitex negundo* in thioacetamide-induced liver fibrosis in male rats. Evid. Based Complement. Alternat. Med. 2013, 1–9.

Kang, H., Koppula, S., 2014. Hepatoprotective effect of *Houttuynia cordata* thunb extract against carbon tetrachloride-induced hepatic damage in mice. Indian J. Pharm. Sci. 76, 267.

Kang, W., Yang, H., Hong, H.J., Han, C.H., Lee, Y.J., 2012. Anti-oxidant activities of kiwi fruit extract on carbon tetrachloride-induced liver injury in mice. Korean J. Vet. Res. 52, 270–280.

Kangralkar, V.A., Patil, S.D., Bandivadekar, R., Nandagaon, V., Burli, S., 2010. Hepatoprotective activity of *Feronia elephantum* fruit extract against paracetamol induced hepatic damage in Wistar rats. Int. J. Pharm. Appl. 1, 46–49.

Kashkooli, R.I., Najafi, S.S., Sharif, F., Hamedi, A., Asl, M.K.H., Kalyani, M.N., Birjandi, M., 2015. The effect of *Berberis vulgaris* extract on transaminase activities in non-alcoholic fatty liver disease. Hepat. Mon. 15, 1–5.

Kaur, G., Jabbar, Z., Athar, M., Alam, M.S., 2006. *Punica granatum* (pomegranate) flower extract possesses potent antioxidant activity and abrogates Fe-NTA induced hepatotoxicity in mice. Food Chem. Toxicol. 44, 984–993.

Kiran, P.M., Raju, A.V., Rao, B.G., 2012. Investigation of hepatoprotective activity of *Cyathea gigantea* (Wall. Ex. Hook.) leaves against paracetamol-induced hepatotoxicity in rats. Asian Pac. J. Trop. Biomed. 2, 352–356.

Kumar, P., 2008. Antioxidant and hepatoprotective activity of tubers of *Momordica tuberosa* Cogn. against CCl_4 induced liver injury in rats. Indian J. Exp. Biol. 46, 510–513.

Kumar, S.S., Mishra, S., 2014. Protective effect of extracts of *Baliospermum montanum* (Willd.) Muell.-Arg. against paracetamol-induced hepatotoxicity-an *in vivo* and *in vitro* study. Anc. Sci. Life 33, 216.

Kumar, R.S., Sivakumar, T., Sivakumar, P., Nethaji, R., Vijayabasker, M., Perumal, P., Gupta, M., Mazumder, U., 2005. Hepatoprotective and in vivo antioxidant effects of *Careya arborea* against carbon tetrachloride induced liver damage in rats. Int. J. Mol. Med. Adv. Sci. 1, 418–424.

Kumar, R., Kumar, S., Patra, A., Jayalakshmi, S., 2009. Hepatoprotective activity of aerial parts of *Plumbago zeylanica* Linn against carbon tetrachloride-induced hepatotoxicity in rats. Int. J. Pharm. Pharm. Sci. 1, 171–175.

Kumar, R.S., Kumar, K.A., Murthy, N.V., 2010. Hepatoprotective and antioxidant effects of *Caesalpinia bonducella* on carbon tetrachloride-induced liver injury in rats. Int. Res. J. Plant Sci. 1, 062–068.

Kumar, K.E., Harsha, K., Sudheer, V., 2013a. In vitro antioxidant activity and in vivo hepatoprotective activity of aqueous extract of *Allium cepa* bulb in ethanol induced liver damage in Wistar rats. Food Sci. Human Wellness 2, 132–138.

Kumar, V., Modi, P.K., Saxena, K., 2013b. Exploration of hepatoprotective activity of aqueous extract of *Tinospora cordifolia*—an experimental study. Asian J. Pharm. Clin. Res. 6, 87–91.

Kumar, N., Choudhary, A., Tiwari, A., Rasal, A., Jetti, R., Rao, C.M., 2017. Evaluation of hepatoprotective effect of aqueous extract of *Schrebera swietenioides* bark against carbon tetrachloride-induced toxicity in Wistar rats. Adv. Sci. Lett. 23, 1917–1920.

Laouar, A., Klibet, F., Bourogaa, E., Benamara, A., Boumendjel, A., Chefrour, A., Messarah, M., 2017. Potential antioxidant properties and hepatoprotective effects of *Juniperus phoenicea* berries against CCl_4 induced hepatic damage in rats. Asian Pac. J. Trop. Biomed. 10, 263–269.

Lata, S., Singh, S., NathTiwari, K., Upadhyay, R., 2014. Evaluation of the antioxidant and hepatoprotective effect of *Phyllanthus fraternus* against a chemotherapeutic drug cyclophosphamide. Appl. Biochem. Biotechnol. 173, 2163–2173.

Lee, B.-H., Huang, Y.-Y., Duh, P.-D., Wu, S.-C., 2012. Hepatoprotection of emodin and *Polygonum multiflorum* against CCl_4-induced liver injury. Pharm. Biol. 50, 351–359.

Li, S., Tan, H.-Y., Wang, N., Zhang, Z.-J., Lao, L., Wong, C.-W., Feng, Y., 2015. The role of oxidative stress and antioxidants in liver diseases. Int. J. Mol. Sci. 16, 26087–26124.

Lima, F.C., Sousa, D.F., Ferreira, J.M., Lima Jr., R.C., Tomé, A.R., Cardoso, J.H.L., Queiroz, M.G.R., Campos, A.R., 2008. *Croton zehntneri* essential oil prevents acetaminophen-induced acute hepatotoxicity in mice. Rec. Nat. Prod. 2, 135–140.

Limdi, J.K., Hyde, G.M., 2003. Evaluation of abnormal liver function tests. Postgrad. Med. J. 79, 307–312.

Lin, S.-C., Chung, T.-C., Lin, C.-C., Ueng, T.-H., Lin, Y.-H., Lin, S.-Y., Wang, L.-Y., 2000. Hepatoprotective effects of *Arctium lappa* on carbon tetrachloride-and acetaminophen-induced liver damage. Am. J. Chin. Med. 28, 163–173.

Lin, H.-M., Tseng, H.-C., Wang, C.-J., Lin, J.-J., Lo, C.-W., Chou, F.-P., 2008. Hepatoprotective effects of *Solanum nigrum* Linn extract against CCl4-iduced oxidative damage in rats. Chem. Biol. Interact. 171, 283–293.

Lina, S.M., Ashab, I., Ishtiaq Ahmed, M., Shahriar, M., 2012. Hepatoprotective activity of *Asteracantha longifolia* (Nees.) extract against anti-tuberculosis drugs induced hepatic damage in Sprague-Dawley rats. Pharmacologyonline 3, 13–19.

Liu, J.-Y., Chen, C.-C., Wang, W.-H., Hsu, J.-D., Yang, M.-Y., Wang, C.-J., 2006. The protective effects of *Hibiscus sabdariffa* extract on CCl4-induced liver fibrosis in rats. Food Chem. Toxicol. 44, 336–343.

Lu, B., Xu, Y., Xu, L., Cong, X., Yin, L., Li, H., Peng, J., 2012. Mechanism investigation of dioscin against CCl4-induced acute liver damage in mice. Environ. Toxicol. Pharmacol. 34, 127–135.

Mahesh, B.U., Shrivastava, S., Pragada, R.R., Naidu, V., Sistla, R., 2014. Antioxidant and hepatoprotective effects of *Boswellia ovalifoliolata* bark extracts. Chin. J. Nat. Med. 12, 663–671.

Maheshwari, D., Kumar, M.Y., Verma, S.K., Singh, V.K., Singh, S.N., 2011. Antioxidant and hepatoprotective activities of phenolic rich fraction of Seabuckthorn (*Hippophae rhamnoides* L.) leaves. Food Chem. Toxicol. 49, 2422–2428.

Mahmood, N., Mamat, S., Kamisan, F., Yahya, F., Kamarolzaman, M., Nasir, N., Mohtarrudin, N., Tohid, S., Zakaria, Z., 2014. Amelioration of paracetamol-induced hepatotoxicity in rat by the administration of methanol extract of *Muntingia calabura* L. leaves. Biomed. Res. Int. 2014, 1–10.

Mahmoodzadeh, Y., Mazani, M., Rezagholizadeh, L., 2017. Hepatoprotective effect of methanolic *Tanacetum parthenium* extract on CCl4-induced liver damage in rats. Toxicol. Rep. 4, 455–462.

Majee, C., Mazumder, R., Choudhary, A.N., 2019. Medicinal plants with anti-ulcer and hepatoprotective activity: a review. Int. J. Pharm. Sci. Res. 10, 1–11.

Mallhi, T.H., Qadir, M.I., Khan, Y.H., Ali, M., 2014. Hepatoprotective activity of aqueous methanolic extract of *Morus nigra* against paracetamol-induced hepatotoxicity in mice. Bangladesh J. Pharmacol. 9, 60–66.

Mandal, A., Bandyopadhyay, S., Chatterjee, M., 1997. *Trianthema portulacastrum* L. reverses hepatic lipid peroxidation, glutathione status and activities of related antioxidant enzymes in carbon tetrachloride-induced chronic liver damage in mice. Phytomedicine 4, 239–244.

Mandal, S.C., Jana, G.K., Das, S., Sahu, R., Venkidesh, R., Dewanjee, S., 2008. Hepatoprotective and antioxidant activities of *Smilax chinensis* L. root. Pharmacologyonline 2, 529–535.

Manjunatha, B., Vidya, S., 2008. Hepatoprotective activity of *Vitex trifolia* against carbon tetrachloride-induced hepatic damage. Indian J. Pharm. Sci. 70, 241.

Mankani, K., Krishna, V., Manjunatha, B., Vidya, S., Singh, S.J., Manohara, Y., Raheman, A.-U., Avinash, K., 2005. Evaluation of hepatoprotective activity of stem bark of *Pterocarpus marsupium* Roxb. Indian J. Pharm. 37, 165.

Maurya, H., Upadhyay, G., 2019. Pharmacological evaluation of *Chrozophora tinctoria* as hepatoprotective potential in CCl4 induced liver damage in rat. Appl. Sci. 19, 303–310.

Miled, H.B., Barka, Z.B., Hallegue, D., Lahbib, K., Ladjimi, M., Tlili, M., Sakly, M., Rhouma, K.B., Ksouri, R., Tebourbi, O., 2017. Hepatoprotective activity of *Rhus oxyacantha* root cortex extract against DDT-induced liver injury in rats. Biomed. Pharmacother. 90, 203–215.

Mimica-Dukic, N., Popovic, M., Jakovljevic, V., Szabo, A., Gašic, O., 1999. Pharmacological studies of *Mentha longifolia* phenolic extracts. II. Hepatoprotective activity. Pharm. Biol. 37, 221–224.

Mohamed, M.A., Eldin, I.M.T., Mohammed, A.-E.H., Hassan, H.M., 2016. Effects of *Lawsonia inermis* L. (henna) leaves' methanolic extract on carbon tetrachloride-induced hepatotoxicity in rats. J. Intercult. Ethnopharmacol. 5, 22.

Mohan, K., Robert, J., 2009. Hepatoprotective effects of *Stevia rebaudiana* Bertoni leaf extract in CCl4-induced liver injury in albino rats. Med. Arom. Plant Sci. Biotechnol. 3, 59–61.

Moshaie-Nezhad, P., Faed Maleki, F., Hosseini, S., Yahyapour, M., Iman, M., Khamesipour, A., 2019. Hepatoprotective and antioxidant effects of *Hedera helix* extract on acetaminophen induced oxidative stress and hepatotoxicity in mice. Biotech. Histochem. 94, 313–319.

Mujeeb, M., Alam Khan, S., Aeri, V., Ali, B., 2011. Hepatoprotective activity of the ethanolic extract of *Ficus carica* Linn. leaves in carbon tetrachloride-induced hepatotoxicityin rats. Iran J. Pharm. Res. 10, 301–306.

Murugesh, K.S., Channabasappa Yeligar, V., Maiti, B.C., Kumar Maity, T., 2005. Hepatoprotective and antioxidant role of *Berberis tinctoria* Lesch leaves on paracetamol induced hepatic damage in rats. Iran. J. Pharmacol. Ther. 4, 64–69.

Nevin, K., Vijayammal, P., 2005. Effect of *Aerva lanata* against hepatotoxicity of carbon tetrachloride in rats. Environ. Toxicol. Pharmacol. 20, 471–477.

Noh, H.M., Ahn, E.M., Yun, J.M., Cho, B.L., Paek, Y.J., 2015. *Angelica keiskei* Koidzumi extracts improve some markers of liver function in habitual alcohol drinkers: a randomized double-blind clinical trial. J. Med. Food 18, 166–172.

Obidah, W., Garba, G.K., Fate, J.Z., Wakawa, H., 2011. Protective effects of *Bixa orellana* seed oil on carbon tetrachloride induced liver damage in rats. Rep. Opin. 3, 92–95.

Oboh, G., 2005. Hepatoprotective property of ethanolic and aqueous extracts of fluted pumpkin (*Telfairia occidentalis*) leaves against garlic-induced oxidative stress. J. Med. Food 8, 560–563.

Okokon, J.E., Oguamanam, W.N., Umoh, E.E., 2017a. Hepatoprotective and nephroprotective activities of *Solenostemon monostachyus* P. Beauv (Lamiaceae) leaf extract. Afr. J. Pharm. Pharmacol. 6, 123–133.

Okokon, J.E., Simeon, J.O., Umoh, E.E., 2017b. Hepatoprotective activity of the extract of *Homalium letestui* stem against paracetamol-induced liver injury. Avicenna J. Phytomed. 7, 27.

Olaleye, M.T., Akinmoladun, A.C., Ogunboye, A.A., Akindahunsi, A.A., 2010. Antioxidant activity and hepatoprotective property of leaf extracts of *Boerhaavia diffusa* Linn against acetaminophen-induced liver damage in rats. Food Chem. Toxicol. 48, 2200–2205.

Omoruyi, S., Enogieru, A., Momodu, O., Ayinde, B., Grillo, B., 2015. Paracetamol-induced liver damage: ameliorative effects of the crude aqueous extract of *Musanga cecropioides*. Niger. J. Health Sci. 15, 2–7.

Osadebe, P.O., Okoye, F.B., Uzor, P.F., Nnamani, N.R., Adiele, I.E., Obiano, N.C., 2012. Phytochemical analysis, hepatoprotective and antioxidant activity of *Alchornea cordifolia* methanol leaf extract on carbon tetrachloride-induced hepatic damage in rats. Asian Pac. J. Trop. Biomed. 5, 289–293.

Palanivel, M., Rajkapoor, B., Kumar, R., Einstein, J., Kumar, E., Kumar, M., Kavitha, K., Kumar, M., Jayakar, B., 2008. Hepatoprotective and antioxidant effect of *Pisonia aculeata* L. against CCl4-induced hepatic damage in rats. Sci. Pharm. 76, 203–216.

Panahi Kokhdan, E., Ahmadi, K., Sadeghi, H., Sadeghi, H., Dadgary, F., Danaei, N., Aghamaali, M.R., 2017. Hepatoprotective effect of *Stachys pilifera* ethanol extract in carbon tetrachloride-induce hepatotoxicity in rats. Pharm. Biol. 55, 1389–1393.

Panahi, Y., Kianpour, P., Mohtashami, R., Atkin, S.L., Butler, A.E., Jafari, R., Badeli, R., Sahebkar, A., 2018. Efficacy of artichoke leaf extract in non-alcoholic fatty liver disease: a pilot double-blind randomized controlled trial. Phytother. Res. 32, 1382–1387.

Panda, V., Kharat, P., Sudhamani, S., 2015. Hepatoprotective effect of the *Macrotyloma uniflorum* seed (horse gram) in ethanol-induced hepatic damage in rats. J. Biol. Active Prod. Nat. 5, 178–191.

Pandey, A., Bigoniya, P., Raj, V., Patel, K., 2011. Pharmacological screening of *Coriandrum sativum* Linn. for hepatoprotective activity. J. Pharm. Bioallied Sci. 3, 435.

Parmar, M., Shah, P., Thakkar, V., Al-Rejaie, S., Gandhi, T., 2013. Hepatoprotective potential of methanolic extract of *Vetiveria zizanioides* roots against carbon tetrachloride induced acute liver damage in rats. Dig. J. Nanomater. Biostruct. 8, 835–844.

Patel, T., Shirode, D., Roy, S.P., Kumar, S., Setty, S.R., 2010. Evaluation of antioxidant and hepatoprotective effects of 70% ethanolic bark extract of *Albizzia lebbeck* in rats. Int. J. Res. Pharm. Sci. 1, 270–276.

Pingale, S.S., 2010. Hepatoprotection by *Acacia catechu* in CCl4 induced liver dysfunction. Int. J. Pharm. Sci. Rev. Res. 1, 150–154.

Prabha, D., Annapoorani, S., 2009. Hepatoprotective effect of *Cynodon dactylon* on CCl4 induced experimental mice. J. Biosci. 17, 27–34.

Prabha, S.P., Ansil, P.N., Nitha, A., Wills, P.J., Latha, M.S., 2012. Preventive and curative effect of methanolic extract of *Gardenia gummifera* Linn. f. on thioacetamide induced oxidative stress in rats. Asian Pac. J. Trop. Dis. 2, 90–98.

Prakash, T., Fadadu, S.D., Sharma, U.R., Surendra, V., Goli, D., Stamina, P., Kotresha, D., 2008. Hepatoprotective activity of leaves of *Rhododendron arboreum* in CCl₄ induced hepatotoxicity in rats. J. Med. Plant Res. 2, 315–320.

Praneetha, P., Rani, V.S., Kumar, B.R., 2011. Hepatoprotective activity of methanolic extract of leaves of *Marsilea minuta* Linn against CCl₄ induced hepatic damage in rats. Global J. Pharmacol. 5, 164–171.

Prince, E.S., Parameswari, P., Mahaboob, K.R., 2011. Protective effect of *Ricinus communis* leaves extract on carbon tetrachloride induced hepatotoxicity in albino rats. Iran. J. Pharm. Res. 7, 269–278.

Pushpalatha, M., Ananthi, T., 2012. Protective effect of *Solanum pubescens* Linn on CCl₄ induced hepatotoxicity in albino rats. Mintage J. Pharm. Med. Sci. 1, 1–3.

Qureshi, A.A., Prakash, T., Patil, T., Swamy, A., Gouda, A.V., 2007. Hepatoprotective and antioxidant activities of flowers of *Calotropis procera* (Ait) R. Br. in CCl₄ induced hepatic damage. Indian J. Exp. Biol. 45, 304–310.

Rabeh, N.M., Aboraya, A.O., Raheem, Z.H., Jebor, A., Mohammed, S.K., Saulawa, L., 2014. Hepatoprotective effect of dill (*Anethum graveolens* L.) and fennel (*Foeniculum vulgare*) oil on hepatotoxic rats. Pak. J. Nutr. 13, 303–309.

Rabiul, H., Subhasish, M., Sinha, S., Roy, M.G., Sinha, D., Gupta, S., 2011. Hepatoprotective activity of *Clerodendron inerme* against paracetamol induced hepatic injury in rats for pharmaceutical product. Int. J. Drug Dev. Res. 3, 118–126.

Rahim, S.M., Taha, E.M., Al-janabi, M.S., Al-douri, B.I., Simon, K.D., Mazlan, A.G., 2014. Hepatoprotective effect of *Cymbopogon citratus* aqueous extract against hydrogen peroxide-induced liver injury in male rats. Afr. J. Tradit. Complement. Altern. Med. 11, 447–451.

Rajesh, M., Latha, M., 2004. Protective activity of *Glycyrrhiza glabra* Linn. on carbon tetrachloride-induced peroxidative damage. Indian J. Pharmacol. 36, 284.

Rajkapoor, B., Venugopal, Y., Anbu, J., Harikrishnan, N., Gobinath, M., Ravichandran, V., 2008. Protective effect of *Phyllanthus polyphyllus* on acetaminophen induced hepatotoxicity in rats. Pak. J. Pharm. Sci. 21, 57–62.

Ramadan, S.I., Shalaby, M., Afifi, N., El-Banna, H., 2011. Hepatoprotective and antioxidant effects of *Silybum marianum* plant in rats. Int. J. Agro Vete. Med. Sci. 5, 541–547.

Ranawat, L., Bhatt, J., Patel, J., 2010. Hepatoprotective activity of ethanolic extracts of bark of *Zanthoxylum armatum* DC in CCl₄ induced hepatic damage in rats. J. Ethnopharmacol. 127, 777–780.

Rao, G.M., Venkateswararao, C., Rawat, A., Pushpangadan, P., Shirwaikar, A., 2005. Antioxidant and antihepatotoxic activities of *Hemidesmus indicus* R. Br. Acta Pharm. Turc. 47, 107–113.

Rašković, A., Milanović, I., Pavlović, N., Ćebović, T., Vukmirović, S., Mikov, M., 2014. Antioxidant activity of rosemary (*Rosmarinus officinalis* L.) essential oil and its hepatoprotective potential. BMC Complement. Altern. Med. 14, 225.

Rathi, M., Baffila, P., Sasikumar, J., Gopalakrishnan, V., 2009. Hepatoprotective activity of ethanolic extract of *Hedyotis corymbosa* on perchloroethylene induced rats. Pharmacologyonline 3, 230–239.

Rejitha, S., Prathibha, P., Indira, M., 2012. Amelioration of alcohol-induced hepatotoxicity by the administration of ethanolic extract of *Sida cordifolia* Linn. Br. J. Nutr. 108, 1256–1263.

Roome, T., Dar, A., Ali, S., Naqvi, S., Choudhary, M.I., 2008. A study on antioxidant, free radical scavenging, anti-inflammatory and hepatoprotective actions of *Aegiceras corniculatum* (stem) extracts. J. Ethnopharmacol. 118, 514–521.

Roy, C.K., Kamath, J.V., Asad, M., 2006. Hepatoprotective activity of *Psidium guajava* Linn. leaf extract. Indian J. Exp. Biol. 44, 305–311.

Sabir, S., Rocha, J., 2008. Antioxidant and hepatoprotective activity of aqueous extract of *Solanum fastigiatum* (false "Jurubeba") against paracetamol-induced liver damage in mice. J. Ethnopharmacol. 120, 226–232.

Sabir, S., Ahmad, S., Hamid, A., Khan, M., Athayde, M., Santos, D., Boligon, A., Rocha, J., 2012. Antioxidant and hepatoprotective activity of ethanolic extract of leaves of *Solidago microglossa* containing polyphenolic compounds. Food Chem. 131, 741–747.

Sadeque, M.Z., Begum, Z.A., 2010. Protective effect of dried fruits of *Carica papaya* on hepatotoxicity in rat. Bangladesh J. Pharmacol. 5, 48–50.

Sahreen, S., Khan, M.R., Khan, R.A., 2011. Hepatoprotective effects of methanol extract of *Carissa opaca* leaves on CCl₄-induced damage in rat. BMC Complement. Altern. Med. 11, 48.

Said, A., Ibrahim, M., Mashi, J., Daha, I., 2017. Hepatoprotective effect of aqueous bark extract of *Bosweillia dalzielii* against paracetamol induced hepatotoxicity in rabbits. J. Adv. Med. Pharm. Sci. 12, 1–11.

Saka, W., Akhigbe, R., Ishola, O., Ashamu, E., Olayemi, O., Adeleke, G., 2011. Hepatotherapeutic effect of *Aloe vera* in alcohol-induced hepatic damage. Pak. J. Biol. Sci. 14, 742.

Salama, S.M., Abdulla, M.A., AlRashdi, A.S., Hadi, A.H.A., 2013a. Mechanism of hepatoprotective effect of *Boesenbergia rotunda* in thioacetamide-induced liver damage in rats. Evid. Based Complement. Alternat. Med. 2013, 1–13.

Salama, S.M., Abdulla, M.A., AlRashdi, A.S., Ismail, S., Alkiyumi, S.S., Golbabapour, S., 2013b. Hepatoprotective effect of ethanolic extract of *Curcuma longa* on thioacetamide induced liver cirrhosis in rats. BMC Complement. Altern. Med. 13, 56.

Saleem, M., Asif, A., Akhtar, M.F., Saleem, A., 2018. Hepatoprotective potential and chemical characterization of *Artocarpus lakoocha* fruit extract. Bangladesh J. Pharmacol. 13, 90–2018.

Samal, P.K., 2013. Hepatoprotective activity of *Ardisia solanacea* in CCl_4 induced Hepatoxic albino rats. Asian J. Res. Pharm. Sci. 3, 79–82.

Sanmugapriya, E., Venkataraman, S., 2006. Studies on hepatoprotective and antioxidant actions of *Strychnos potatorum* Linn. seeds on CCl_4-induced acute hepatic injury in experimental rats. J. Ethnopharmacol. 105, 154–160.

Sannigrahi, S., Mazumder, U.K., Pal, D., Mishra, S.L., 2009. Hepatoprotective potential of methanol extract of *Clerodendrum infortunatum* Linn. against CCl_4 induced hepatotoxicity in rats. Pharmacogn. Mag. 5, 394.

Saral, Ö., Yildiz, O., Aliyazicioğlu, R., Yuluğ, E., Canpolat, S., Öztürk, F., Kolayli, S., 2016. Apitherapy products enhance the recovery of CCL_4-induced hepatic damages in rats. Turk. J. Med. Sci. 46, 194–202.

Savaş, N., 2014. Karaciğer fonksiyon testi bozukluğuna yaklaşım. J. Turk. Fam. Physician 5, 1–7.

Sengottuvelu, S., Duraisami, S., Nandhakumar, J., Duraisami, R., Vasudevan, M., 2008. Hepatoprotective activity of *Camellia sinensis* and its possible mechanism of action. Iran. J. Pharmacol. Ther. 7, 9–14.

Shahjahan, M., Sabitha, K., Jainu, M., Devi, C.S., 2004. Effect of *Solanum trilobatum* against carbon tetra chloride induced hepatic damage in albino rats. Indian J. Med. Res. 120, 194–198.

Shahrzad, K., Mahya, N., Fatemeh, T.B., Maryam, K., Mohammadreza, F.B., Jahromy, M.H., 2014. Hepatoprotective and antioxidant effects of *Salvia officinalis* L. hydroalcoholic extract in male rats. Chin. Med. 5, 130–136.

Shama, I., Marwa, I., 2013. *Kigelia africana* fruits' extracts anti hepato-toxic effects on male Wistar rats liver destruction induced by CCL_4. Asian J. Med. Sci. 5, 26–32.

Shankar, N.G., Manavalan, R., Venkappayya, D., Raj, C.D., 2008. Hepatoprotective and antioxidant effects of *Commiphora berryi* (Arn) Engl bark extract against CCl_4-induced oxidative damage in rats. Food Chem. Toxicol. 46, 3182–3185.

Shanmugasundaram, P., Venkataraman, S., 2006. Hepatoprotective and antioxidant effects of *Hygrophila auriculata* (K. Schum) Heine Acanthaceae root extract. J. Ethnopharmacol. 104, 124–128.

Sharma, V., Singh, M., 2014. Attenuation of *N*-nitrosodimethylamine induced hepatotoxicity by *Operculina turpethum* in Swiss Albino mice. Iran. J. Basic Med. Sci. 17, 73.

Shastri, S.L., Krishna, V., Ravishnakar, B., Vinay Kumar, N.M., Chethan Kumara, G.P., 2017. Antioxidant and hepatoprotective potential of *Mammea suriga* aqueous extract against CCl_4 induced hepatotoxicity in rat models. World J. Pharm. Res. 6, 1396–1409.

Shen, X., Tang, Y., Yang, R., Yu, L., Fang, T., Duan, J.-A., 2009. The protective effect of *Ziziphus jujube* fruit on carbon tetrachloride-induced hepatic injury in mice by anti-oxidative activities. J. Ethnopharmacol. 122, 555–560.

Shenoy, K.A., Somayaji, S., Bairy, K., 2001. Hepatoprotective effects of *Ginkgo biloba* against carbon tetrachloride induced hepatic injury in rats. Indian J. Pharm. 33, 260–266.

Shirani, M., Raeisi, R., Heidari-Soureshjani, S., Asadi-Samani, M., Luther, T., 2017. A review for discovering hepatoprotective herbal drugs with least side effects on kidney. J. Nephropharmacol. 6, 38–48.

Shokrzadeh, M., Chabra, A., Ahmadi, A., Naghshvar, F., Habibi, E., Salehi, F., Assadpour, S., 2015. Hepatoprotective effects of *Zataria multiflora* ethanolic extract on liver toxicity induced by cyclophosphamide in mice. Drug Res. 65, 169–175.

Shyamal, S., Latha, P., Shine, V., Suja, S.R., Rajasekharan, S., Devi, T.G., 2006. Hepatoprotective effects of *Pittosporum neelgherrense* Wight & Arn., a popular Indian ethnomedicine. J. Ethnopharmacol. 107, 151–155.

Siddique, N.A., Mujeeb, M., Najmi, A.K., Aftab, A., Aslam, J., 2011. Free radical scavenging and hepatoprotective activity of *Aegle marmelos* (Linn.) Corr leaves against carbon tetrachloride. Int. J. Clin. Pharmacol. 2, 1–6.

Šimánek, V., Škottová, N., Bartek, J., Psotova, J., Kosina, P., Balejova, L., Ulirhova, J., 2001. Extract from *Silybum marianum* as a nutraceutical: a double-blind placebo-controlled study in healthy young men. Czech J. Food Sci. 19, 106–110.

Singab, A.N.B., Youssef, D.T., Noaman, E., Kotb, S., 2005. Hepatoprotective effect of flavonol glycosides rich fraction from Egyptian *Vicia calcarata* desf. against CCl_4-induced liver damage in rats. Arch. Pharm. Res. 28, 791–798.

Singh, D., Gupta, R., 2011. Hepatoprotective activity of methanol extract of *Tecomella undulata* against alcohol and paracetamol induced hepatotoxicity in rats. Life Sci. Med. Res. 26, 1–8.

Singh, D., Arya, P., Aggarwal, V., Gupta, R., 2014. Evaluation of antioxidant and hepatoprotective activities of *Moringa oleifera* Lam. leaves in carbon tetrachloride-intoxicated rats. Antioxidants 3, 569–591.

Sreepriya, M., Devaki, T., Balakrishna, K., Apparanantham, T., 2001. Effect of *Indigofera tinctoria* Linn on liver antioxidant defense system during D-galactosamine I endotoxin-induced acute hepatitis in rodents. Indian J. Exp. Biol. 39, 181–184.

Srivastava, A., Shivanandappa, T., 2010. Hepatoprotective effect of the root extract of *Decalepis hamiltonii* against carbon tetrachloride-induced oxidative stress in rats. Food Chem. 118, 411–417.

Suneetha, B., Pavan Kumar, P., Prasad Kvsrg, V.S., 2011. Hepatoprotective and antioxidant activities of methanolic extract of *Mimosa pudica* roots against carbon tetrachloride induced hepatotoxicity in albino rats. Int. J. Pharm. 1, 46–53.

Syed, S.N., Rizvi, W., Kumar, A., Khan, A.A., Moin, S., Ahsan, A., 2014. *In vitro* antioxidant and *in vivo* hepatoprotective activity of leave extract of *Raphanus sativus* in rats using CCL_4 model. Afr. J. Tradit. Complement. Altern. Med. 11, 102–106.

Tahmasebi, M., Sadeghi, H., Nazem, H., Kokhdan, E., Omidifar, N., 2018. Hepatoprotective effects of *Berberis vulgaris* leaf extract on carbon tetrachloride-induced hepatotoxicity in rats. J. Educ. Health Promot. 7, 147.

Takate, S., Pokharkar, R., Chopade, V., Gite, V., 2010. Hepato-protective activity of the aqueous extract of *Launaea intybacea* (Jacq) Beauv against carbon tetrachloride-induced hepatic injury in albino rats. J. Pharm. Sci. Technol. 2, 247–251.

Talluri, M.R., Gummadi, V.P., Battu, G.R., 2018. Chemical composition and hepatoprotective activity of *Saponaria officinalis* on paracetamol-induced liver toxicity in rats. Pharmacognosy J. J10, 1196–1201.

Tamilarasi, R., Sivanesan, D., Kanimozhi, P., 2012. Hepatoprotective and antioxidant efficacy of *Anethum graveolens* Linn in carbon tetrachloride induced hepatotoxicity in albino rats. J. Chem. Pharm. Res. 4, 1885–1888.

Tang, X.-H., Gao, L., Gao, J., Fan, Y.-M., Xu, L.-Z., Zhao, X.-N., Xu, Q., 2004. Mechanisms of hepatoprotection of *Terminalia catappa* L. extract on D-galactosamine-induced liver damage. Am. J. Chin. Med. 32, 509–519.

Tasduq, S., Kaisar, P., Gupta, D., Kapahi, B., Jyotsna, S., Maheshwari, H., Johri, R., 2005. Protective effect of a 50% hydroalcoholic fruit extract of *Emblica officinalis* against anti-tuberculosis drugs induced liver toxicity. Phytother. Res. 19, 193–197.

Thiesen, L.C., da Silva, L.M., Santin, J.R., Bresolin, T.M.B., de Andrade, S.F., de Medeiros Amorim, C., Merlin, L., de Freitas, R.A., Niero, R., Netz, D.J.A., 2017. Hepatoprotective effect of *Maytenus robusta* Reiss extract on CCl_4-induced hepatotoxicity in mice and HepG2 cells. Regul. Toxicol. Pharmacol. 86, 93–100.

Thirumalai, T., David, E., Therasa, S.V., Elumalai, E., 2011. Restorative effect of *Eclipta alba* in CCl_4 induced hepatotoxicity in male albino rats. Asian Pac. J. Trop. Dis. 1, 304–307.

Tiwari, B.K., Khosa, R., 2009. Hepatoprotective and antioxidant effect of *Sphaeranthus indicus* against acetaminophen-induced hepatotoxicity in rats. J. Pharm. Sci. Res. 1, 26–30.

Tonkiri, A., Essien, E., Akaninwor, J., 2014. Evaluation of hepatoprotective and in vivo antioxidant activity of the methanolic stem extract of *Costus afer* (Bush Cane) in alcohol induced liver cirrhosis in rats. J. Biol. Food Sci. Res. 3, 29–34.

Trivedi, N.P., Rawal, U., 2001. Hepatoprotective and antioxidant property of *Andrographis paniculata* (Nees) in BHC induced liver damage in mice. Indian J. Exp. Biol. 39, 41–46.

Tsai, J.-C., Peng, W.-H., Chiu, T.-H., Huang, S.-C., Huang, T.-H., Lai, S.-C., Lai, Z.-R., Lee, C.-Y., 2010. Hepatoprotective effect of *Scoparia dulcis* on carbon tetrachloride induced acute liver injury in mice. Am. J. Chin. Med. 38, 761–775.

Türel, I., Özbek, H., Erten, R., Öner, A.C., Cengiz, N., Yilmaz, O., 2009. Hepatoprotective and anti-inflammatory activities of *Plantago major* L. Indian J. Pharm. 41, 120.

Uduman, T.S., Sundarapandian, R., Muthumanikkam, A., Kalimuthu, G., Parameswari, S., Vasanthi Srinivas, T., Karunakaran, G., 2011. Protective effect of methanolic extract of *Annona squamosa* Linn in isoniazid-rifampicin induced hepatotoxicity in rats. Pak. J. Pharm. Sci. 24, 129–134.

Ulganathan, I., Divya, D., Radha, K., Vijaykumar, T., Dhanaraju, M., 2010. Protective effect of *Luffa acutangula* (var) *amara* against carbon tetrachloride-induced hepatotoxicity in experimental rats. Res. J. Biol. Sci. 5, 615–624.

Upadhyay, R., Pandey, N.D., Narvi, S.S., Verma, A., Ahmed, B., 2010. Antihepatotoxic effect of *Feronia limonia* fruit against carbon tetrachloride induced hepatic damage in albino rats. Chin. Med. 1, 18.

Upadhyay, G., Malik, J., Joshi, R., Lakshmayya, S.U., 2017. Hepatoprotective potential of lyophilized hydro-alcoholic extract of *Roylea elegans* Wall. against CCl_4 and PCM induced hepatotoxicity in Wistar rats. Ann. Pharmacol. Pharm. 2, 1045.

Uroko, R.I., Agbafor, A., Nwuke, C.P., Uhuo, E.N., Nweje-Anyalowu, P.C., Orjiakor, C.A., 2019. Hepatoprotective and curative effects of methanol extract of *Funtumia africana* leaves against carbon tetrachloride-induced liver damage in rats. Drugs 3, 4.

Urrutia-Hernández, T.A., Santos-López, J.A., Benedí, J., Sánchez-Muniz, F.J., Velázquez-González, C., la O-Arciniega, D., Jaramillo-Morales, O.A., Bautista, M., 2019. Antioxidant and hepatoprotective effects of *Croton hypoleucus* extract in an induced-necrosis model in rats. Molecules 24, 2533.

Vadivu, R., Krithika, A., Biplab, C., Dedeepya, P., Shoeb, N., Lakshmi, K., 2008. Evaluation of hepatoprotective activity of the fruits of *Coccinia grandis* Linn. Int. J. Health Res. 1, 163–168.

Vaidya, A.B., Antarkar, D.S., Doshi, J.C., Bhatt, A.D., Ramesh, V.V., Vora, P.V., Perissond, D.D., Baxi, A.J., Kale, P.M., 1996. *Picrorhiza kurroa* (Kutaki) Royle *ex* Benth as a hepatoprotective agent-experimental & clinical studies. J. Postgrad. Med. 42, 105–108.

Venkatanarasimhan, M., Reddy, G.A., Pawar, S., Pandian, J.J., 2014. Hepatoprotective effect of methanolic extract of *Coldenia procumbens* Linn against D-galactosamine induced acute liver damage in rats. Pharma Sci. Monit. 5, 13–18.

Venukumar, M., Latha, M., 2002. Hepatoprotective effect of the methanolic extract of *Curculigo orchioides* in CCl_4. Indian J. Pharm. 34, 269–275.

Verma, P.K., Raina, R., Sultana, M., Prawez, S., Jamwal, N., 2013. Hepatoprotective mechanisms of *Ageratum conyzoides* L. on oxidative damage induced by acetaminophen in Wistar rats. Free Radicals Antioxid. 3, 73–76.

Wegwu, M.O., Didia, B.C., 2007. Hepatoprotective effects of *Garcinia kola* seed against hepatotoxicity induced by carbon tetrachloride in rats. Biokemistri 19, 17–21.

Wills, P., Asha, V., 2006. Protective effect of *Lygodium flexuosum* (L.) Sw. (Lygodiaceae) against D-galactosamine induced liver injury in rats. J. Ethnopharmacol. 108, 116–123.

Xin-Hua, W., Chang-Qing, L., Xing-Bo, G., Lin-Chun, F., 2001. A comparative study of *Phyllanthus amarus* compound and interferon in the treatment of chronic viral hepatitis B. Southeast Asian J. Trop. Med. Public Health 32, 140–142.

Yaeesh, S., Jamal, Q., Khan, A.u., Gilani, A.H., 2006. Studies on hepatoprotective, antispasmodic and calcium antagonist activities of the aqueous-methanol extract of *Achillea millefolium*. Phytother. Res. 20, 546–551.

Yahya, F., Mamat, S., Kamarolzaman, M., Seyedan, A., Jakius, K., Mahmood, N., Shahril, M., Suhaili, Z., Mohtarrudin, N., Susanti, D., 2013. Hepatoprotective activity of methanolic extract of *Bauhinia purpurea* leaves against paracetamol-induced hepatic damage in rats. Evid. Based Complement Alternat. Med. 2013, 1–10.

Yalcin, A., Yumrutas, O., Kuloglu, T., Elibol, E., Parlar, A., Yilmaz, İ., Pehlivan, M., Dogukan, M., Uckardes, F., Aydin, H., 2017. Hepatoprotective properties for *Salvia cryptantha* extract on carbon tetrachloride-induced liver injury. Cell. Mol. Biol. (Noisy-le-Grand) 63, 56–62.

Yam, M.F., Basir, R., Asmawi, M.Z., Ismail, Z., 2007. Antioxidant and hepatoprotective effects of *Orthosiphon stamineus* Benth. standardized extract. Am. J. Chin. Med. 35, 115–126.

Yang, J., Li, Y., Wang, F., Wu, C., 2010. Hepatoprotective effects of apple polyphenols on CCl_4-induced acute liver damage in mice. J. Agric. Food Chem. 58, 6525–6531.

Yar, H.S., Ismail, D.K., Alhmed, M.N., 2012. Hepatoprotective effect of *Carthamus tinctorius* L. against carbon tetrachloride induced hepatotoxicity in rats. Pharmacie Globale 3, 1–5.

Yousuf, F., Devaraj, E., Narayan, V., 2019. Asteraceae: a review of hepatoprotective plant principles. Drug Invent. Today 11, 22–24.

Yusufoglu, H.S., Soliman, G.A., Foudah, A.I., Abdelkader, M.S., Alam, A., Salkini, M.A., 2018. Anti-inflammatory and hepatoprotective potentials of the aerial parts of *Silene villosa* Caryophyllaceae methanol extract in rats. Trop. J. Pharm. Res. 17, 117–125.

Zangeneh, M.M., Zangeneh, A., Tahvilian, R., Moradi, R., Zhaleh, H., Amiri-Paryan, A., Bahrami, E., 2018. Hepatoprotective and hematoprotective effects of *Falcaria vulgaris* aqueous extract against CCl_4-induced hepatic injury in mice. Comp. Clin. Pathol. 27, 1359–1365.

Zargar, S., 2014. Protective effect of *Trigonella foenum-graecum* on thioacetamide induced hepatotoxicity in rats. Saudi J. Biol. Sci. 21, 139–145.

Zeng, H., Li, D., Qin, X., Chen, P., Tan, H., Zeng, X., Li, X., Fan, X., Jiang, Y., Zhou, Y., 2016. Hepatoprotective effects of *Schisandra sphenanthera* extract against lithocholic acid-induced cholestasis in male mice are associated with activation of the pregnane × receptor pathway and promotion of liver regeneration. Drug Metab. Dispos. 44, 337–342.

Zhang, Q., Hu, X., Hui, F., Song, Q., Cui, C., Wang, C., Zhao, Q., 2017. Ethanol extract and its dichloromethane fraction of *Alpinia oxyphylla* Miquel exhibited hepatoprotective effects against CCl_4-induced oxidative damage in vitro and *in vivo* with the involvement of Nrf2. Biomed. Pharmacother. 91, 812–822.

Zhu, C.S., Liu, K., Wang, J.L., Li, J.F., Liu, M.F., Hao, N., Lin, Y.X., Xiao, Z.F., 2018. Antioxidant activities and hepatoprotective potential of *Dracocephalum rupestre* Hance extract against CCl_4-induced hepatotoxicity in Kunming mice. J. Food Biochem. 42, 1–8.

CHAPTER 14

Plant extracts with putative hepatotoxicity activity

Palaniappan Saravanapriya and Kasi Pandima Devi
Department of Biotechnology, Alagappa University [Science Campus], Karaikudi, Tamil Nadu, India

14.1 Introduction

Drugs obtained from plant extracts are used both in their crude form and as commercial extracts to treat various diseases. Mostly in developing countries, parts of the plants such as the leaves, seeds, roots, and bark are used to prepare crude herbal drugs as therapeutic remedies. The components of some of the combination drugs prepared in some developing countries such as China, Thailand, and India remain unknown and contain impurities such as arsenic, lead, and mercury, which cause harmful effects. In developed countries, herbal products are available in the form of tablets or capsules and are often used to treat certain diseases. Overall, people are interested in improving their health through the intake of herbal and dietary supplements (HDS), which is becoming popular all over the world. People who take HDS are believed to be very secure without any problems with their long-term health (Ekor, 2014). Worldwide, medicinal products produced from plants grow rapidly and large numbers of products are launched into the market. However, their safety effects are also gradually compromised (Table 14.1).

Traditional medicine compliments the patient's welfare and also the value of their life when compared to allopathic treatment, which has made herbal medicine popular among people. Even though some herbal remedies have favorable efficacy and are used effectively, most of them are still unproven scientifically and their use is overlooked. Some of the medicinal plants act as hepatoprotective agents and protect against liver damage. For example, polyphenolic compounds present in plants have the ability to eliminate free radicals and act as excellent antioxidants (Sreelatha et al., 2009). Some of the reported hepatoprotective plants are *Andrographis paniculata* (Burm.f.) Nees., *Hygrophila auriculata* Schumach., *Rhinacanthus nasuta* L., Kurz., *Flaveria trinervia* (Spreng.) C. Mohr., *Bauhinia racemosa* Lam., *Emblica officinalis L.*, *Cassia fistula L.*, *Solanum nigrum L.*, etc. (Adewusi and Afolayan, 2010). Universally, the use of traditional medicinal plants is popular, although some plants cause hepatotoxicity.

Influence of Nutrients, Bioactive Compounds, and Plant Extracts in Liver Diseases. https://doi.org/10.1016/B978-0-12-816488-4.00002-4

Table 14.1: Toxic dosage of the plant extracts in different model systems.

SI no.	Name of the plants	Toxic dosage of plant extracts		References
		Model	LD50	
1	*Atractylis gummifera* **Linnaeus**	· Mice (oral) · Rat (oral)	> 2000 mg/kg 1000 mg/kg	Bouabid et al. (2019) Haouzi et al. (2002)
2	*Morinda citrifolia* **Linnaeus**	· Rats	2000 mg/kg	Srikanth and Muralidharan (2009)
3	*Camellia sinensis* **Linnaeus**	· Rats	2500 mg/kg	Hsu et al. (2011)
4	*Aloe indica* **Linnaeus**	· Swiss albino mice · Humans	1000 mg/kg 120 mg/kg	Guo and Mei (2016) Kwack et al. (2009)
5	*Teucrium chamaedrys* **Linnaeus**	· Rats	2000 mg/kg	Tanira et al. (1996)
6	*Chelidonium majus* **Linnaeus**	· Rats	10 mg/kg	Ulrichova et al. (1996)
7	*Methysticum rhizoma* **G.Forst**	· Test animals · Humans	300-400 mg/kg > 300 mg/day	Meyer (1962) Ulbricht et al. (2002)
8	*Larrea tridentata* **(Sess. & Moc. ex DC.) Cov.**	· Mice	75 mg/kg	Ladd (2013)
9	*Mentha pulegium* Linnaeus	· Swiss-Webster mice	500 mg/kg	Gordon et al. (1982)
10	*Amanita phalloides* **(Vaill. ex Fr. :Fr.)**	· Mice · Beagles	1 mg/kg 85 mg/kg	Zheleva et al. (2007) Vogel et al. (1984)
11	*Viscumalbum* **Linnaeus**	· Mice	4.18 ± 0.96 g/kg	Ohiri et al. (2003)
12	*Xanthium strumarium* **Linnaeus**	· Mice · Rats	2000 mg/kg 30.0 g/kg	Akarte et al. (2009) Xue et al. (2014a)
13	*Scutellaria biacalensis* Georgi	· Rats	2500 mg/kg	Yan et al. (2018)
14	*Callilepis laureola* DC.,	· Hep G2 cells	6.7 mg/mL	Popat et al. (2001)
15	*Valeriana officinalis* **Linnaeus**	· Human Hepatoma cells (HG2P128) · Rats	20 mg/mL 18.6 g/kg	Vo et al. (2003)
16	*Hypericum perforatum* **Linnaeus**	· Wistar rats	100 mg/kg /day	Gregoretti et al. (2004)
17	*Cascara sagrada* **DC**	· Rats	3700 mg/kg	Mahady (2004)
18	*Cassia acutifolia* **Delile**	· Mice	4000 mg/kg	Westendorf (1993)
19	*Actaea racemosa* **Linnaeus**	· HepG2 cells · Rats	75 µg/ mL 1000 mg/kg	Lüde et al. (2007)
20	*Echinaceae purpurea* **Linnaeus**	· Humans	1500 mg/day	Kocaman et al. (2008)

Generally, hepatotoxicity is caused by infections, autoimmune diseases, and the excessive intake of acetaminophen and alcohol. In general, most hepatotoxic chemicals affect and damage liver cells by causing the oxidative degradation of lipids while also inducing other oxidative damage (Ullah and Ahmad, 2014). Hepatotoxins are generally defined as chemical compounds that may originate from foods, pharmaceuticals, and medicinal plants that cause toxicity to the liver (Thompson et al., 2017). Troglitazone is an example for drug-induced hepatotoxicity that helps to treat type II diabetes and can also be useful to treat nonalcoholic fatty liver disease to reduce the liver enzyme levels (Caldwell et al., 2001). However, the use of the drug was discontinued after the potential for fulminant hepatitis was unambiguously confirmed (Smith, 2003).

Sometimes problems may occur with the herbal product even on prescribing the regulations on its usage. In some cases, if the patient's herbal medication is not disclosed, there could be a delay in identifying the toxicity induced by herbs. Though there are no precise medical tests to diagnose herbal hepatotoxicity, if there is any form of liver injury such as necrotic lesions or vascular injury, especially veno-occlusive disease (VOD), with regional necrosis, steatosis, or bile duct injury, herbal hepatotoxicity can be suspected (Stedman, 2002). Many studies reported that the use of active phytoconstituents has no adverse side effects. Therefore, the hepatotoxicity of certain medications only becomes evident after they have been exposed to a significant number of patients. Even then, the hepatotoxicity of herbal drugs still remains unnoticed because consumers and prescribers do not understand the causal relationship immediately. In addition, there are no regulations to access herbal drugs in many countries, where these drugs are available at affordable prices (Stickel et al., 2005). The reports on herbal toxicity are also not widely known to users because only isolated case reports and small case series were noted.

Among 80%–100% of cases related to hepatotoxicity occur in women due to *Larrea tridentata* (Sess. & Moc. ex DC.) Cov., *Teucrium chamaedrys* L., and *Chelidonium majus* L. The plant *Teucrium chamaedrys* L. is promoted primarily as a drug for reducing weight; hence it has prompted the tendency of women to use these drugs. However, the gender-based difference reported on the use of plant-based drugs raises a contradictory concern (Kessler et al., 2001). Overall, the investigation of plant extracts with putative hepatotoxicity has become a promising area for developing standardized, regulated, and novel phytopharmaceuticals to alleviate illness.

14.2 General concepts of hepatotoxicity

The liver, which performs various vital functions such as detoxification, bile secretion, and the metabolism of carbohydrates, protein, fats, and lipids, is also involved in various biochemical pathways. The diseases that affect the normal functions of the liver are termed hepatic diseases, and they are a chief health problem worldwide. Out of the different liver diseases, hepatotoxicity is the toxic damage to the liver caused by certain toxic chemical compounds categorized as hepatotoxins. It begins with mild liver damage and progresses to jaundice. Sufferers may need liver transplantation due to liver failure, and sometimes this ends in death. It is characterized by an increased level of alanine aminotransferase or alkaline phosphatase without concomitant raised levels of serum bilirubin. Hepatotoxicity is caused by a number of agents such as drugs, alcohol consumption, and even the improper intake of nutritional supplements and herbal drugs. In particular, herbal drugs used over the long term result in hepatotoxicity, which can range from changes in the levels of the liver enzymes at a mild level to severe liver disease resulting in liver damage (Anand and Lal, 2016). The diagnosis of a person for herbal hepatotoxicity is desired because there are no diagnostic biomarkers to distinctly detect herbal hepatotoxicity when compared to the detection of other types of hepatic diseases. Consequently, the diagnosis needs awareness concerning its putative incidence and information, essential to eliminating all other sources for liver injury (Larson et al., 2005; Zimmerman, 1999). RUCAM (Roussel Uclaf Causality Assessment Method) is a quantitative and effective tool to diagnose liver damage by HILI (herb-induced liver injury) and DILI (drug-induced liver injury) (Frenzel and Teschke, 2016). This is a diagnostic method of hepatotoxicity based on clinical and biochemical parameters used to calculate the scores, in which higher scores denote an increased chance of liver injury. Worldwide, RUCAM is widely used as an assessment method to analyze liver injury caused by CAM (complementary and alternative medicine) by calculating to what extent the levels of the enzymes alkaline phosphatase (ALP) and alanine transaminase (ALT) have increased over the upper normal limit (calculated as N). The R values are calculated by taking the ratio of ALT and ALP. Depending upon whether the R values are above 5, above 2, or between 2 and 5, the severity of the disease is determined (Danan and Teschke, 2016).

14.2.1 Types of hepatotoxicity

The levels of ALP and ALT can be used to categorize what type of liver injury a patient has, it may be a mild form of cholestatic injury if the ALP levels are elevated or it may be a more severe form of hepatocellular damage if the ALT levels are elevated (Hussaini and Farrington, 2007). Hepatic injury can be classified as hepatocellular, cholestasis, or a mixed-type injury depending on the R ratio (ALT/ULN)/(ALP/ULN) (ULN—upper limits of normal ranges) (Lin et al., 2019). If the R ratio is greater than 5, less than 2, or between 2 and 5, it indicates hepatocellular, cholestasis, or a mixed-type liver injury, respectively. In addition, a liver injury due to hepatotoxin is characterized by two forms, idiosyncratic injury or intrinsic (Uetrecht, 2007, 2008) (Fig. 14.1).

14.2.1.1 Idiosyncratic form of liver injury

Idiosyncratic DILI is a rare adverse drug reaction independent of the dose that sometimes results in severe hepatic failure or even death. The most common causes are the metabolism of drugs, prolonged use of drugs by aged people, increased risk from the unknown quality of HDS, and environmental factors (Yamashita et al., 2017). Drug metabolism by the liver

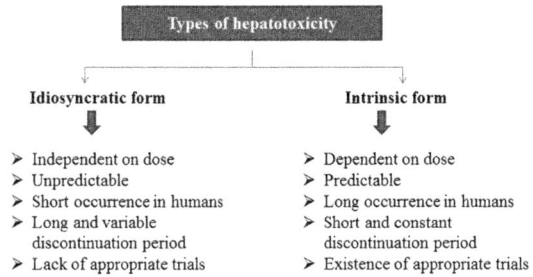

Fig. 14.1
Type of hepatotoxicity.

involves biotransformation by phase I metabolic reactions, which involves oxidation as well as hydrolytic and reduction reactions, and phase II, which involves conjugation reactions (Zimmerman, 1999; Knowles et al., 2000; Pessayre, 1995). The development of toxic reactive metabolites during liver metabolism combined with the involvement of native and adaptive immunity are involved in the development of liver injuries. An increase in eosinophils by 25%–30% in the peripheral blood and hypersensitive characteristics such as fever in DILI patients supports that this type of liver injury is also immunologically mediated (Björnsson et al., 2007; Ibáñez et al., 2002).

It has been presumed that most of the herbs associated with hepatotoxicity cases are possibly idiosyncratic. An example of idiosyncratic hepatotoxicity is the use of *Piper methysticum* with the common name of kava, a herb with psychotropic effects indigenous to Polynesia (Teschke and Eickhoff, 2015). Studies carried out in patients with kava-induced liver toxicity have shown that the plant induces idiosyncratic toxicity through its metabolites and is not immunologically mediated, as no hypersensitivity reactions were observed. Because the type of toxicity induced by kava is idiosyncratic, it cannot be reproduced in any in vivo model system such as experimental animals, which makes it difficult to study its pathogenesis (Teschke et al., 2008).

14.2.1.2 Intrinsic form of liver injury

Unlike the idiosyncratic form, which is nonpredictable, the intrinsic type of liver injury is dose-dependent and predictable. The different causative factors include genetic factors, inflammatory stress, and environmental factors. Drugs that act as intrinsic hepatotoxic agents mainly target the liver and induce injury to it. Among the hepatotoxic agents, an overdose of the antipyretic drug acetaminophen (APAP) causes serious liver pathogenesis. The reactive metabolites of APAP that are formed by the action of the drug-metabolizing enzyme cytochrome P450 are normally removed by conjugation with glutathione. But during an APAP overdose, there will not be effective removal through conjugation, so the accumulated metabolites react with the cellular components and induce hepatic necrosis.

The inflammatory stress developed involves the activation of nonparenchymal cells, the development of oxidative stress, mitochondrial dysfunction, and other factors (Roth and Ganey, 2010). An example of intrinsic hepatotoxicity in the case of herbal drug use includes the intake of *Teucrium chamaedrys* L., *Mentha pulegium*, and pyrrolizidine alkaloids, which depends on the dose. The intrinsic type of liver injury is reproducible in animals, so the toxicity of Germander (*Teucrium chamaedrys*) could be studied in mice. The metabolism of the diterpenoids present in the germander by the cytochrome P4503A enzyme produces toxic metabolites that are normally removed through conjugation with glutathione. The depletion of glutathione levels occurs during an overdose, wherein the metabolites bind to the cellular proteins and induce hepatic cell death. The identification of autoantibodies in the serum of patients who had a germander overdose proposes that the plant induces immunoallergic hepatic injury (Larrey and Faure, 2011; Thomassen et al., 1992).

14.2.2 Causes of hepatotoxicity

Liver is an important organ that carries out vital functions in the body, so to maintain a person's health, it is important that the liver functions are normal in that person. But a variety of factors such as environmental pollutants, alcohol consumption, improper drug usage, etc., cause damage to the liver such as fat accumulation, inflammation, hepatitis, and other serious liver diseases (Subramoniam and Pushpangadan, 1999).

14.2.2.1 Hepatotoxicity induced by drugs

The liver may get damaged by the intake of some therapeutic drugs when used for a prolonged period, even upon administration within the treatment limits. More than 900 drugs have been involved in inducing liver damage, which is the major reason for discontinuing the use of these drugs (Ostapowicz et al., 2002). In addition, it becomes a problem to pharmaceutical industries because the drugs have to be withdrawn from the market and simultaneously doctors have to be properly informed about withdrawing the drug because continued treatment may lead to hepatic disease and sometimes death. Although a number of liver injuries can be caused by medications, only a few of these injuries can actually cause death. Cytolytic hepatitis is the most common one induced by drugs. It is often triggered by the formation of cytochrome P450-mediated reactive metabolites that target the liver constituents and can cause harmful, immunoallergic reactions or autoimmune hepatitis (Pessayre and Larrey, 1988). Paracetamol, chlorpromazine, isoniazid, and amoxicillin-clavulanate are some examples of the reported causes of hepatotoxicity induced by drugs (Zimmerman, 2000; Weber et al., 2003). Paracetamol (acetaminophen), which is an over-the-counter drug, is the therapeutically active metabolite of acetanilide and phenacetin used for its analgesic and antipyretic properties. Also, paracetamol is primarily hepatotoxic and nephrotoxic in a variety of laboratory animals. Mice and hamsters are particularly sensitive to the drug's hepatotoxic effects, comparable to their effect in humans (Lubek et al., 1988).

14.2.2.2 Hepatotoxicity induced by viruses

The viruses that have been identified in humans as causing liver damage are hepatitis viruses A, B, C, D, E, and G, and sometimes the transfusion-transmitted (TT) viruses are also involved in inducing hepatitis (Zuckerman, 1996). When compared to the other viruses, HBV (hepatitis B virus) and HCV (hepatitis C virus) are the most common type of viruses found to cause chronic hepatitis and even hepatocellular carcinoma (HCC) in patients. Clinical evaluations of hepatitis patients with these viruses have revealed that patients can be asymptomatic or symptomatic or can also exhibit fulminant hepatic failure more commonly in HBV patients, where the hepatic function is severely affected. In addition, the immune system of the host acts against the viral proteins produced by the hepatitis viruses in the hepatocytes, which is the major contributor for liver injury sometimes when compared to the cytopathic effects caused by the viruses. Liver injury by the immune system is mainly caused by the cytotoxic T cells, which are produced specifically against the viral antigens. The activation of these cells induces the apoptosis of the affected hepatocytes and causes liver injury (Nakamoto and Kaneko, 2003; Arias et al., 2011).

14.2.3 Mechanisms of hepatotoxicity

Important functions of the liver are the production of bile acids and the excretion of toxins such as bilirubin (Fig. 14.2). Cholestasis occurs when hepatocytes and bile ducts are damaged by drugs. The mechanism of hepatotoxicity involves bile acid accumulation as well as activation of both parenchymal and nonparenchymal cells.

14.2.3.1 Bile acid accumulation

Bile acids (cholic acid and chenodeoxycholic), which are produced by the catabolism of cholesterol, help not only in the absorption of nutrients but also in the excretion of toxic metabolites. They also help in regulating the metabolism of lipids, glucose, and energy in the cells by acting as signaling molecules. These acids activate the signaling mechanism by binding to the bile acid receptors such as FXR (farnesoid X receptor) and Gpbar-1, also called TGR5 (membrane G protein-coupled bile acid receptor). Though bile acids are important to maintain the homeostasis of the liver, if their levels are not maintained, they accumulate in the liver and cause injury. For example, the accumulation of hydrophobic bile acids such as deoxycholic acid damages the liver by acting as an inflammatory agent (Chiang, 1998, 2004, 2013). In the liver disease called cholestasis, the target genes of FXR are not regulated, which causes a reduction in the flow of bile acids leading to accumulation (Trauner et al., 1998).

14.2.3.2 Activation of parenchymal cells

Most of the metabolic functions are performed by hepatocytes, which are the parenchymal cells that make up as much as 80% of the liver mass. Hepatocytes express the essential proteins such as albumin (the abundantly present circulating plasma protein), transporters, modulators of immune complexes, and inflammation. Additionally, hepatocytes perform

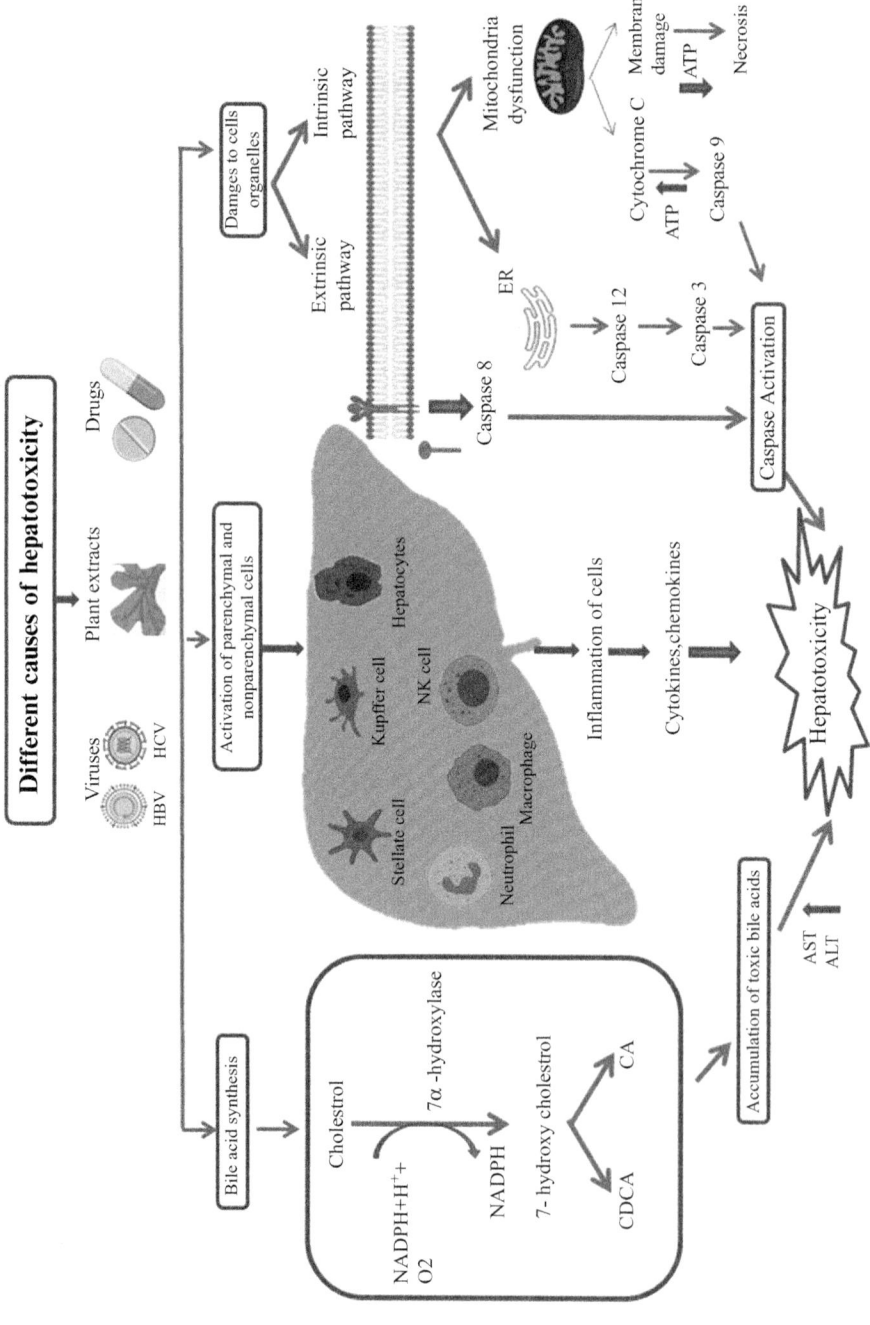

Fig. 14.2

Different mechanisms of hepatotoxicity.

pH regulation essential for urea synthesis and ammonia detoxication. The remaining 20% of the liver mass consists of nonparenchymal cells (NPC), which are made of Kupffer cells, endothelial cells, stellate cells (called ito cells), leukocytes, and sinusoidal cells called pit cells. Most of the activities are focused on the hepatocyte, a parenchymal cell that develops the hepatotoxicity. Apart from damage to the hepatocytes, NPCs are also damaged as a secondary response, which can significantly worsen the initial damage (Michalopoulos, 2007; Tanaka et al., 2011).

14.2.3.3 Activation of nonparenchymal cells

Kupffer cells, which constitute up to about 20% of NPC, are the resident macrophages of the liver that are involved in immunomodulation and phagocytosis while protecting against biochemical attack. When the Kupffer cells are activated, they release reactive oxygen and nitrogen species, proteases, and metabolites of lipids such as prostaglandins (Decker, 1990; Wang et al., 1993). Apart from these molecules, various inflammatory cytokines such as TNF-α, interferon α/β, and IL-1 and IL-6 are also secreted by the activated Kupffer cells (Decker, 1990). Experimentally, it has been reported that Kupffer cells are activated by endotoxin and xenobiotics such as ethanol, acetaminophen, and carbon tetrachloride (Tsukamoto, 2002). The significance of Kupffer cells was understood in experimental studies in which the cells were inactivated by the compound gadolinium chloride. Depletion of the cells using these compounds was able to protect the liver against hepatotoxic agents, which signifies the importance of Kupffer cells in inducing liver damage (Tsukamoto, 2002).

The activation of the nonparenchymal cell sinusoidal endothelial cell present in the liver develops liver fibrosis and hepatitis (Ni et al., 2017). During pathological conditions, type I collagen synthesis is activated in stellate cells, which can be identified from the collagen deposition in histological sections taken from patients with liver fibrosis and cirrhosis (Jaeschke et al., 2002). Under normal conditions, these cells act as a major storage place for vitamin A, however, when they are activated, the levels of vitamin A in the cells are depleted. The cells will then attain altered phenotypes and start synthesizing collagen. In addition, the activated stellate cells produce many other ECM (extracellular matrix) proteins, which leads to liver fibrosis (Bataller and Brenner, 2005).

14.3 Hepatotoxicity induced by plant extracts and mushrooms

Plant extracts contain a combination of chemical compositions in which the type of ingredient and the presence of any impurities are generally not known. Because these extracts might contain some harmful hepatotoxins, studying the risk of hepatotoxicity from plant extracts is more important during drug development (Nadir et al., 2000). Hepatotoxicity induced by different herbal plants (Fig. 14.3) is explained below.

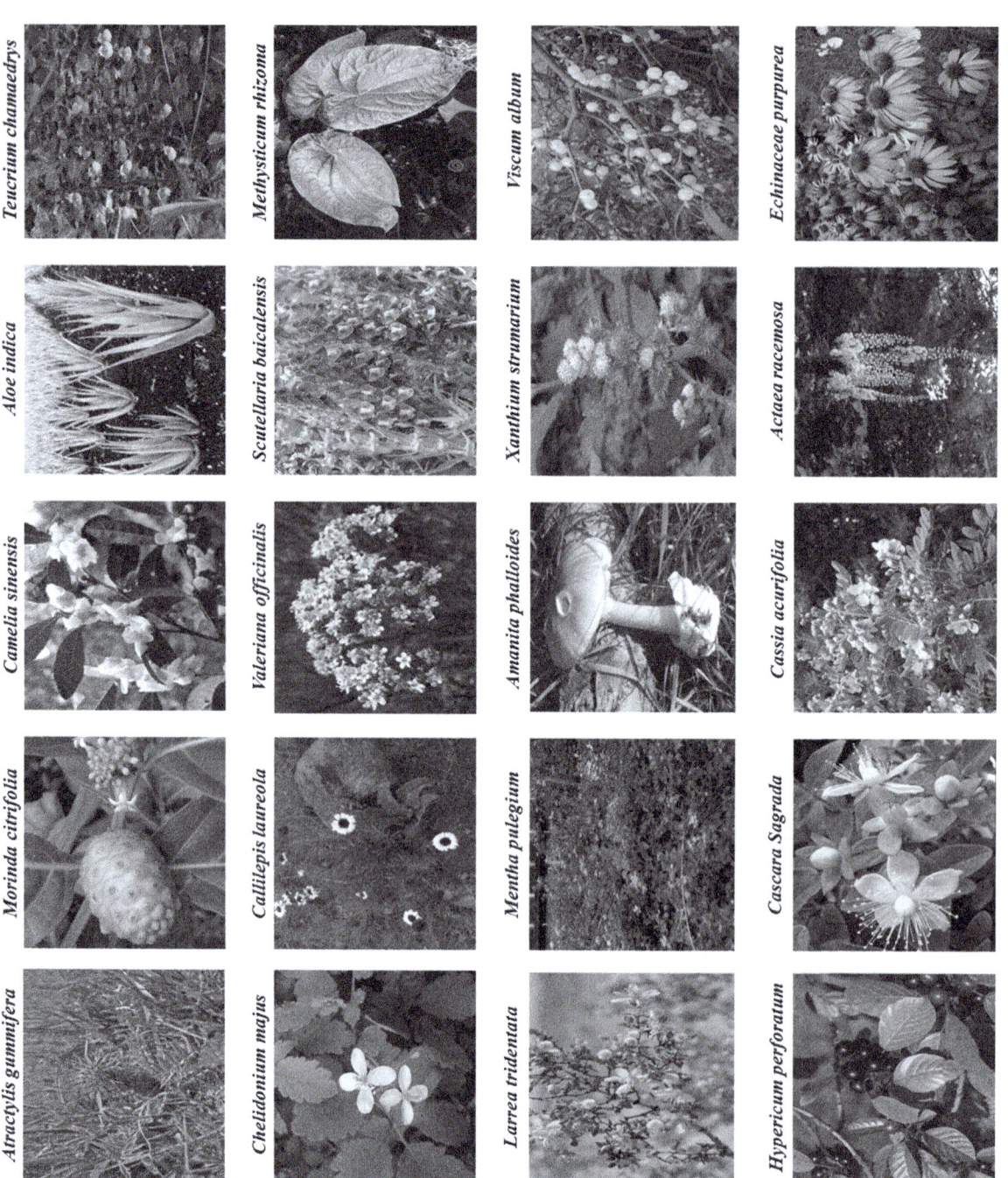

Fig. 14.3

Plants with potential hepatotoxic effect.

14.3.1 Atractylis gummifera L.

Atractylis gummifera is a thorny herb commonly known as blue thistle, chamaelon, or bird lime that belongs to the family Asteraceae. It is found worldwide but is particularly present in abundance in Mediterranean regions. The herb has been used for various treatments due to its diuretic, emetic, purgative, and antipyretic properties. The plant secretes a glue-like substance that is used in making chewing gum (Larrey, 1997). During springtime, the intake of *A. gummifera* is unsafe due to the accumulation of toxins in the roots or when the plant is confused with wild artichoke. The toxicity of *A. gummifera* is due to diterpenoid glycosides such as atractyloside and carboxyatractyloside, which are inhibitors of the Krebs cycle and other mitochondrial functions (Daniele et al., 2005). These glycosides prevent ATP synthesis by blocking ADP transport through the mitochondrial membrane, which causes energy deprivation in the cells due to the nonavailability of glucose, resulting in cell death (Stewart and Steenkamp, 2000). There are no specific pharmacological treatments available for the toxicity of *A. gummifera*, and all existing treatments are symptomatic. New therapeutic methods may come from immunotherapy research. Bouabid et al. (2019) reported the acute toxicity of *A. gummifera,* and the LD 50 was 2000 mg/kg for mice and 1000 mg/kg for rats. But the toxicity of the plant depends on the part of the plant ingested and its preparation as well as the dose (Vallejo et al., 2009). In a case report, a 7-year-old boy accidentally took an extract of *A. gummifera* and was admitted to the hospital in stage II of a coma. The patient developed jaundice while the liver increased in size, the liver marker enzymes increased, intrahepatic cholestasis developed, and unfortunately the patient died after 8 days. This report cautioned that accidental intake may be suicidal to humans (Georgiou et al., 1988).

14.3.2 Morinda citrifolia L.

Morinda citrifolia, commonly known as the noni berry, is used to prepare the health drink called NONI juice. It is used in Polynesian herbal remedies to treat diseases such as cancer, gastric ulcers, depression, etc. Although it is used in various treatments, sometimes the ingestion of this health drink causes acute hepatotoxicity, mainly caused by two components identified in the plant. The first group includes anthraquinones such as morindone, nordamnacanthal, rubiadin, rubiadin-1-methyl ether, and anthraquinone glycosides, which induces hepatotoxicity dose-dependently. The other group of compounds includes coumarins such as scopoletin, which are candidates for hepatotoxicity independent of the dose (Wang et al., 2002). The toxicity of *M. citrifolia* was studied in mice in which the mortality and change in physiological behaviors were observed at higher doses at different time intervals (Younos et al., 1990). A case report of a 14-year-old boy revealed that he suffered from acute hepatotoxicity upon the intake of a drink that had noni berries (Elizabeth et al., 2011). Another case report is of a 45-year-old patient with an unexceptional medical history due to extremely high transaminases and lactate dehydrogenase; he took no medicines on a habitual basis. In diagnosis, no proof was observed for viral hepatitis and no malformations were detected. Toxicity due to NONI intake was revealed after the patient confessed the intake of NONI juice for precautionary reasons. Liver biopsy samples revealed liver toxicity, but after the discontinuation of NONI juice, the transaminase levels were standardized and attained normal limits after 1 month (Millonig et al., 2005).

14.3.3 Camellia sinensis L.

Green tea is a commonly used dietary supplement that has been consumed worldwide for many years due to its antioxidant and weight loss benefits. Although green tea extract has benefits, there has been rising concern with reference to possible hepatotoxicity leading to severe liver failure (Mazzanti et al., 2009; Stickel et al., 2011). Green tea derived from the leaves of *Camellia sinensis* over long-term use induces hepatotoxicity with a recovery time of about 2 months. In some cases, there is an interaction between the ingredients due to the mixed preparation of green tea, which induces severe liver damage with a recovery time of about 10 months (Mazzanti et al., 2015). Epigallocatechin-3-gallate (EGCG), which is the main constituent in green tea, induced toxicity in cultured rat hepatocytes (Schmidt et al., 2005). Studies in experimental animals and mammalian cells have shown that EGCG undergoes oxidative metabolism, glucuronidation at various positions, and methylation by catechol-*O*-methyltransferase (Lu et al., 2003). A case report regarding green tea extract intake is discussed hereafter. The case report is of a 76-year-old man who drank tea extracts as a routine practice. He was reported with jaundice, weight loss, and subacute hepatitis. A diagnosis revealed that the prolonged intake of green tea as a dietary supplement is the major cause of liver inflammation. After 7 months, due to reduced consumption of green tea, moderate improvement in his health was observed, and based on histology data it was observed that the hepatitis was cured (Vanstraelen et al., 2008).

14.3.4 Aloe vera L.

Aloe vera has been used for centuries and is cultivated worldwide for its therapeutic benefits such as antiinflammatory and antibacterial properties. It is also grown as an ornamental plant. It has been taken in the form of topical and oral therapeutics produced from its fleshy leaves. Although it has therapeutic benefits, sometimes the intake of *Aloe vera* is correlated with diarrhea, kidney dysfunction, electrolyte imbalance, erythema, and phototoxicity. The aloe leaf gel consists of amino acids, polysaccharides, minerals, organic acids, and phenolic compounds. It also contains anthrones, C-glycosides, and anthraquinones such as aloe-emodin, aloesin, aldehydes, and ketones (Boudreau and Beland, 2006). Among these compounds, the most toxic is emodin, and the overconsumption of emodin elevated the liver enzyme concentration. When the compound was administered to mice at concentrations of 40 and 80 μM, a decrease in the viability of the hepatocytes to about 45% was observed

(Dong et al., 2016). Based on the animal studies, the consumption level for a 60 kg adult was estimated at 24 mg/kg/day (Calitz et al., 2015). A case report of a 35-year-old woman revealed that the patient suffered from heavy blood loss during surgery based on the antiplatelet effect due to the possible interaction between the drug sevoflurane, which causes platelet aggregation, and *Aloe vera*. Also, the hepatotoxicity of *Aloe vera* was determined by the Roussel Uclaf Causality Assessment Method, in which patients with high scores may suffer from liver injury. Due to this herb-drug interaction, it was suggested that the herbal medicines with antiplatelet capacity should be terminated before anesthesia and surgery (Lee et al., 2004). Another case report is of a 73-year-old female who was taking capsules containing *Aloe vera to* treat constipation. The liver markers of hepatotoxicity returned to normal levels in the patient after the discontinuation of oral *Aloe vera* (Bottenberg et al., 2007).

14.3.5 Teucrium chamaedrys L.

This plant, which is commonly called germander, belongs to the family Labiatae. It has been perceived to have choleretic and antiseptic properties since ancient times. It was commonly taken in tea, through capsules, and as an addition to liquors to lose weight. It was approved in France in 1986, but was later banned there in 1992 in France. It was also banned in Italy in 1996 and Belgium in 1997 because hepatotoxicity was observed in germander intake (Savvidou et al., 2007). Out of its different components such as glycosides, flavonoids, and saponins, the hepatotoxic compounds were identified as the diterpenoids, including Teucrin A and Teuchmaedryn A. The xenobiotic metabolizing enzyme cytochrome P450 3A4 oxidizes these diterpenoids into the reactive metabolite epoxide that is detoxified by the glutathione present in the cells. When the levels of cellular glutathione are depleted, the reactive metabolites formed will cause damage to the liver. The recommended dose of germander is 600–1600 mg/day; however when taken over a period of 2 months, this causes hepatoxicity. Though specific symptoms were not observed, patients had adverse hepatocellular changes, including jaundice and changes in liver marker enzymes (Lin et al., 2019; Laliberte and Villeneuve, 1996).

In the case reports of two patients (one with a previous history of hepatitis B infection), it was shown that the intake of *T. chamaedrys* decoctions led to complaints of nausea and asthenia, without any clinical observation of a rise in liver marker enzymes. The enzyme levels were found to be elevated after a 5-month follow-up; however, the patients denied the intake of any drug that was known to induce hepatotoxicity. After a few days, they agreed that they took a decoction containing a plant, which was botanically identified as *T. chamaedrys*. The Naranjo scale calculation also revealed that the patients had possibly developed an ADR (adverse drug reaction) due to *T. chamaedrys* and the drug had induced a secondary immune response in the patients. The liver markers were normalized after the intake of the herb was discontinued, and the patients recovered completely (Savvidou et al., 2007).

14.3.6 Chelidonium majus L.

Greater celandine is often used to treat biliary disorders, gastrointestinal problems, and irritable bowel syndrome. The plant *Greater celandine* consists of isoquinoline alkaloids such as chelerythrine, berberine, coptisine, sanguinarine, protopine, and allocryptopine, which inhibit mitochondrial enzymes such as succinate and NADH dehydrogenase (Barreto et al., 2003). In vivo studies reported that sanguinarine or chelerythrine, when administered at 10 mg/kg of body weight in adult rats through i.p. injection, resulted in necrotic liver damage (Ulrichová et al., 1996). Hepatotoxicity was also reported in two patients, who completely improved after the withdrawal of *Greater celandine* (Stickel et al., 2003). *C. majus*-induced hepatotoxicity was reported in a 42-year-old woman who was admitted to the hospital due to severe hepatitis. It was found that the patient consumed a herbal product containing the combination of *greater celandine* and Curcuma root, which was prescribed by an alternative therapist for skin complaints. The patient recovered after stopping the consumption of greater celandine and within 2 months, the liver function also returned to normal (Crijns et al., 2002).

14.3.7 Piper methysticum G. Forst

Kava, which is the pepper plant *Piper methysticum,* is consumed as an alcoholic beverage in the South Pacific islands as a psychotropic remedy. The plant is also used to treat anxiety ailments and depression. Some reports show possible cases of hepatotoxicity caused by the intake of various commercial products produced from kava (Jussofie et al., 1994; Davies et al., 1992). The consumption of kava is generally considered to be safe and also has some side effects such as symptoms of hair loss and yellowish skin discoloration, collectively known as kavaism (Norton and Ruze, 1994). The hepatotoxicity of kava has not been clearly explained, but it consists of some possible hepatotoxic components such as flavokavain B, pipermethystine (an alkaloid), and contaminating mold consisting of hepatotoxins (Teschke, 2010; Teschke et al., 2011). It was recommended that the hepatotoxicity of kava is partially curable by quality control and avoiding combined intake. Meanwhile, it was observed that hepatoxicity occurs mainly due to the consumption of more than 250 mg of kava lactones/day (Teschke et al., 2008; Teschke and Schulze, 2010).

The case report of a patient with hepatotoxicity due to the consumption of kava-containing tablets is explained below. A 14-year-old female was admitted to the hospital due to hepatitis with symptoms of nausea and vomiting for 10 days. She admitted taking 2 tablets per day of Tension Tamer (Celestial Seasonings) tablets containing 100 mg of kava extract for anxiety. After diagnosis, the liver functions continued to worsen with increased bilirubin, AST, and ALT levels and 70% hepatocellular necrosis confirmed by liver biopsy. After the eighth day of admission, the left lateral segment was removed through an orthotopic liver transplant. Seven months after liver transplantation, the patient was healthy and the liver function was within normal levels (Humberston et al., 2003). Another case report is of a 39-year-old woman who was admitted to a hospital with a history of increased liver enzyme levels due to kava consumption. The patient's liver enzyme levels were normalized after 1 week with the cessation of all medicines. Again, the liver enzymes increased due to the ingestion of kava after 2 weeks. Acute hepatitis was confirmed by a liver biopsy. The patient's transaminase levels were within normal levels after the consumption of kava was stopped again (Strahl et al., 1998).

14.3.8 Larrea tridentata *(Sess. & Moc. ex DC.) Cov.*

Chapparal is a shrubland plant growing in deserts found commonly in North America and Mexico. It is commonly referred to as "creosote bush" or "greasewood" and is taken in the form of tea after grinding the leaves; it is also used as a herbal remedy to treat various diseases such as bronchitis, the common cold, and muscle pain (Sheikh et al., 1997). Chapparal is commercially available as tablets, capsules, and ointments and is sold for its suspected antiinflammatory and blood-purifying capacities. It is popularly consumed as a liver tonic and is also used to treat skin diseases. Additionally, chaparral has led to increased awareness that acceptable weight loss and antioxidant properties may inhibit the aging process; it is also used as an alternative medicine in the treatment of AIDS (Kassler et al., 1991). Because the plant induced renal and hepatic toxicity, based on safety concerns, the drug was removed from the GRAS (Generally Recognized As Safe) list by the US Food and Drug Administration (FDA).

The leaves of the plant consist of the phenolic compound NGDA (nordihydroguaiaretic acid). This compound at a concentration of 50 and 75 μM acts as a lipoxygenase inhibitor and reduced the prolactin action on the biosynthesis of the protein casein, RNA, and lipids. Because the inhibition of prolactin will affect mammary gland development, it is not safe to be consumed by women during pregnancy and lactation (Rillema, 1984). The compound acted as a selective 5 and 15 lipoxygenase inhibitor in human leukocytes and platelets (Salari et al., 1984). It is reported that 18 patients with hepatotoxicity due to chapparal were reported, 13 of whom exhibited liver damage and complete liver failure from mild hepatitis to cirrhosis (Sheikh et al., 1997).

A case report describes a 27-year-old Hispanic male admitted to the hospital with symptoms of nausea, vomiting, diarrhea, and abdominal pain due to hepatitis. He confessed the ingestion of chaparral in a dose of 3–7 capsules per day over the past year; however, the recommended dose is 2 capsules per day. After diagnosis, a liver biopsy indicated that necrosis and periportal inflammation occurred due to hepatocellular injury. The patient was hospitalized for transplantation, and after 6 weeks the liver function was within normal levels. The patient was advised to avoid chaparral, alcohol, and other hepatotoxic drugs. The long-term use of chaparral in higher doses causes acute hepatotoxicity and such prolonged use should be standardized (Grant et al., 1998). Another case report of a 22-year-old woman with hepatotoxicity showed that the patient ingested chaparral to increase milk secretion during breastfeeding after the delivery of a healthy newborn. After diagnosis, severe hepatitis and hepatic fibrosis were confirmed in the patient due to the herb intake (Kauma et al., 2004).

14.3.9 Mentha pulegium L.

Pennyroyal, which is commonly known as squaw mint, mosquito plant, and pudding grass, belongs to the family Lamiaceae. It has been taken in the form of tea or oil as well as used as an aromatic stimulant (Gunby, 1979). It has mainly been used as an abortifacient that has been concomitant with acute hepatotoxicity and death (Gordon and Khojasteh, 2015). The toxicity of pennyroyal is supposed to be primarily from a cytochrome P450 oxidized metabolite of pulegone known as menthofuran. Also, pulegone significantly reduces glutathione as measured in the plasma and liver, making glutathione unavailable to remove the toxic metabolite menthofuran, which subsequently causes liver damage (Thomassen et al., 1990). Many case reports support the adverse side effects of these supplements. An 8-week-old boy with pennyroyal oil toxicity was reported as a case study due to the ingestion of 120 mL of tea prepared from a mint plant containing pennyroyal oil. After diagnosis, the infant was reported with fulminant liver failure affected by menthofuran. Another case report is of a 6-month-old Spanish baby who had liver failure with acute epileptic encephalopathy due to the consumption of aspirin and 90 mL of tea prepared from the domestic mint plant for his congestion and colic. He tested for both pulegone and menthofuran (Bakerink et al., 1996).

14.3.10 Amanita phalloides (Vaill. ex Fr.: Fr.)

This plant, which is called the death cap or a toadstool, is a toxic mushroom causing severe poisoning in humans. The classes of cyclic peptide toxins found in this plant are amatoxins, phallotoxins, and virotoxins, in which the second position of the indole ring of the tryptophan of these toxic peptides is substituted by a sulfur atom. Among these toxins, the amatoxins are considered to be highly toxic with an LD_{50} of 0.4–0.8 mg/kg in mice, but it takes nearly 2–8 days to cause death. Phallotoxins and virotoxins are considered to be comparatively less toxic with an LD_{50} of 1–20 mg/kg in mice; however they have a rapid response time as they cause death within 2–5 h of drug intake (Vetter, 1998). α-Amanitin, which is the most toxic amatoxin, is absorbed in the gastrointestinal tract and inhibits the enzyme RNA polymerase II, thus causing a deficiency in protein synthesis. It also induces necrosis and further damages the liver and kidney (Santi et al., 2012). In humans, it was reported that 6.3 mg of α-amanitin was excreted in the feces over a period of 24 h; this quantity was found to be lethal (Jaeger et al., 1993). A case study report a 72-year-old female and her 45-year-old son who were admitted to the hospital with symptoms of nausea, diarrhea, and abdominal pain due to the consumption of a wild mushroom they harvested. After diagnosis, it was reported that both had increased liver enzyme levels due to *A. phalloides* poisoning (Ward et al., 2013). Another case report showed a 64-year-old woman who was admitted with acute hepatic failure after the consumption of the *A. phalloides* of a wild mushroom picked from her garden. She had symptoms of nausea, diarrhea, and intestinal pain. After diagnosis, it was found that the wild mushroom that contained α-amanitin had induced hepatotoxicity, and a liver transplant was required (Özçay et al., 2006).

14.3.11 Viscum album L.

The European mistletoe is an obligate hemiparasitic plant commonly called *Viscum album*; it is not commercially available. Conventionally, it is used as an antispasmodic, calmative, and abortifacient agent. The American mistletoe called *Phoradendron tomentosum* is commercially available for the purpose of Christmas decoration. It is also available in the name of Detensyl for treating hypertension. That contains 100 mg of smashed leaves, stems, and berries of viscum in addition to dried calf viscera. Although it has beneficial effects, the dose is limited and the prolonged use of leaves and berries causes systemic poisoning and leads to death (Hall et al., 1986). The plant consists of a galactoside-specific plant lectin known as *Viscum album* agglutinin-I (VAA-I), which inhibits protein synthesis. It increased the section of proinflammatory cytokines in human peripheral blood mononuclear cells, and also induced apoptosis in human monocytes, lymphocytes, and murine thymocytes (Hostanska et al., 1995, 1996). It also contains other compounds such as abrin and ricin in the seeds and modeccin in the roots and seeds. Similar to lectin, ricin also is a potent toxin with an LD_{50} of 3 µg/kg in mice (Stirpe et al., 1980). A case study was reported in a paper of a 49-year-old woman who was admitted with vomiting, depression, and pain in the right hypochondrium. The liver enzyme levels showed hepatitis and after treatment, she recovered. However, after 2 years the patient was admitted with the same symptoms and ailments. The cause was discovered to be the consumption of a herbal medicine containing kelp, skullcap, and mistletoe. After diagnosis, it was found that the reason for illness was the consumption of mistletoe-containing tablets. Although it is used in herbal preparations, long-term use may cause hepatitis (Harvey and Colin-Jones, 1981).

14.3.12 Xanthium strumarium L.

It is an annual plant commonly known as rough cocklebur, common cocklebur, or woolgarie bur belonging to the family Asteraceae. It is used in conventional Chinese medicine for treating nasal ailments and headaches (Wang et al., 2011). The major hepatotoxic components found in water extracts of the fruits are atractyloside (a diterpenoid glycoside); carboxyatractyloside, which is more toxic than atractyloside; and 4′-desulphate-atractyloside (Xue et al., 2014). The compounds increased the level of low-density lipoprotein, choline, lactate, acetate, and acetone in the plasma of Wistar male rats. Also decreased levels of glucose and valine in plasma and increased levels of the enzymes ALT, AST, and ALP in serum were found in the treated rats, which showed that the mechanism of toxicity is related to the lipid and energy metabolism. Compared with the control, the liver tissues of the treated rats at doses of 30 g/kg revealed the hepatic injury, which was characterized by central vein necrosis, severe hepatocellular degeneration, vacuolation of cytoplasm, and degeneration of fat. A case report on a 25-year-old women who was admitted to the hospital with a mental disorder and was reactive only to pain stimuli due to consumption revealed the intake of herbal tea 7 days before. Clinical reports showed elongated blood clotting, hypoglycemia, increased liver and kidney enzymes, and abnormal liver function. As per the advice of the herbal practitioner, the patient was drinking herbal tea containing *Xanthium strumarium* that had a dry weight of about 30–40 g to treat an infertility problem. After treatment, the patient recovered after 7 days and the liver enzymes became normalized within 3 months (Saidi and Mofidi, 2009).

14.3.13 Scutellaria biacalensis *Georgi*

Scutellaria baicalensis with the common name Chinese skullcap is also known as huangqin, baikal, and scutellaria; it belongs to the mint family and is used as a relaxant (Burnett et al., 2007). The herbal supplement prepared with Chinese skullcap is used to treat arthritis in the United States. After taking this supplement, hepatotoxicity has been reported; however, there are no reported cases of hepatotoxicity for glucosamine, chondroitin, or black catechu in previous cases (Linnebur et al., 2010). *S. baicalensis* consists of flavonoids including wogonin, baicalein, oroxylin, and wogonoside. Studies in HepG2 cells reported that baicalin is cytotoxic and induces hepatotoxicity. However, it is not yet clear if this is because of the plant extract alone or if other liver toxic components are involved. But the prolonged treatment of this extract in rats has caused some changes in electrolyte and lipid levels (Khanal et al., 2012). When this plant extract was given to male and female rats at a dose of 2500 mg/kg/day, it showed some inflammation in the liver tissue but did not produce toxicity in other organs. However, the prolonged use of this drug may cause hepatotoxicity. Therefore, to ensure the safety of the drug, the levels of serum glucose, lipids, and electrolytes in the liver and heart should be observed (Yan et al., 2018). A case study involved a patient who was admitted with herb-induced liver injury due to the consumption of Chinese skullcap as a supplement for arthritis. There was a progressive link between the ingestion of the supplement and the start of symptoms as well as respiratory infiltrates concurrently with the hepatotoxicity. When the patient discontinued the herb intake, both the liver and respiratory problems completely recovered after a few weeks (Dhanasekaran et al., 2013). Another case report is of a 78-year-old woman who presented with symptoms of hepatitis and cholestasis due to the consumption of a herbal supplement named "Move Free Advanced" to treat arthritis. The herbal supplement contained Chinese skullcap that induced hepatotoxicity (Yang et al., 2012).

14.3.14 Callilepis laureola *DC.*

This herbaceous perennial is native to eastern South Africa and belongs to the Compositae family. In Zulu, an ethnic group of South Africa, *C. laureola* is generally called "impila," meaning health. Traditionally, impila is used to treat abdominal problems, infertility, cough, and worm infection (Popat et al., 2001). Studies have found that atractyloside, a toxic diterpenoid glycoside isolated from impila, may undergo alteration in the liver, leading to toxic effects due to the production of active radicals (Ohermann et al., 1973). The compound may cause apoptosis by inducing the opening of the mitochondrial transition pore, the release of cytochrome C, and caspase activation (Yang and Cortopassi, 1998). The mechanism of cytotoxicity induced by impila in vitro in Hep G2cells includes the reduction of cellular total glutathione, which plays a major role in detoxifying exogenous and endogenous compounds and also acts as a reducing agent in free radical metabolism. The extract at a concentration of 6.7 mg/mL induced 100% toxicity in the cells (Popat et al., 2001). Most of the children up to 12 years with impila toxication were diagnosed with hypoglycemia as well as liver and kidney dysfunctions. In a case report of a 21-year-old mother and her 18-month-old daughter, a toxic reaction was observed due to the consumption of impila. The mother died because of hepatotoxicity, although the child recovered (Steenkamp et al., 1999).

14.3.15 Valeriana officinalis *L.*

It is a perennial flowering plant belonging to the Valerianaceae family that is native to North America, Europe, and Asia. Valerian is the dried root of *V. officinalis* that has been used to treat insomnia, depression, and anxiety since ancient times. The chemical composition of this plant consists of valeric acid (sesquiterpenes), valepotriates (iridoids), and alkaloids. The roots and rhizomes of this plant contain 0.2%–2.8% of essential oils comprising sesquiterpenes, which are mostly related to the biological or pharmacological effects of valerian. It is mainly used as a sleeping pill and the distinctive dose as a sleeping pill is 300–600 mg/day (Cohen and Del Toro, 2008; Patočka and Jakl, 2010). In a case report, a 27-year-old female was reported with valeriana hepatotoxicity due to the consumption of 1 capsule of valerian root extract for 3 months. She recovered after the cessation of herbal medicine (Cohen and Del Toro, 2008). Valeriana-induced hepatotoxicity was reported in another 50-year-old Caucasian woman who consumed the root tea for 3 weeks. Histological analysis revealed necrosis in the hepatocytes and altered transaminase levels. The report cautions the public that the herb has the ability to establish acute hepatitis (Vassiliadis et al., 2009).

14.3.16 Hypericum perforatum *L.*

It is a perennial herb commonly known as St. John's Wort (SJW) that is native to Europe. Traditionally, St. John's Wort extract is prepared from the aerial part of the herb. It has been in use for more than 200 years to treat various medical ailments such as insomnia, respiratory problems, adenosis, trauma, insect and snake bites, scabies, and cancer. Primarily, SJW has been used as an antidepressant and has developed as one of the best retailing antidepressant agents (Izzo, 2004; Ernst, 2002; Singh, 2005). The plant extracts consist of hypericin and pseudohypericin, which are believed to be the main constituents with potential toxicity that induces cytochrome P450 enzymes as well as P-glycoprotein. The plant extract was given to rats at a dose of 100 mg/kg/day. Microscopical studies were performed and showed severe renal and hepatic damage (Gregoretti et al., 2004). Additionally, SJW interacted with other drugs and caused severe concerns such as a decrease of blood cyclosporine levels causing serotonin syndrome when treated along with serotonin reuptake inhibitors. In a case report, a 36-year-old patient required liver transplantation due to the interaction between the cyclosporine drug (175 mg) twice per day and SJW. The patient had taken *H. perforatum* tablets (900 mg) twice a day as an antianxiety drug along with the cyclosporine drug. The patient presented with acute hepatitis due to the reduced level of cyclosporine (Karliova et al., 2000).

14.3.17 Cascara sagrada *DC.*

Cascara sagrada is commonly known as bitter bark or sacred bark and belongs to the Rhamnaceae family; it is indigenous to the northwestern United States. It acts as a laxative to treat constipation. The bark extract of cascara consist of a mixture of constituents, including anthracenes (10%–20% of glycosides and 80%–90% C-glycosides), emodins, oxanthrone, barbaolin, chyrosophanol, linoleic, rhamnol, and myristic and syringic acids. Among these compounds, anthracene glycoside was previously identified to cause chronic hepatitis (Awang, 2009). The consumption of *Cascara sagrada* in higher doses is not recommended for more than 6 days because it has been concomitant with the development of hepatitis. In a case report, a 48-year-old man was admitted with abdominal pain and jaundice due to the consumption of *Cascara sagrada* for 3 days. After 1 week, the liver biopsy showed acute portal inflammation and hydro peritoneum. Intracanalicular biliary stasis was also seen, with increasing bile ducts enclosed by provocative cells. The patient recovered after the cessation of cascara intake (Nadir et al., 2000).

14.3.18 Cassia acutifolia *Delile*

Cassia acutifolia, which is commonly known as Sennaalexandrina, is found in Egypt and has different species. For example, the species cultivated in other countries such as India are *Cassia acutifolia* Delile and *Cassia alata* Linn in tropical America. It is an ornamental shrub that belongs to the Fabaceae family and is mostly cultivated in tropical countries. It is used as herbal tea made from senna pods and leaves, which are widely used as laxatives (Beuers et al., 1991). The plant extract of the different species consists of many active anthraquinones, including sennosides, torosaols I and II (bitetrahydroanthracene derivative), chrysophanol, aloe-emodin diathrone diglucoside, rhein, and rhein glucosides. The pods of *C. senna* consist of anthraquinone derivatives such as rhein-8-monoglucoside and aglycone sennidin (Dave and Ledwani, 2012). Among the above-mentioned senna species, *C. angustifolia* has been related to hepatotoxicity (Andrade et al., 2019). The hepatotoxin anthraquinone glycosides present in senna are known as sennosides. The long-term use of senna as a herbal tea may be concomitant with various symptoms that include dehydration and chronic diarrhea. Acute hepatotoxicity was reported in a case where huge quantities of senna fruits were consumed as herbal tea. A 52-year-old woman who developed severe liver failure and kidney damage required intensive care treatment due to the consumption of herbal tea for more than 3 years made from a tea bag that contained 70 g of dry senna fruits. The severity of liver failure was revealed by the increase in the prothrombin level and the development of encephalitis. Liver transplantation was carried out, but the patient finally recovered with supportive treatment. The senna samples identified in the patient's house revealed the presence of 2.2% of hydroxyanthracene glycosides (sennoside B). Therefore, through the Naranjo probability scale, the hepatoxicity in the patient was linked with senna intake (Vanderperren et al., 2005).

14.3.19 Actaea racemosa L.

This plant, which is native to the United States and Canada, is commonly known as black cohosh, black snakeroot, and fairy candle; it belongs to the family Ranunculaceae. Traditionally, it is used for treating renal disorders, gynecological disorders, arthritis, and throat infection. It has also been used to cure symptoms related to menopause. Black cohosh consists of triterpene glycosides that act as a hepatoprotective and salicylates and alkaloids that are hepatotoxic. In human breast cancer cells, rhizome extracts and constituents have been shown to cause programmed cell death and cell cycle arrest (Hostanska et al., 2004). Additionally, it consists of some catechols such as piscidic acid, fukiic acid esters, and caffeic acid, which has antioxidant properties (Takahira et al., 1998). The catechols are converted to toxic electrophilic quinones through metabolic or chemical activation. The toxicity is exhibited by the quinones through the arylation of cellular proteins and DNA or redox cycling leading to the production of free radicals (Bolton et al., 2000). Black cohosh consumption has been linked to autoimmune hepatitis in a 69-year-old female patient, who was taking 150 mg/ day of black cohosh to treat her hot flashes. A clinical examination revealed an elevated liver function test and the histology of the liver showed chronic inflammation. The causality assessment revealed a score of 10 points, which implies that the drug is highly probable in initiating hepatotoxicity. The analysis of the other biochemical parameters suggested that the intake of black cohosh can induce autoimmune hepatitis (Franco et al., 2017).

14.3.20 Echinaceae purpurea L.

Echinaceae purpurea is commonly known as the purple cone flower or the hedgehog cone flower, and it belongs to the family Asteraceae that is indigenous to midwestern North America (Barrett, 2003). Conventionally, Echinacea species have been used to treat snake bites, diphtheria, dysentery, and cancer (Wills et al., 2000). Nowadays, *E. purpurea* is used to treat influenza, common colds, and bronchitis; it is also used as an immunostimulant. Echinacea spp. consists of active constituents such as arabinogalactan, echincoside, echinacin, verbascoside, cynarin, borneol, bornylacetate, acidic arabinorhamnogalactan, cichoric acid, pyrrolizide alkaloids tussilagine, isotussilagine, and isobutylamides (Tharun et al., 2017). The hepatotoxicity of Echinacea typically occurs due to prolonged use of more than 8 weeks and is related to the use of drugs such as anabolic steroids, ketoconazole, methotrexate, and amiodarone (Miller, 1998). A 45-year-old man's was diagnosed with fatigue and jaundice. The patient consumed Echinacea root extract in the dose of 1500 mg/day to treat the symptoms of flu and had no history of other medicines. After diagnosis, it was reported that the biological parameters showed increased levels of alanine aminotransferase, aspartate aminotransferase, and alkaline phosphatase; the bilirubin levels and liver biopsy showed hepatitis. After discontinuation of Echinaceae extract, the biological parameter was normal within a month (Kocaman et al., 2008).

14.4 Conclusion

In Ayurvedic and Chinese traditional medicines, many medicinal products produced from plants are used to relieve diseases. These medical methods have been practiced for centuries to treat a variety of illnesses. Some medicinal plants have been identified as hepatoprotective agents to treat liver damage while there are a few plants that trigger hepatic damage. Hepatotoxicity is a condition that starts with the development of jaundice from moderate liver damage and may involve liver transplantation due to liver failure or sometimes even death. Studying the risk of hepatotoxicity from plant extracts is important because the components present in many plants are not known. Also, when the plants are used as a combination drug containing different plant extracts, it may contain some harmful impurities that can cause toxicity. Hence, before new drugs are launched into the market, we need to carry out accurate testing to reveal the safety and efficiency of the product. Further, the effectiveness of the product needs to be examined through human trials to establish that the product will have the demanded effect. In this context, the exploration of plant extracts with putative hepatotoxicity has to be taken up for the development of phytopharmaceuticals to cure illnesses.

Acknowledgments

The authors wish to acknowledge the (i) Alagappa University Bioinformatics Infrastructure Facility (DBT, BT/BI/25/012/2012,BIF), (ii) DST-FIST (SR/FST/LSI-639/2015(C)), (iii) UGC-SAP (F.5-1/2018/DRS-II(SAP-II)), (iv) DST-PURSE (SR/PURSE Phase 2/38 (G), (v) RUSA 2.0 [F.24-51/2014-U, Policy (TN Multi-Gen), Dept of Edn, GoI], and (vi) the University Science Instrumentation Centre (USIC), Alagappa University.

References

Adewusi, E.A., Afolayan, A.J., 2010. A review of natural products with hepatoprotective activity. J. Med. Plant Res. 4 (13), 1318–1334.

Akarte, A.S., Bhagat, V.C., Deshmukh, P.T., Disle, C., 2009. Evaluation of antinociceptive effect of *Xanthium strumarium* Linn. leaves extract in Swiss albino mice. Int. J. Green Pharm. 3 (2).

Anand, K., Lal, U.R., 2016. Hepatitis and medicinal plants: an overview. J. Pharmacogn. Phytochem. 5 (6), 408–415.

Andrade, R.J., Aithal, G.P., Björnsson, E.S., Kaplowitz, N., Kullak-Ublick, G.A., Larrey, D., Karlsen, T.H., European Association for the Study of the Liver, 2019. EASL clinical practice guidelines: drug-induced liver injury. J. Hepatol. 70 (6), 1222–1261.

Arias, I.M., Wolkoff, A.W., Boyer, J.L., Shafritz, D.A., Fausto, N., Alter, H.J., Cohen, D.E. (Eds.), 2011. The Liver: Biology and Pathobiology. John Wiley & Sons.

Awang, D.V.C., 2009. Tyler's Herbs of Choice: the Therapeutic Use of Phytomedicinals, third ed. Pharmaceutical Products Press/CRC Press, Florida.

Bakerink, J.A., Gospe, S.M., Dimand, R.J., Eldridge, M.W., 1996. Multiple organ failure after ingestion of pennyroyal oil from herbal tea in two infants. Pediatrics 98 (5), 944–947.

Barreto, M.C., Pinto, R.E., Arrabaça, J.D., Pavão, M.L., 2003. Inhibition of mouse liver respiration by *Chelidonium majus* isoquinoline alkaloids. Toxicol. Lett. 146 (1), 37–47.

Barrett, B., 2003. Medicinal properties of Echinacea: a critical review. Phytomedicine 10 (1), 66–86.

Bataller, R., Brenner, D.A., 2005. Liver fibrosis. J. Clin. Invest. 115, 209–218.

Beuers, U., Spengler, U., Pape, G., 1991. Hepatitis after chronic abuse of senna. Lancet 337 (8737), 372–373.

Björnsson, E., Kalaitzakis, E., Olsson, R., 2007. The impact of eosinophilia and hepatic necrosis on prognosis in patients with drug-induced liver injury. Aliment. Pharmacol. Ther. 25 (12), 1411–1421.

Bolton, J.L., Trush, M.A., Penning, T.M., Dryhurst, G., Monks, T.J., 2000. Role of quinones in toxicology. Chem. Res. Toxicol. 13 (3), 135–160.

Bottenberg, M.M., Wall, G.C., Harvey, R.L., Habib, S., 2007. Oral *Aloe vera*-induced hepatitis. Ann. Pharmacother. 41 (10), 1740–1743.

Bouabid, K., Lamchouri, F., Hamid, T., Faouzi, M.E.A., 2019. Inventory of poisonings and toxicological studies carried out on *Atractylis gummifera* L.: a review. Plant Sci. Today 6 (4), 457–464.

Boudreau, M.D., Beland, F.A., 2006. An evaluation of the biological and toxicological properties of *Aloe barbadensis* (miller), Aloe vera. J. Environ. Sci. Health C 24 (1), 103–154.

Burnett, B.P., Jia, Q., Zhao, Y., Levy, R.M., 2007. A medicinal extract of *Scutellaria baicalensis* and *Acacia catechu* acts as a dual inhibitor of cyclooxygenase and 5-lipoxygenase to reduce inflammation. J. Med. Food 10 (3), 442–451.

Caldwell, S.H., Hespenheide, E.E., Redick, J.A., Iezzoni, J.C., Battle, E.H., Sheppard, B.L., 2001. A pilot study of a thiazolidinedione, troglitazone, in nonalcoholic steatohepatitis. Am. J. Gastroenterol. 96 (2), 519–525.

Calitz, C., Du Plessis, L., Gouws, C., Steyn, D., Steenekamp, J., Muller, C., Hamman, S., 2015. Herbal hepatotoxicity: current status, examples, and challenges. Expert Opin. Drug Metab. Toxicol. 11 (10), 1551–1565.

Chiang, J.Y., 1998. Regulation of bile acid synthesis. Front. Biosci. 3, d176–d193.

Chiang, J.Y., 2004. Regulation of bile acid synthesis: pathways, nuclear receptors, and mechanisms. J. Hepatol. 40 (3), 539–551.

Chiang, J.Y., 2013. Bile acid metabolism and signaling. Compr. Physiol. 3 (3), 1191–1212.

Cohen, D.L., Del Toro, Y., 2008. A case of valerian-associated hepatotoxicity. J. Clin. Gastroenterol. 42 (8), 961–962.

Crijns, A.P., De Smet, P.A., van den Heuvel, M., Schot, B.W., Haagsma, E.B., 2002. Acute hepatitis after use of a herbal preparation with greater celandine (*Chelidonium majus*). Ned. Tijdschr. Geneeskd. 146 (3), 124.

Danan, G., Teschke, R., 2016. RUCAM in drug and herb induced liver injury: the update. Int. J. Mol. Sci. 17 (1), 14.

Daniele, C., Dahamna, S., Firuzi, O., Sekfali, N., Saso, L., Mazzanti, G., 2005. *Atractylis gummifera* L. poisoning: an ethnopharmacological review. J. Ethnopharmacol. 97 (2), 175–181.

Dave, H., Ledwani, L., 2012. A review on anthraquinones isolated from Cassia species and their applications. Indian J. Nat. Prod. Resour. 3 (3), 291–319.

Davies, L.P., Drew, C.A., Duffield, P., Johnston, G.A., Jamieson, D.D., 1992. Kava pyrones and resin: studies on GABAA, GABAB and benzodiazepine binding sites in rodent brain. Pharmacol. Toxicol. 71 (2), 120–126.

Decker, K., 1990. Biologically active products of stimulated liver macrophages (Kupffer cells). Eur. J. Biochem. 192 (2), 245–261.

Dhanasekaran, R., Owens, V., Sanchez, W., 2013. Chinese skullcap in move free arthritis supplement causes drug induced liver injury and pulmonary infiltrates. Case Rep. Hepatol., 2013.

Dong, X., Fu, J., Yin, X., Cao, S., Li, X., Lin, L., Huyiligeqi and Ni, J., 2016. Emodin: a review of its pharmacology, toxicity and pharmacokinetics. Phytother. Res. 30 (8), 1207–1218.

Ekor, M., 2014. The growing use of herbal medicines: issues relating to adverse reactions and challenges in monitoring safety. Front. Pharmacol. 4, 177.

Elizabeth, L.Y., Sivagnanam, M., Ellis, L., Huang, J.S., 2011. Acute hepatotoxicity after ingestion of Morinda citrifolia (Noni Berry) juice in a 14-year-old boy. J. Pediatr. Gastroenterol. Nutr. 52 (2), 222.

Ernst, E., 2002. The risk—benefit profile of commonly used herbal therapies: Ginkgo, St. John's Wort, Ginseng, Echinacea, Saw Palmetto, and Kava. Ann. Intern. Med. 136 (1), 42–53.

Franco, D.L., Kale, S., Lam-Himlin, D.M., Harrison, M.E., 2017. Black cohosh hepatotoxicity with autoimmune hepatitis presentation. Case Rep. Gastroenterol. 11 (1), 23–28.

Frenzel, C., Teschke, R., 2016. Herbal hepatotoxicity: clinical characteristics and listing compilation. Int. J. Mol. Sci. 17 (5), 588.

Georgiou, M., Sianidou, L., Hatzis, T., Papadatos, J., Koutselinis, A., 1988. Hepatotoxicity due to *Atractylis gummifera*-L. J. Toxicol. Clin. Toxicol. 26 (7), 487–493.

Gordon, P., Khojasteh, S.C., 2015. A decades-long investigation of acute metabolism-based hepatotoxicity by herbal constituents: a case study of pennyroyal oil. Drug Metab. Rev. 47 (1), 12–20.

Gordon, W.P., Forte, A.J., McMurtry, R.J., Gal, J., Nelson, S.D., 1982. Hepatotoxicity and pulmonary toxicity of pennyroyal oil and its constituent terpenes in the mouse. Toxicol. Appl. Pharmacol. 65 (3), 413–424.

Grant, K.L., Boyer, L.V., Erdman, B.E., 1998. Chaparral-induced hepatotoxicity. Integr. Med. 1 (2), 83–87.

Gregoretti, B., Stebel, M., Candussio, L., Crivellato, E., Bartoli, F., Decorti, G., 2004. Toxicity of *Hypericum perforatum* (St. John's Wort) administered during pregnancy and lactation in rats. Toxicol. Appl. Pharmacol. 200 (3), 201–205.

Gunby, P., 1979. Plant known for centuries still causes problems today. JAMA 241 (21), 2246–2247.

Guo, X., Mei, N., 2016. *Aloe vera*: a review of toxicity and adverse clinical effects. J. Environ. Sci. Health C 34 (2), 77–96.

Hall, A.H., Spoerke, D.G., Rumack, B.H., 1986. Assessing mistletoe toxicity. Ann. Emerg. Med. 15 (11), 1320–1323.

Harvey, J., Colin-Jones, D.G., 1981. Mistletoe hepatitis. Br. Med. J. (Clin. Res. Ed.) 282 (6259), 186–187.

Hostanska, K., Hajto, T., Spagnoli, G.C., Fischer, J., Lentzen, H., Herrmann, R., 1995. A plant lectin derived from *Viscum album* induces cytokine gene expression and protein production in cultures of human peripheral blood mononuclear cells. Nat. Immun. 14 (5–6), 295–304.

Hostanska, K., Hajto, T., Weber, K., Fischer, J., Lentzen, H., Sütterlin, B., Saller, R., 1996. A natural immunity-activating plant lectin, *Viscum album* agglutinin-I, induces apoptosis in human lymphocytes, monocytes, monocytic THP-1 cells and murine thymocytes. Nat. Immun. 15 (6), 295–311.

Hostanska, K., Nisslein, T., Freudenstein, J., Reichling, J., Saller, R., 2004. *Cimicifuga racemosa* extract inhibits proliferation of estrogen receptor-positive and negative human breast carcinoma cell lines by induction of apoptosis. Breast Cancer Res. Treat. 84 (2), 151–160.

Haouzi, D., Cohen, I., Vieira, H.L.A., Poncet, D., Boya, P., Castedo, M., Vadrot, N., Belzacq, A.S., Fau, D., Brenner, C., Feldmann, G., 2002. Mitochondrial permeability transition as a novel principle of hepatorenal toxicity in vivo. Apoptosis 7 (5), 395–405.

Hsu, Y.W., Tsai, C.F., Chen, W.K., Huang, C.F., Yen, C.C., 2011. A subacute toxicity evaluation of green tea (*Camellia sinensis*) extract in mice. Food Chem. Toxicol. 49 (10), 2624–2630.

Humberston, C.L., Akhtar, J., Krenzelok, E.P., 2003. Acute hepatitis induced by kava kava. J. Toxicol. Clin. Toxicol. 41 (2), 109–113.

Hussaini, S.H., Farrington, E.A., 2007. Idiosyncratic drug-induced liver injury: an overview. Expert Opin. Drug Saf. 6 (6), 673–684.

Ibáñez, L., Pérez, E., Vidal, X., Laporte, J.R., 2002. Prospective surveillance of acute serious liver disease unrelated to infectious, obstructive, or metabolic diseases: epidemiological and clinical features, and exposure to drugs. J. Hepatol. 37 (5), 592–600.

Izzo, A.A., 2004. Drug interactions with St. John's Wort (*Hypericum perforatum*): a review of the clinical evidence. Int. J. Clin. Pharmacol. Ther. 42 (3), 139–148.

Jaeger, A., Jehl, F., Flesch, F., Sauder, P., Kopferschmitt, J., 1993. Kinetics of amatoxins in human poisoning: therapeutic implications. J. Toxicol. Clin. Toxicol. 31 (1), 63–80.

Jaeschke, H., Gores, G.J., Cederbaum, A.I., Hinson, J.A., Pessayre, D., Lemasters, J.J., 2002. Mechanisms of hepatotoxicity. Toxicol. Sci. 65 (2), 166–176.

Jussofie, A., Schmiz, A., Hiemke, C., 1994. Kavapyrone enriched extract from *Piper methysticum* as modulator of the GABA binding site in different regions of rat brain. Psychopharmacology 116 (4), 469–474.

Karliova, M., Treichel, U., Malagò, M., Frilling, A., Gerken, G., Broelsch, C.E., 2000. Interaction of *Hypericum perforatum* (St. John's Wort) with cyclosporin A metabolism in a patient after liver transplantation. J. Hepatol. 33 (5), 853–855.

Kassler, W.J., Blanc, P., Greenblatt, R., 1991. The use of medicinal herbs by human immunodeficiency virus-infected patients. Arch. Intern. Med. 151 (11), 2281–2288.

Kauma, H., Koskela, R., Mäkisalo, H., Autio-Harmainen, H., Lehtola, J., Höckerstedt, K., 2004. Toxic acute hepatitis and hepatic fibrosis after consumption of chaparral tablets. Scand. J. Gastroenterol. 39 (11), 1168–1171.

Kessler, R.C., Davis, R.B., Foster, D.F., Van Rompay, M.I., Walters, E.E., Wilkey, S.A., Kaptchuk, T.J., Eisenberg, D.M., 2001. Long-term trends in the use of complementary and alternative medical therapies in the United States. Ann. Intern. Med. 135 (4), 262–268.

Khanal, T., Kim, H.G., Choi, J.H., Park, B.H., Do, M.T., Kang, M.J., Yeo, H.K., Kim, D.H., Kang, W., Jeong, T.C., Jeong, H.G., 2012. Protective role of intestinal bacterial metabolism against baicalin-induced toxicity in HepG2 cell cultures. J. Toxicol. Sci. 37 (2), 363–371.

Knowles, S.R., Uetrecht, J., Shear, N.H., 2000. Idiosyncratic drug reactions: the reactive metabolite syndromes. Lancet 356 (9241), 1587–1591.

Kocaman, O., Hulagu, S., Senturk, O., 2008. Echinacea-induced severe acute hepatitis with features of cholestatic autoimmune hepatitis. Eur. J. Intern. Med. 19 (2), 148.

Kwack, S.J., Kim, K.B., Lee, B.M., 2009. Estimation of tolerable upper intake level (UL) of active aloe. J. Toxic. Environ. Health A 72 (21 – 22), 1455–1462.

Ladd, J.M., 2013. Synthesis of nordihydroguaiaretic acid derivatives via suzuki and stille cross-coupling reactions and subsequent raney nickel desulfurization and reduction. Doctoral dissertation, Middle Tennessee State University.

Laliberte, L., Villeneuve, J.P., 1996. Hepatitis after the use of germander, a herbal remedy. CMAJ 154 (11), 1689.

Larrey, D., 1997. Hepatotoxicity of herbal remedies. J. Hepatol. 26, 47–51.

Larrey, D., Faure, S., 2011. Herbal medicine hepatotoxicity: a new step with development of specific biomarkers. J. Hepatol. 54 (4), 599–601.

Larson, A.M., Polson, J., Fontana, R.J., Davern, T.J., Lalani, E., Hynan, L.S., Reisch, J.S., Schiødt, F.V., Ostapowicz, G., Shakil, A.O., Lee, W.M., 2005. Acetaminophen-induced acute liver failure: results of a United States multicenter, prospective study. Hepatology 42 (6), 1364–1372.

Lee, A., Chui, P.T., Aun, C.S., Gin, T., Lau, A.S., 2004. Possible interaction between sevoflurane and Aloe vera. Ann. Pharmacother. 38 (10), 1651–1654.

Lin, N.H., Yang, H.W., Su, Y.J., Chang, C.W., 2019. Herb induced liver injury after using herbal medicine: a systemic review and case-control study. Medicine 98 (13).

Linnebur, S.A., Rapacchietta, O.C., Vejar, M., 2010. Hepatotoxicity associated with chinese skullcap contained in move free advanced dietary supplement: two case reports and review of the literature. Pharmacotherapy 30 (7), 750.

Lu, H., Meng, X., Li, C., Sang, S., Patten, C., Sheng, S., Hong, J., Bai, N., Winnik, B., Ho, C.T., Yang, C.S., 2003. Glucuronides of tea catechins: enzymology of biosynthesis and biological activities. Drug Metab. Dispos. 31 (4), 452–461.

Lubek, B.M., Avaria, M., Basu, P.K., Wells, P.G., 1988. Pharmacological studies on the in vivo cataractogenicity of acetaminophen in mice and rabbits. Toxicol. Sci. 10 (4), 596–606.

Lüde, S., Török, M., Dieterle, S., Knapp, A.C., Kaeufeler, R., Jäggi, R., Spornitz, U., Krähenbühl, S., 2007. Hepatic effects of *Cimicifuga racemosa* extract *in vivo* and *in vitro*. Cell. Mol. Life Sci. 64 (21), 2848–2857.

Mahady, G.B., 2004. *Cascara sagrada* (*Rhamnus purshiana*). In: Encyclopedia of Dietary Supplements (Online). CRC Press, p. 89.

Mazzanti, G., Menniti-Ippolito, F., Moro, P.A., Cassetti, F., Raschetti, R., Santuccio, C., Mastrangelo, S., 2009. Hepatotoxicity from green tea: a review of the literature and two unpublished cases. Eur. J. Clin. Pharmacol. 65 (4), 331–341.

Mazzanti, G., Di Sotto, A., Vitalone, A., 2015. Hepatotoxicity of green tea: an update. Arch. Toxicol. 89 (8), 1175–1191.

Meyer, H.J., 1962. Pharmakologie der wirksamen prinzipien des Kawa-Rhizoms (*Piper methysticum* Forst). Arch. Int. Pharmacodyn. Ther. 138 (3–4), 505.

Michalopoulos, G.K., 2007. Liver regeneration. J. Cell. Physiol. 213 (2), 286–300.

Miller, L.G., 1998. Herbal medicinals: selected clinical considerations focusing on known or potential drug-herb interactions. Arch. Intern. Med. 158 (20), 2200–2211.

Millonig, G., Stadlmann, S., Vogel, W., 2005. Herbal hepatotoxicity: acute hepatitis caused by a Noni preparation (*Morinda citrifolia*). Eur. J. Gastroenterol. Hepatol. 17 (4), 445–447.

Nadir, A., Reddy, D., Van Thiel, D.H., 2000. *Cascara sagrada*-induced intrahepatic cholestasis causing portal hypertension: case report and review of herbal hepatotoxicity. Am. J. Gastroenterol. 95 (12), 3634–3637.

Nakamoto, Y., Kaneko, S., 2003. Mechanisms of viral hepatitis induced liver injury. Curr. Mol. Med. 3 (6), 537–544.

Ni, Y., Li, J.M., Liu, M.K., Zhang, T.T., Wang, D.P., Zhou, W.H., Hu, L.Z., Lv, W.L., 2017. Pathological process of liver sinusoidal endothelial cells in liver diseases. World J. Gastroenterol. 23 (43), 7666.

Norton, S.A., Ruze, P., 1994. Kava dermopathy. J. Am. Acad. Dermatol. 31 (1), 89–97.

Ohermann, H., Spiteller, G., Hoyer, G.A., 1973. Struktur eines aus Menschenharn isolierten C19-terpenoids—2β-hydroxy-15-oxoatractylan-4α-carbonsäure. Chem. Ber. 106 (11), 3506–3518.

Ohiri, F.C., Esimone, C.O., Nwafor, S.V., Okoli, C.O., Ndu, O.O., 2003. Hypoglycemic properties of *Viscum album* (Mistletoe) in alloxan-induced diabetic animals. Pharm. Biol. 41 (3), 184–187.

Ostapowicz, G., Fontana, R.J., Schiødt, F.V., Larson, A., Davern, T.J., Han, S.H., McCashland, T.M., Shakil, A.O., Hay, J.E., Hynan, L., Crippin, J.S., 2002. Results of a prospective study of acute liver failure at 17 tertiary care centers in the United States. Ann. Intern. Med. 137 (12), 947–954.

Özçay, F., Baskin, E., Özdemir, N., Karakayali, H., Emiroglu, R., Haberal, M., 2006. Fulminant liver failure secondary to mushroom poisoning in children: importance of early referral to a liver transplantation unit. Pediatr. Transplant. 10 (2), 259–265.

Patočka, J., Jakl, J., 2010. Biomedically relevant chemical constituents of *Valeriana officinalis*. J. Appl. Biomed. 8 (1), 11–18.

Pessayre, D., 1995. Role of reactive metabolites in drug-induced hepatitis. J. Hepatol. 23, 16–24.

Pessayre, D., Larrey, D., 1988. Acute and chronic drug-induced hepatitis. Baillieres Clin. Gastroenterol. 2 (2), 385–422.

Popat, A., Shear, N.H., Malkiewicz, I., Stewart, M.J., Steenkamp, V., Thomson, S., Neuman, M.G., 2001. The toxicity of *Callilepis laureola*, a South African traditional herbal medicine. Clin. Biochem. 34 (3), 229–236.

Qu, G.J., Dong, X.Q., Wang, Y.Z., Liu, N.N., Liu, S.M., 2010. Research of acute toxicity of total alkaloids of *Chelidonium majus* in rats. Chin. J. Vet. Drug 9.

Rillema, J.A., 1984. Effect of NDGA, a lipoxygenase inhibitor, on prolactin actions in mouse mammary gland explants. Prostaglandins Leukot. Med. 16 (1), 89–94.

Roth, R.A., Ganey, P.E., 2010. Intrinsic versus idiosyncratic drug-induced hepatotoxicity—two villains or one? J. Pharmacol. Exp. Ther. 332 (3), 692–697.

Saidi, H., Mofidi, M., 2009. Toxic effect of *Xanthium strumarium* as an herbal medicine preparation. EXCLI J. 8, 115–117.

Salari, H., Braquet, P., Borgeat, P., 1984. Comparative effects of indomethacin, acetylenic acids, 15-HETE, nordihydroguaiaretic acid and BW755C on the metabolism of arachidonic acid in human leukocytes and platelets. Prostaglandins Leukot. Med. 13 (1), 53–60.

Santi, L., Maggioli, C., Mastroroberto, M., Tufoni, M., Napoli, L., Caraceni, P., 2012. Acute liver failure caused by *Amanita phalloides* poisoning. Int. J. Hepatol. 2012.

Savvidou, S., Goulis, J., Giavazis, I., Patsiaoura, K., Hytiroglou, P., Arvanitakis, C., 2007. Herb-induced hepatitis by *Teucrium polium* L.: report of two cases and review of the literature. Eur. J. Gastroenterol. Hepatol. 19 (6), 507–511.

Schmidt, M., Schmitz, H.J., Baumgart, A., Guedon, D., Netsch, M.I., Kreuter, M.H., Schmidlin, C.B., Schrenk, D., 2005. Toxicity of green tea extracts and their constituents in rat hepatocytes in primary culture. Food Chem. Toxicol. 43 (2), 307–314.

Sheikh, N.M., Philen, R.M., Love, L.A., 1997. Chaparral-associated hepatotoxicity. Arch. Intern. Med. 157 (8), 913–919.

Singh, Y.N., 2005. Potential for interaction of kava and St. John's Wort with drugs. J. Ethnopharmacol. 100 (1–2), 108–113.

Smith, M.T., 2003. Mechanisms of troglitazone hepatotoxicity. Chem. Res. Toxicol. 16 (6), 679–687.

Sreelatha, S., Padma, P.R., Umadevi, M., 2009. Protective effects of *Coriandrum sativum* extracts on carbon tetrachloride-induced hepatotoxicity in rats. Food Chem. Toxicol. 47 (4), 702–708.

Srikanth, J., Muralidharan, P., 2009. Antiulcer activity of *Morinda citrifolia* Linn fruit extract. J. Sci. Res. 1 (2), 345–352.

Stedman, C., 2002. Herbal hepatotoxicity. Semin. Liver Dis. 22 (2), 195–206.

Steenkamp, V., Stewart, M.J., Zuckerman, M., 1999. Detection of poisoning by Impila (*Callilepis laureola*) in a mother and child. Hum. Exp. Toxicol. 18 (10), 594–597.

Stewart, M.J., Steenkamp, V., 2000. The biochemistry and toxicity of atractyloside: a review. Ther. Drug Monit. 22 (6), 641–649.

Stickel, F., Pöschl, G., Seitz, H.K., Waldherr, R., Hahn, E.G., Schuppan, D., 2003. Acute hepatitis induced by greater celandine (*Chelidonium majus*). Scand. J. Gastroenterol. 38 (5), 565–568.

Stickel, F., Patsenker, E., Schuppan, D., 2005. Herbal hepatotoxicity. J. Hepatol. 43 (5), 901.

Stickel, F., Kessebohm, K., Weimann, R., Seitz, H.K., 2011. Review of liver injury associated with dietary supplements. Liver Int. 31 (5), 595–605.

Stirpe, F., Legg, R.F., Onyon, L.J., Ziska, P., Franz, H., 1980. Inhibition of protein synthesis by a toxic lectin from *Viscum album* L. (mistletoe). Biochem. J. 190 (3), 843–845.

Strahl, S., Ehret, V., Dahm, H.H., Maier, K.P., 1998. Necrotizing hepatitis after taking herbal remedies. Dtsch. Med. Wochenschr. 123 (47), 1410–1414.

Subramoniam, A., Pushpangadan, P., 1999. Development of phytomedicines for liver disease. Indian J. Pharmacol. 31 (3), 166.

Takahira, M., Kusano, A., Shibano, M., Kusano, G., Miyase, T., 1998. Piscidic acid and fukiic acid esters from *Cimicifuga simplex*. Phytochemistry 49 (7), 2115–2119.

Tanaka, M., Itoh, T., Tanimizu, N., Miyajima, A., 2011. Liver stem/progenitor cells: their characteristics and regulatory mechanisms. J. Biochem. 149 (3), 231–239.

Tanira, M.O.M., Wasfi, I.A., Homsi, M.A., Bashir, A.K., 1996. Toxicological effects of *Teucrium stocksianum* after acute and chronic administration in rats. J. Pharm. Pharmacol. 48 (10), 1098–1102.

Teschke, R., 2010. Kava hepatotoxicity: pathogenetic aspects and prospective considerations. Liver Int. 30 (9), 1270–1279.

Teschke, R., Eickhoff, A., 2015. Herbal hepatotoxicity in traditional and modern medicine: actual key issues and new encouraging steps. Front. Pharmacol. 6, 72.

Teschke, R., Schulze, J., 2010. Risk of kava hepatotoxicity and the FDA consumer advisory. JAMA 304 (19), 2174–2175.

Teschke, R., Schwarzenboeck, A., Hennermann, K.H., 2008. Kava hepatotoxicity: a clinical survey and critical analysis of 26 suspected cases. Eur. J. Gastroenterol. Hepatol. 20 (12), 1182–1193.

Teschke, R., Qiu, S.X., Lebot, V., 2011. Herbal hepatotoxicity by kava: update on pipermethystine, flavokavain B, and mould hepatotoxins as primarily assumed culprits. Dig. Liver Dis. 43 (9), 676–681.

Tharun, G., Ramana, G., Sandhya, R., Shravani, M., 2017. Phytochemical and pharmacological review on Echinacea. J. Pharm. Res. 11 (3), 249–256.

Thomassen, D., Slattery, J.T., Nelson, S.D., 1990. Menthofuran-dependent and independent aspects of pulegone hepatotoxicity: roles of glutathione. J. Pharmacol. Exp. Ther. 253 (2), 567–572.

Thomassen, D., Knebel, N., Slattery, J.T., McClanahan, R.H., Nelson, S.D., 1992. Reactive intermediates in the oxidation of menthofuran by cytochromes P-450. Chem. Res. Toxicol. 5 (1), 123–130.

Thompson, M., Jaiswal, Y., Wang, I., Williams, L., 2017. Hepatotoxicity: treatment, causes and applications of medicinal plants as therapeutic agents. J. Phytopharmacol. 6 (3), 186–193.

Trauner, M., Meier, P.J., Boyer, J.L., 1998. Molecular pathogenesis of cholestasis. N. Engl. J. Med. 339 (17), 1217–1227.

Tsukamoto, H., 2002. Redox regulation of cytokine expression in Kupffer cells. Antioxid. Redox Signal. 4 (5), 741–748.

Uetrecht, J., 2007. Idiosyncratic drug reactions: current understanding. Annu. Rev. Pharmacol. Toxicol. 47, 513–539.

Uetrecht, J., 2008. Idiosyncratic drug reactions: past, present, and future. Chem. Res. Toxicol. 21 (1), 84–92.

Ulbricht, C., Basch, E., Paul, H., David, S., Samuel, B., Boon, H., Ulbricht, C., Tsouronis, C., Rogers, A., Bent, S., Ernst, E., 2002. Kava monograph: a clinical decision support tool. J. Herb. Pharmacother. 2 (4), 65–91.

Ullah, A., Ahmad, M., 2014. Hepatoprotective activity of *Chenopodium murale* in carbon tetrachloride-induced hepatic damage in rabbits. Bangladesh J. Pharmacol. 9 (1), 118–123.

Ulrichová, J., Walterová, D., Vavrečková, C., Kamarád, V., Šimánek, V., 1996. Cytotoxicity of benzo[c] phenanthridinium alkaloids in isolated rat hepatocytes. Phytother. Res. 10 (3), 220–223.

Vallejo, J.R., Peral, D., Gemio, P., Carrasco, M.C., Heinrich, M., Pardo-de-Santayana, M., 2009. *Atractylis gummifera* and *Centaurea ornata* in the Province of Badajoz (Extremadura, Spain)—ethnopharmacological importance and toxicological risk. J. Ethnopharmacol. 126 (2), 366–370.

Vanderperren, B., Rizzo, M., Angenot, L., Haufroid, V., Jadoul, M., Hantson, P., 2005. Acute liver failure with renal impairment related to the abuse of senna anthraquinone glycosides. Ann. Pharmacother. 39 (7–8), 1353–1357.

Vanstraelen, S., Rahier, J., Geubel, A.P., 2008. Jaundice as a misadventure of a green tea (*Camellia sinensis*) lover: a case report. Acta Gastro-Enterol. Belg. 71 (4), 409–412.

Vassiliadis, T., Anagnostis, P., Patsiaoura, K., Giouleme, O., Katsinelos, P., Mpoumponaris, A., Eugenidis, N., 2009. Valeriana hepatotoxicity. Sleep Med. 10 (8), 935.

Vetter, J., 1998. Toxins of *Amanita phalloides*. Toxicon 36 (1), 13–24.

Vo, L.T., Chan, D., King, R.G., 2003. Investigation of the effects of peppermint oil and valerian on rat liver and cultured human liver cells. Clin. Exp. Pharmacol. Physiol. 30 (10), 799–804.

Vogel, G., Tuchweber, B., Trost, W., Mengs, U., 1984. Protection by silibinin against *Amanita phalloides* intoxication in beagles. Toxicol. Appl. Pharmacol. 73 (3), 355–362.

Wang, J.F., Komarov, P., Degroot, H., 1993. Luminol chemiluminescence in rat macrophages and granulocytes: the role of $NO, O_2^- - /H_2O_2$, and HOCl. Arch. Biochem. Biophys. 304 (1), 189–196.

Wang, M.Y., West, B.J., Jensen, C.J., Nowicki, D., Su, C., Palu, A.K., Anderson, G., 2002. *Morinda citrifolia* (Noni): a literature review and recent advances in Noni research. Acta Pharmacol. Sin. 23 (12), 1127–1141.

Wang, Y., Han, T., Xue, L.M., Han, P., Zhang, Q.Y., Huang, B.K., Zhang, H., Ming, Q.L., Peng, W., Qin, L.P., 2011. Hepatotoxicity of kaurene glycosides from *Xanthium strumarium* L. fruits in mice. Pharmazie 66 (6), 445–449.

Ward, J., Kapadia, K., Brush, E., Salhanick, S.D., 2013. Amatoxin poisoning: case reports and review of current therapies. J. Emerg. Med. 44 (1), 116–121.

Weber, L.W., Boll, M., Stampfl, A., 2003. Hepatotoxicity and mechanism of action of haloalkanes: carbon tetrachloride as a toxicological model. Crit. Rev. Toxicol. 33 (2), 105–136.

Westendorf, J., 1993. Anthranoid derivatives—Cassia species. In: Adverse Effects of Herbal Drugs 2. Springer, Berlin, Heidelberg, pp. 125–128.

Wills, R.B., Bone, K., Morgan, M., 2000. Herbal products: active constituents, modes of action and quality control. Nutr. Res. Rev. 13 (1), 47–77.

Xue, L.M., Zhang, Q.Y., Han, P., Jiang, Y.P., Yan, R.D., Wang, Y., Rahman, K., Jia, M., Han, T., Qin, L.P., 2014. Hepatotoxic constituents and toxicological mechanism of *Xanthium strumarium* L. fruits. J. Ethnopharmacol. 152 (2), 272–282.

Yamashita, Y.I., Imai, K., Mima, K., Nakagawa, S., Hashimoto, D., Chikamoto, A., Baba, H., 2017. Idiosyncratic drug-induced liver injury: a short review. Hepatol. Commun. 1 (6), 494–500.

Yan, Y., Yong, Z., Chunying, L., Yushi, Z., Yang, B., Yalan, Y., Chen, P., Lianmei, W., Aihua, L., 2018. Potential chronic liver toxicity in rats orally administered an ethanol extract of Huangqin (Radix *Scutellariae baicalensis*). J. Tradit. Chin. Med. 38 (2), 242–256.

Yang, J.C., Cortopassi, G.A., 1998. dATP causes specific release of cytochrome C from mitochondria. Biochem. Biophys. Res. Commun. 250 (2), 454–457.

Yang, L., Aronsohn, A., Hart, J., Jensen, D., 2012. Herbal hepatoxicity from Chinese skullcap: a case report. World J. Hepatol. 4 (7), 231.

Younos, C., Rolland, A., Fleurentin, J., Lanhers, M.C., Misslin, R., Mortier, F., 1990. Analgesic and behavioural effects of *Morinda citrifolia*. Planta Med. 56 (05), 430–434.

Zheleva, A., Tolekova, A., Zhelev, M., Uzunova, V., Platikanova, M., Gadzheva, V., 2007. Free radical reactions might contribute to severe alpha amanitin hepatotoxicity—a hypothesis. Med. Hypotheses 69 (2), 361–367.

Zimmerman, H.J., 1999. Hepatotoxicity: The Adverse Effects of Drugs and Other Chemicals on the Liver. Lippincott Williams & Wilkins.

Zimmerman, H.J., 2000. Drug-induced liver disease. Clin. Liver Dis. 4 (1), 73–96.

Zuckerman, A., 1996. Alphabet of hepatitis viruses. Lancet 347 (9001), 558–559.

Index

Note: Page numbers followed by *f* indicate figures and *t* indicate tables.

A

Abdominal ultrasound, 111
Abutilon indicum, 148–149
Acacia catechu, 228–241*t*
Acacia mellifera, 31
Acalypharacemosa, 228–241*t*
Acantholimongilliati, 228–241*t*
Acetaminophen, 185, 263
Achilleamillefolium, 228–241*t*
Acrocarpusfraxinifolius, 228–241*t*
Actaearacemosa, 260*t*, 268*f*, 279
Actinidiadeliciosa, 228–241*t*
Acute aflatoxicosis, 109
Acyl-CoA, 166
Acyl-CoA binding protein (ACBP),
    166
ADH6 gene, 65
Adipocytokines, 62–64
Adiponectin, 64
Aegicerascorniculatum, 228–241*t*
Aeglemarmelos, 228–241*t*
Aervalanata, 228–241*t*
Aflatoxicosis, 109
Aflatoxins (AF), 108
Ageratum conyzoides, 228–241*t*
ALA. *See* Alpha-linolenic acid
    (ALA)
Alanine aminotransferase, 142,
    144–145
Alanine transaminase, 242,
    261–262
Albizzialebbeck, 228–241*t*
Alchorneacordifolia, 228–241*t*
Alcohol, 57
    consumption, 148
    as depressant, 66
    hepatocellular carcinoma and,
        109

metabolism and oxidative stress,
    58–61
Alcohol dehydrogenase (ADH), 59
Alcoholic fatty liver disease
    (AFLD), 130–131, 194
Alcoholic hepatitis, 57
Alcoholic liver disease
    adipocytokines in, 62–64
    chemokines in, 62–64
    cytokines in, 62–64
    genetic alterations in developing,
        61–62
    herbal medicines, 71, 74*t*
        Hoveniadulcis, 73–74
        Hypericumperforatum, 71
        Morusnigra, 73
        Panax ginseng, 72
        Piper methysticum, 73
        Puerarialobata, 71–72
        Salvia miltiorrhiza, 72
        Tabernantheiboga, 72
        Taraxacumcoreanum, 73
    sex differences, 64–65
    treatment, 66–67
        choline/betaine, 68
        cyanidanol-3, 70
        folate, 68
        prebiotics, 67
        silibinin, 69
        vitamin supplementation, 68
    vitamin E, 184
Alcohol-induced liver injury, 134
Alcoholism, 58–59
Aldehyde dehydrogenase (ALDH),
    59
Alkaline phosphatase (ALP),
    144–145, 242, 261–262
Alkaloids, hepatitis B virus, 32
Allium cepa, 228–241*t*

Allium sativum, 96
Allopurinol, 185
Aloe vera, 228–241*t*, 268*f*, 270–271
α-amanitin, 274–275
Alpha-1-antitrypsin deficiency, 109
Alpha fetoprotein (AFP), 113
Alpha-linolenic acid (ALA),
    161–164
    conversion to EPA and DHA,
        165, 165*f*
Alpha-lipoic acid, 218, 219*f*
Alpiniaoxyphylla, 228–241*t*
Amanita phalloides, 117, 260*t*,
    268*f*, 274–275
Amatoxins, 274–275
American Diabetes Association diet
    (ADA), 88–90
2-Amino-5-guanidino-pentanoic
    acid, 195
Ampelopsis grossedentata, 94
Anastatin A, 5–9*t*
Anastatin B, 5–9*t*
Andrographispaniculata, 228–241*t*
Anethumgraveolens, 228–241*t*
Angelica keiskei, 228–241*t*,
    243–245*t*
Angiomyolipoma, 106, 108*t*
Angiotensin-converting enzyme
    inhibitors, 221–222
Annonasquamosa, 228–241*t*
Anoectochilusformosanus,
    228–241*t*
Anthocyanins, NAFLD treatment,
    93–94
Anthraquinones, 269–270
Anticarcinogenic activity
    Ganodermalucidum, 22
    naringenin, 117–118
    resveratrol, 107–108

Antimitochondrial antibodies
(AMAs), 132
Antioxidant enzymes, 86–87
minerals in, 214–215
Antiproliferative activity,
Cyphomandrabetacea, 119
Antiviral activity
Ganodermalucidum
peptidoglycan, 22
glycyrrhizin, 64
Oenanthejavanica, 23
phenolic acids, 29
Phyllanthusamarus, 24
Apigenin, 5–9*t*, 48*t*, 49
Aquilariaagallocha, 228–241*t*
Arctiumlappa, 228–241*t*
Ardisiasolanacea, 228–241*t*
Arginine, 193
functional links with liver, 196
hepatoprotective functions,
196–197
metabolism, 195
structural characteristics, 195
Aromatic amino acids (AAs),
134–135
Arsenic compounds, 110
Artemisia aucheri, 228–241*t*
Artemisia capillaris, 228–241*t*
Artemisinin, 31
Artocarpuslakoocha, 228–241*t*
Ascorbic acid. *See* Vitamin C
Asiaticoside, 28
Aspalathuslinearis, 228–241*t*
Asparagus racemosus, 228–241*t*
Asparagus racemosus (AR),
148–149
Aspartate aminotransferase, 142
Aspartate transaminase, 242
Asteracanthalongifolia, 228–241*t*
Atractylisgummifera, 260*t*, 268*f*,
269
Atractyloside, 275–276
Azadirachtaindica, 228–241*t*
Azimatetracantha, 228–241*t*

B

Bacopamonnieri, 228–241*t*
Baliospermummontanum, 228–241*t*
Bauhinia purpurea, 228–241*t*
Bayberry, 97

Behenic acid, 163*f*
Benign tumors, 106
Berberine, 5–9*t*
cancer treatment, 119, 120*t*
chemical structure, 91*f*
NAFLD treatment, 92
Berberistinctoria, 228–241*t*
Berberis vulgaris, 91*f*, 228–241*t*,
243–245*t*
Beta-carotene, 217, 217*f*
Betaine, 60, 200–202, 211, 211*f*
Betulinic acid, in HBV, 27–28
Bile acid, accumulation, 265
Bile duct, 105
cystadenocarcinoma, 107, 108*t*
cystadenoma, 106, 108*t*
Bioactive compounds, 5–9*t*
in chronic liver disease (CLD),
132–134
Bioactive peptides, antitumor
activities, 121
Biotransformation, 144
Bixaorellana, 228–241*t*
Boehmerianivea, 26–27
Boehmerianivea root extract
(BNE), 26–27
Boerhaaviadiffusa, 228–241*t*
Boesenbergia rotunda, 228–241*t*
Boswelliadalzielii, 228–241*t*
Boswelliaovalifoliolata, 228–241*t*
Branched chain amino acids
(BCAAs), 134–135
Buteamonosperma, 149–150

C

Caesalpiniabonducella, 228–241*t*
Caffeic acid, 30
Caffeine, 5–9*t*
Cajanuscajan, 228–241*t*
Callilepislaureola, 260*t*, 268*f*, 277
Calotropisprocera, 228–241*t*
Camellia sinensis, 95–96, 228–
241*t*, 243–245*t*, 260*t*, 268*f*,
270
Capparisspinosa, 228–241*t*
Caprylic acid, 163*f*
Carbamazepine (CBZ), 214
Carbon tetrachloride (CCl₄), 214
Careyaarborea, 228–241*t*
Carica papaya, 228–241*t*

Carissa carandas, 228–241*t*
Carissa opaca, 228–241*t*
Carissa spinarum, 228–241*t*
Carthamustinctorius, 228–241*t*
Cascara sagrada, 260*t*, 268*f*, 278
Cassia acutifolia, 260*t*, 268*f*,
278–279
Cassia fistula, 150, 228–241*t*
Catechin, 30
in chronic liver diseases,
132–133, 133*f*
Catechol-*O*-methyltransferase, 270
Catechols, 279
Caudatin, 28
Cell activation, hepatotoxicity
mechanisms
nonparenchymal, 267
parenchymal, 265–267
Celosia argentea, 228–241*t*
Cepharanthine, 31
Chelidoniummajus, 260*t*, 268*f*, 272
Chemokines, alcoholic liver
disease, 62–64
Chemotherapy, 119–121
Chenopodium album, 228–241*t*
Chinese grass. *See Boehmerianivea*
Chlorogenic acid, 29
Cholangiocarcinoma (CCA),
intrahepatic, 107, 108*t*
Cholangiography, 130
Choline, 60, 193, 210, 211*f*
alcoholic disease treatment, 68
dietary sources, 200–202, 201*t*
effect on liver health, 203–204
metabolism, 202–203
metabolites, 200–202
Chronic aflatoxicosis, 109
Chronic hepatitis C, 45
Chronic liver disease (CLD), 129
bioactive compounds in,
132–134
hepaticsteatosis, 130–131
liver fibrosis, 132
nutritional support in, 134–135
plant extracts in, 132–134
primary biliary cirrhosis (PBC),
131–132, 131*f*
primarysclerosing cholangitis
(PSC), 129–130
progression of, 3–4, 3*f*

Chrozophoratinctoria, 228–241t
Cichoriumintybus, 228–241t
Cinnamomumverum, 95
Cinnamomumzeylanicum,
228–241t
Cinnamon, NAFLD treatment, 95
Cirrhosis, 3, 57
cancer and, 107–108
Citrus maxima, 228–241t
Clausenaexcavata, 31
Clavulanic acid, 146f
Clerodendruminfortunatum, 228–241t
Clonorchissinensis, 110
Cocciniagrandis, 228–241t
Coenzyme Q10, 219, 220f
Colchicine, 5–9t
Coldeniaprocumbens, 228–241t
Colocasiaesculenta, 228–241t
Color Doppler sonography, 111
Combined hepatocellular
and cholangiocarcinoma,
107, 108t
Commiphoraberryi, 228–241t
Computed tomography (CT),
hepatic cancer, 111
Copper, 214
Coriandrumsativum, 228–241t
Corilagin, hepatitis C treatment,
48t, 50–51
Corydalis saxicola, 32
Costunolide lactone, 31
Costus after, 228–241t
Covalently closed circular DNA
(CCC DNA), 20
Crassocephalumcrepidioides,
228–241t
Croton hypoleucus, 228–241t
Croton zehntneri, 228–241t
Curculigoorchioides, 228–241t
Curcuma longa, 23–24, 228–241t
pharmacological activities, 23–24
Curcuma xanthorrhiza, 228–241t
Curcumin, 5–9t, 133–134,
219–220, 220f
cancer and, 116–117, 120t
NAFLD treatment, 94
Cyanidanol-3, 70
Cyatheagigantea, 228–241t
Cyclooilivil-4'-*O*-β-
Dglucopyranoside, 28

Cymbopogoncitratus, 228–241t
Cynanchumauriculatum, 28
Cynarascolymus, 228–241t,
243–245t
Cynodondactylon, 228–241t
CYP2A5, 60
CYP2E1, 59–60
CYP450 enzymes, 141–142
Cyperusarticulatus, 228–241t
Cyphomandrabetacea, 119
CYP isozymes, 64
Cystadenocarcinoma, bile duct, 107
Cystadenoma, bile duct, 106
Cytokines, in alcoholic liver
disease, 62–64
Cytolytic hepatitis, 264
Cytosolic Cu-Zn dismutase (Cu-
ZnSOD), 214

D

Daidzein, 71
Daidzin, 71
Dauricumidine, 32
Decalepishamiltonii, 228–241t
Dehydroapocavidine, 32
Dehydrocavidine, 32
Dehydrodiconiferyl alcohol, 26
Dehydrozingerone, 26
Dehygroisoapocavadine, 32
Delonixregia, 228–241t
Dendritic cells (DCs), 1
Dendrocnidesinuata, 228–241t
Dendrophthoepentandra, 228–241t
Detoxification, 146–147
DHA. *See* Docosahexaenoic acid
(DHA)
Dietary choline, 202
Diffuse liver diseases (DLDs), 3
Digital subtraction angiography
(DSA), hepatic cancer, 112
Dihydrochelerythrine, 32
Dihydromyricetin, NAFLD
treatment, 94
1,25-Dihydroxyvitamin D, 178
Directly acting antiviral drugs
(DAAs), 42, 47t
Docosahexaenoic acid (DHA),
161–165
Docosapentaenoic acid (DPA),
162–164

Dopamine, 66
Dracocephalumrupestre, 228–241t
Drug-induced hepatotoxicity
(DIH), 141
epidemiological aspects, 147
mechanisms, 141–142, 145–147
natural compounds and plant
extracts in, 148–150
risk factors, 145–147
Drug-induced liver injury (DILI),
261–262
acetaminophen, 147
external/environmental factors
and risk for, 147t
paracetamol (PCM), 147
Drugs, hepatotoxic, 264
Duck HBV (DHBV), 28–29

E

Echinaceaepurpurea, 260t, 268f,
279–280
Ecliptaalba, 228–241t
Eicosapentaenoic acid (EPA),
161–164
Elettariacardamomom, 95
Ellagic acid, 5–9t
Emblicaofficinalis, 228–241t
Emodin, 270–271
Enicostemmaaxillare, 228–241t
Enzymatic defence, 86–87
Enzyme immunosorbent assay
(EIA), 44
EPA. *See* Eicosapentaenoic acid
(EPA)
Epaltesdivaricata, 228–241t
Epicatechin (EC), 30
Epicatechin- 3-gallate (ECG), 30
Epigallocatechin-3-gallate (EGCG),
5–9t, 30, 270
hepatitis C treatment, 48–49,
48t
Erythromycin, 146f
Esculetin, 5–9t
Ethanol extract, *Rheum palmatum*,
22
Euphorbia antiquorum, 228–241t
Eurosil 85, 185
Evodiafargesii, 31
Extracellular superoxide dismutase
(EcSOD), 214

F

Falcaria vulgaris, 228–241t
Fatty acid, 161
Fatty acid binding proteins (FABP), 166
Fatty liver disease. *See* Hepatic steatosis
Fatty liver index (FLI), 88–90
Feroniaelephantum, 228–241t
Feronialimonia, 228–241t
Fibrocytes, 64
Fibrosis
  monounsaturated fats in, 170
  omega-3 fatty acids in, 170
Ficuscarica, 228–241t
Flacourtiaindica, 228–241t
Flavanolignans, 217
  Silybummarianum, 69, 75
Flavonoids, antiviral activity, 32
Focal liver diseases (FLDs), 3
Focal nodular hyperplasia (FNH), 106, 108t
Foeniculumvulgare, 228–241t
Folate, alcoholic disease treatment, 68
Folic acid, 60–61
Forsythiaside A, 5–9t
Framingham Risk Score (FRS), 88–90
Fraxinusrhynchophylla, 228–241t
Free fatty acids (FFA), 166
Fumariaindica, 228–241t
Funtumiaafricana, 228–241t

G

Gallic acid, 5–9t
Gammaglutamyltransferase (GGT), 242
Ganodermalucidum, 22
  antiviral and anticarcinogenic activity, 22
  components of, 22
Garcinia kola, 228–241t
Gardenia gummifera, 228–241t
Gardenia jasminoides, 118
Garlic, NAFLD treatment, 96
Geniposide, 5–9t
  cancer, 118, 120t
Gingerol, 5–9t
Ginkgo biloba, 228–241t

Glutathione, 212–213, 213f
Glutathione peroxidase (GSH-Px), 215
Glutathione sulfate (GS), 209
Glycyrrhetinic acid (GA), 28
Glycyrrhizaglabra, 28, 97, 115, 228–241t, 243–245t
Glycyrrhizic acid, 5–9t
Glycyrrhizin, 5–9t, 28
  cancer, 115–116, 120t
Green cardamom seed, 95
Green tea, 270
  NAFLD treatment, 95–96
  polyphenols in, 30
Gundeliatourenfortii, 228–241t

H

HBV. *See* Hepatitis B virus (HBV)
Hedera helix, 228–241t
Hedyotiscorymbosa, 228–241t
Helioxanthinanalogs, 29
Helioxanthine (HE-145), 28
Hemangioma, 3
Hemidesmusindicus, 228–241t
Hemochromatosis, 3, 109
Hepacivirus, 42
Hepatic cancer, 105
  benigntumors, 106
  causes, 107–111, 108t
  chemotherapy, 119–121
  computed tomography (CT), 111
  digital subtraction angiography (DSA), 112
  liver puncture biopsy, 113
  magnetic resonance imaging (MRI), 111–112
  malignanttumors, 106–107
  natural product based remedies, 115f, 120t
  pathological diagnosis, 113
  positron emission tomography (PETCT), 112
  prevention, 114
  serological molecular markers, 113
  single photon emission computed tomography (SPECT), 112–113
  treatment
    advanced stage, 114

    berberine, 119
    cereal-derived proteins and peptides, 119–121
    curcumin, 116–117
    early stage, 114
    geniposide, 118
    glycyrrhizin, 115–116
    intermediate stage, 114
    naringenin, 117–118
    oxymatrine/kwoninone, 118–119
    resveratrol, 116
    rhein, 117
    salvianolic acid B, 118
    silymarin, 117
    tetrandrine, 119
    wogonin, 116
  ultrasonography, 111
Hepatic carcinoma, 105
Hepatic encephalopathy, 142–143
Hepatic hemangioma, 106, 108t
Hepatic lesions, 195
Hepatic steatosis, 130–131
Hepatic stellate cells (HSCs), 1, 63
Hepatitis, 142–143
  alcoholic, 57
Hepatitis A virus (HAV), 107
Hepatitis B virus (HBV), 3, 19
  alkaloids, 32
  carcinoma and, 107
  Curcuma longa, 23–24
  Ganodermalucidum, 22
  life cycle, 20
  lignans, 28–29
  Oenanthejavanica, 23
  phenolic acids, 29–30
  Phyllanthusamarus, 24
  Phyllanthusniruri, 24–26
  polyphenols, 30–32
  Rheum palmatum, 20–22
  terpenoids, 27–28
  vitamin E in, 184
Hepatitis C, 41, 51
  diagnosis, 43
  enzymeimmunosorbent assay, 44
  etiology, 42
  liver biopsy, 45
  prevention, 46
  recombinantimmunoblot assays (RIBA), 44

RNA detection, 45
screening, 46
serology, 43–44
signs and symptoms, 42–43
treatment
corilagin, 50–51
epigallocatechin-3-gallate
(EGCG), 48–49
honokiol, 49
3-hydroxy caruilignan C
(3-HCL-C), 49
IFN-α, 46
ladanein, 49, 50*f*
luteolin and apigenin, 49
naringenin, 48
plumbagin, 50
quercetin, 48
silymarin, 47, 48*t*
Hepatitis C virus (HCV), 3, 41
carcinoma and, 107
genotypes and serotypes, 43
transmission, 41
Hepatitis E virus (HEV), 107
Hepatoblastoma, 107, 108*t*
Hepatocellular adenoma, 106,
108*t*
Hepatocellular carcinoma (HCC),
41, 106, 194
monounsaturated fats in, 170
omega-3 fatty acids in, 170
transition from normal liver to,
169*f*
Hepatocytes, 1, 105, 142–143,
265–267
Hepatolithiasis, 110
Hepatoprotective agents
natural
alpha-lipoic acid, 218, 219*f*
beta-carotene, 217, 217*f*
betaine, 211, 211*f*
choline, 210, 211*f*
coenzyme Q10, 219, 220*f*
curcumin, 219–220, 220*f*
glutathione, 212–213, 213*f*
lycopene, 216, 216*f*
melatonin, 212, 212*f*
minerals in antioxidant
enzymes, 214–215
N-acetylcysteine (NAC),
213–214, 214*f*

S-adenosyl-l-methionine
(SAM), 211, 212*f*
silymarin, 217–218, 218*f*
ursodeoxycholic acid
(UDCA), 210, 210*f*
vitamins C, 215, 216*f*
vitamins E, 215, 215*f*
plants as, 151–153*t*
synthetic
angiotensin-converting
enzyme inhibitors, 221–222
pentoxifylline, 221
Hepatoprotective plants, clinical
trials, 242, 243–245*t*
Hepatotoxic agents, 145, 146*f*
Hepatotoxicity, 142–144
causes of, 264–265
concepts of, 261–267
drug metabolic pathways of liver,
144
drugs
associated with, 144, 145*t*
induced by, 264
mechanisms of, 265–267, 266*f*
bile acid accumulation, 265
nonparenchymal cell
activation, 267
parenchymal cell activation,
265–267
plant extracts and mushrooms,
induced by
Actaearacemosa, 279
Aloe vera, 270–271
Amanita phalloides, 274–275
Atractylisgummifera, 269
Callilepislaureola, 277
Camellia sinensis, 270
Cascara sagrada, 278
Cassia acutifolia, 278–279
Chelidoniummajus, 272
Echinaceaepurpurea, 279–280
Hypericumperforatum,
277–278
Larreatridentata, 273–274
Menthapulegium, 274
Morindacitrifolia, 269–270
Piper methysticum, 272–273
Scutellariabaicalensis, 276
Teucriumchamaedrys, 271
Valerianaofficinalis, 277

Viscum album, 275
Xanthium strumarium,
275–276
types of, 262–264
idiosyncratic form, 262–263,
263*f*
intrinsic form, 263–264, 263*f*
viruse induced, 265
Hepatotoxins, 261
Herbal and dietary supplements
(HDS), 259
Herbal medicines, alcoholism, 71,
74*t*
Herpetosperin B, 31
Herpetospermumcaudigerum, 31
Hesperidin, 121
Hesperidin-induced paraptosis,
121–122
Hibiscus sabdariffa, 228–241*t*,
243–245*t*
High-density lipoprotein (HDL),
177
Hippophaerhamnoides, 72, 74*t*,
228–241*t*
Homaliumletestui, 228–241*t*
Homeostatic model assessment
of insulin resistance
(HOMA-IR), 88–90
Honokiol, hepatitis C treatment,
48*t*, 49
Hoveniadulcis, 73–74, 74*t*
Hybrid lignans, 28
3-Hydroxy caruilignan C
(3-HCL-C), 48*t*, 49
Hydroxysafflor yellow A, 5–9*t*
25-Hydroxyvitamin D (25-OHD),
178
Hygrophilaspinosa, 228–241*t*
Hyperforin, 71
Hypericumperforatum, 71, 74*t*,
228–241*t*, 260*t*, 268*f*,
277–278
Hyperlipidemia, 83–84
Hypervitaminosis, 68
Hypomethylation, 61

I

Iatrogenic diseases, 141
Ibogaine, 72
Ichnocarpusfrutescens, 228–241*t*

Idiosyncratic DILI, 262–263
IL-8, 64
IL-10, 62
Immunomodulating substance,
    Ganodermalucidum, 22
Indigoferaaspalathoides, 228–241*t*
Indigoferatinctoria, 228–241*t*
Infants, HBV infection, 19–20
Inflammation, cancer and, 110
Inflammatory bowel disease, cancer
    and, 110
Insulin resistance, NAFLD and,
    85*t*, 86
Intercellular adhesion molecule-1
    (ICAM-1), 63
Interferon α (IFN-α), 30
    for hepatitis C, 46
Intrahepatic cholangiocarcinoma
    (CCA), 107, 108*t*
Intrinsic hepatotoxicity, 263–264,
    263*f*
Ipomoea aquatica, 228–241*t*
Isoniazid, 150

J

Japanese raisin tree, 73–74
Juniperusphoenicea, 228–241*t*

K

Kaempferol 3-*O*-glucoside, 5–9*t*
Kaempferol 3-*O*-rutinoside, 5–9*t*
Kavapyrones, 73
Kigeliaafricana, 228–241*t*
Kotronen index, 88–90
Kupffer cells, 1, 63, 267

L

Lactones, 31
    in*Swertiamileensis*, 31
Ladanein, hepatitis C treatment,
    48*t*, 49, 50*f*
Laggeraalata, 29
Larreatridentata, 268*f*, 273–274
Launaeaintybacea, 228–241*t*
Lawsoniainermis, 228–241*t*
Leptin, 86
Licorice, NAFLD treatment, 97
Lignanhelioxanthin, 29
Lignans, 28–29
Limoniumtetragonum, 134

Linghzi, 22
Linoleic acid, 163*f*
Lipid peroxidation, 209
Lipotoxicity, 87
Liver, 175, 193
    blood supply, 2
    cancer, 193
    damage, 143, 227
    diseases, 3–4
    drug metabolic pathways, 144
    functions of, 2*f*
    nonparenchymal cells, 1
    parenchymal cells, 1
    prooxidants in, 209
Liver cirrhosis, 41
Liver fibrosis, 132
Liver flukes, cancer and, 110
Liver injury
    idiosyncratic form of, 262–263,
        263*f*
    intrinsic form of, 263–264, 263*f*
Liver puncture biopsy, 113
Low-density lipoproteins (LDL),
    177
Luffaacutangula, 228–241*t*
Luteolin, 49
Lycopene, 216, 216*f*
Lygodiumflexuosum, 228–241*t*

M

Macrotylomauniflorum, 228–241*t*
Macrovesicularsteatosis, 45
Magnesium lithospermate B, 118
Magnetic resonance imaging
    (MRI), hepatic cancer,
    111–112
Malignant tumors, 106–107
Malnutrition, 134
Mammeasuriga, 228–241*t*
Manganese superoxide dismutase
    (MnSOD), 214
Marrubiumperegrinum,ladanein, 49
Marrubiumvulgare, 228–241*t*
Marsileaminuta, 228–241*t*
Matrine, 5–9*t*
Matrix metalloproteinases (MMPs),
    121–122
Maytenusrobusta, 228–241*t*
Mediterranean diet, and NAFLD,
    88–90, 97

Melatonin, 212, 212*f*
Menthalongifolia, 228–241*t*
Menthapulegium, 260*t*, 268*f*, 274
Metadoxin, 70
Methotrexate, 196
Milk thistle, in chronic liver
    diseases, 133
Miltironediterpene, 72
Mimosa pudica, 228–241*t*
Minerals, in antioxidant enzymes,
    214–215
Momordicadioica, 228–241*t*
Momordica tuberose, 228–241*t*
Monounsaturated fats
    in fibrosis, 170
    in hepatocellular carcinoma
        (HCC), 170
    metabolism of, 166
    innonalcoholic fatty liver disease
        (NAFLD), 166
    innonalcoholicsteatohepatitis
        (NASH), 169
Monounsaturated fatty acids
    (MUFA), 162
    chemical structures of, 163*f*,
        166
    classification, 166
    in liver diseases, 168–169, 168*t*
    sources, 166
Morindacitrifolia, 260*t*, 268*f*,
    269–270
Moringaoleifera, 228–241*t*
Morusnigra, 73, 74*t*, 228–241*t*
Multiple parallel hits hypothesis,
    84–85
Muntingiacalabura, 228–241*t*
Murrayakoenigii, 228–241*t*
Musangacecropioides, 228–241*t*
Myofibroblasts, 64

N

N-acetylcysteine (NAC), 213–214,
    214*f*
NAFLD. *See* Nonalcoholic fatty
    liver disease (NAFLD)
NAFLD Activity Score (NAS), 93
Naringenin
    for cancer, 117–118, 120*t*
    hepatitis C treatment, 48, 48*t*
Naringin, 121

Natural compounds, in drug-induced hepatotoxicity, 148–150
Nelumbonucifera, 228–241t
Neo- and nor-lignans, 28
Neohesperidin, 121
Neoplasia, 61
Niacin. See Vitamin B₃
Nicotine-activated MMPs, 121–122
Nigella sativa, 228–241t
Nirtetralin B, 28–29
Nitrosamines, cancer and, 110
N,N-dimethyltryptamine N12-oxide, 31
Nonalcoholic fatty liver disease (NAFLD), 83–84, 130–131, 193–195, 242
  anthocyanins, 93–94
  bayberry, 97
  berberine, 92
  cinnamon, 95
  classification of, 83–84
  curcumin, 94
  dihydromyricetin, 94
  garlic, 96
  green cardamom seed, 95
  green tea, 95–96
  licorice, 97
  mediterranean diet and, 88–90, 97
  monounsaturated fats in, 166
  olive oil, 96–97
  omega-3 fatty acids in, 166
  oxidative stress and lipotoxicity, 86–87
  pathogenesis and progression, 84–86
  prevalence, 83–84
  progression of, 83–84, 84f
  resveratrol, 90–92
  Rhododendron oldhamii leaf extract on, 133
  risk factors, 85t
  silybin, 92–93
  silymarin, 93
  vitamin C in, 176
  vitamin D deficiency and, 179
  vitamin E in, 183
Nonalcoholicsteatohepatitis (NASH), 83–84

curcumin in, 133–134
  monounsaturated fats in, 169
  omega-3 fatty acids in, 169
  vitamin E in, 182–184
Nonenzymatic antioxidants, 86–87
Nonenzymatic defence, 86–87
Nonesterify fatty acids (NEFAs), 86
Nonparenchymal cells (NPC), hepatotoxicity mechanisms, 267
Nordihydroguaiaretic acid (NGDA), 273
Nucleic acid testing (NAT), for HCV, 43–44
Nucleus[t]ide, 30
Nutrients, 5–9t

O

3,4-*O*-dicaffeoylquinic acid, 29
3,5-*O*-dicaffeoylquinic acid, 29
Oenanthejavanica, 23
  biological activities, 23
  hepatitis B treatment, 23
Oldenlandiaumbellata, 228–241t
Oleic acid, 163f
Oligomericlignans, 28
Olive oil, NAFLD treatment, 96–97
Omega-3 fatty acids, 161–162
  chemistry, 162–165
  classification, 162–165, 164f
  in fibrosis, 170
  in hepatocellular carcinoma (HCC), 170
  metabolism of, 166
  innonalcoholic fatty liver disease (NAFLD), 166
  innonalcoholicsteatohepatitis (NASH), 169
  sources, 166
  synthesis of, 165f
Operculinaturpethum, 228–241t
Opisthorchisviverrini, 110
Opuntiaficus-indica, 228–241t
Oral contraceptives, cancer and, 109
OraQuick HCV Rapid Antibody Test, 44
Orthosiphonstamineus, 228–241t
Orychophragmusviolaceus, 228–241t

Oval cells (OCs), 1
Oxaliplatin (OXA), 213
Oxidative stress, 209
Oxymatrine, 32
  cancer treatment, 118–119, 120t

P

Panax ginseng, 228–241t, 243–245t
  alcoholic disease treatment, 72, 74t
Paracetamol, 264
Paracetamol, drug-induced liver injury, 147
Paraptosis, 121–122
Parenchymal cells, hepatotoxicity mechanisms, 265–267
Parkinsoniaaculeata, 228–241t
PegIFN-α2a, 46
Pentoxiyfylline, 221
Peptides, anticancer-associated, 121
Peptidoglycans, *Ganodermalucidum*, 22
Pergulariadaemia, 228–241t
Peroxisome proliferator activated receptor (PPAR-γ), 86
Petromyzonmarinus (lamprey), 31
Phenolic acids
  in*Artemisia capillaris*, 29
  HBV infection, 29
Phoenix dactylifera, 228–241t
Phosphatidylcholine, 202
Phosphatidyl-ethanolamine methyltransferase, 60
Phyllanthin, 5–9t
Phyllanthusamarus, 24, 243–245t
  hepatoprotective effect, 24, 25f
Phyllanthusfraternus, 228–241t
Phyllanthusniruri, 24–26, 228–241t
  bioactive components, 25–26
  Boehmerianivea, 26–27
  for HBV infections, 25–26
Phyllanthuspolyphyllus, 228–241t
Physalisperuviana, 228–241t
Picrorhizakurroa, 228–241t, 243–245t
Pimpinellaanisum, 228–241t
Piper methysticum, 73, 74t, 263, 272–273
Piper nigrum, 94
Pisoniaaculeata, 228–241t

Pistacialentiscus, 228–241*t*

Pit cells, 1, 63

Pittosporumneelgherrense, 228–241*t*

Plantago major, 228–241*t*

Plant extracts, 5–9*t*
    in chronic liver disease (CLD), 132–134
    in drug-induced hepatotoxicity, 148–150
    hepatotoxicity induced by, 267–280, 268*f*
    toxic dosage of, 260*t*

Plants
    withhepatoprotective activity, 227–242, 228–241*t*
    ashepatoprotective agents, 151–153*t*

Plumbagin, hepatitis C treatment, 48*t*, 50

Plumbagoindica, 50

Plumbagozeylanica, 228–241*t*

Polyamines, 196

Polygonummultiflorum, 228–241*t*

Polygonumorientale, 228–241*t*

Polyphenols
    in*Acacia mellifera*, 31
    in green tea, 30
    hepatitis treatment, 30–32
    pharmacological effects, 30

Polysaccharides, in *Ganodermalucidum*, 22

Polyunsaturated fatty acid (PUFA)
    chemical structures of, 163*f*
    in liver diseases, 168–169, 168*t*

Portulacaoleracea, 228–241*t*

Positron emission tomography (PETCT), hepatic cancer, 112

Poulsen lesions, 45

Prebiotics, alcoholic disease treatment, 67

PREDIMED-Malaga trial, 88–90

Primary biliary cirrhosis (PBC), 131–132, 131*f*

Primary liver cancers (PLC), 106

Primary NAFLD, 83–84

Primary sclerosing cholangitis (PSC), 129–130

curcumin in, 133–134

Prunusamygdalus, 228–241*t*

Psidiumguajava, 148, 228–241*t*

Pterocarpusmarsupium, 228–241*t*

Puerarialobata, 71–72, 74*t*

Puerarin, 71

Pulsatillachinensis, 27

Punicagranatum, 228–241*t*

Pyrazinamide, 146*f*

Pyridoxine, 70

Pyrones, kava, 73

Pyrrolidone-carboxylate ion, 70

Pyruspashia, 228–241*t*

Q

Quercetin, hepatitis C treatment, 48, 48*t*

R

Radical oxygen species (ROS), 86–87

Raphanussativus, 228–241*t*

Reactive metabolic species (RMS), 144

Reactive nitrogen species (RNS), 141–142

Reactive oxygen species (ROS), 141–142, 175, 182

Recombinant immunoblot assays (RIBA), 44

Resveratrol, 5–9*t*, 70
    cancer, 116, 120*t*
    chemical structure, 91*f*
    nonalcoholic fatty liver disease (NAFLD), 90–92

Rhein, cancer treatment, 117, 120*t*

Rheum palmatum, 20–22

Rheum rhabarbarum, 117

Rhododendron arboreum, 228–241*t*

Rhusoxyacantha, 228–241*t*

Ribavirin, 41, 46

Ricinuscommunis, 228–241*t*

Rifampicin, 146*f*, 150

Rosmarinusofficinalis, 228–241*t*

RousselUclaf Causality Assessment Method (RUCAM), 261–262

Royleaelegans, 228–241*t*

Rubiacordifolia, 228–241*t*

S

S-adenosyl-methionine (SAM), 60, 211, 212*f*

Salvia cryptantha, 228–241*t*

Salviaemiltiorrhizae, 118

Salvia miltiorrhiza, 72, 74*t*

Salvianolic acid B, 5–9*t*
    cancer treatment, 118, 120*t*

Salvia officinalis, 228–241*t*

Saponariaofficinalis, 228–241*t*

Sarmentosin, 5–9*t*

Saturated fatty acid, 163*f*

Schisandrachinensis, 28, 228–241*t*

Schisandrasphenanthera, 228–241*t*

Schisandrin B, 5–9*t*

Schreberaswietenioides, 228–241*t*

Scopariadulcis, 228–241*t*

Scutellariabaicalensis, 260*t*, 268*f*, 276

Scutellaria radix, 116
    wogonin, 32

Secondary NAFLD, 83–84

Selenium (Se), 215

Serum bilirubin (SBLN), 144

Sidarhombifolia, 228–241*t*

Silenevillosa, 228–241*t*

Silibinin/silybin, 5–9*t*, 47, 69
    NAFLD treatment, 92–93

Silybummarianum, 228–241*t*, 243–245*t*
    flavanolignanes, 69, 75

Silymarin, 5–9*t*, 143–144, 217–218, 218*f*
    antifibrotic effect of, 133
    cancer, 117, 120*t*
    hepatitis C treatment, 47, 48*t*
    NAFLD treatment, 93

Single photon emission computed tomography (SPECT), 112–113

Sinusoidal endothelial cells (SEC), 63

Sirtuin-1, 95

Smilax chinensis, 228–241*t*

Smoking, cancer and, 110

Smooth muscle cells (SMCs), 1

Solanumfastigiatum, 228–241*t*

Solanumnigrum, 228–241*t*

Solanumpubescens, 228–241*t*
Solanumtrilobatum, 228–241*t*
Solanumxanthocarpum, 228–241*t*
Solenostemonmonostachyus, 228–241*t*
Solidagomicroglossa, 228–241*t*
Sophoraalopecuraides, 118–119
*Sophora japonica,*oxymatrine, 32
Sphaeranthusindicus, 228–241*t*
Squalamine, 31
Stachyspilifera, 228–241*t*
Steatohepatitis, 60–61
Steatosis, 214
Stellate cells, 63
*Stephaniace-pharantha,*cepharanthine, 31
Stephaniatetrandra, 119
Stevia rebaudiana, 228–241*t*
St. John's wort, 71
Strychnospotatorum, 228–241*t*
Swerilactones, 31
Swertiachiravita, 28
Swertiamileensis, lactones in, 31
Swetia patens, 26
Swieteniamacrophylla, 49
Sylimarin, alcoholic disease treatment, 69
Syzygiumaromaticum, 228–241*t*

T

Tabernantheiboga, 72, 74*t*
Tageteslucida, 228–241*t*
Taiwaniacryptomerioides, 28
Tamarindusindica, 228–241*t*
Tanacetumparthenium, 228–241*t*
Taraxacumcoreanum, 73
Taurine, 193
  biological functions, 197–198
  chemical structure, 197–198
  effects in liver disease, 199, 200*t*
  as therapeutic agent, 198–199
Tecomellaundulata, 228–241*t*
Telfairiaoccidentalis, 228–241*t*
Terminaliacatappa, 228–241*t*
Terpenoids, for HBV infection, 27–28
Tetrandrine, cancer treatment, 119, 120*t*

Teucriumchamaedrys, 260*t*, 268*f*, 271
Thespesia lampas, 228–241*t*
Thioctic acid. *See* Alpha-lipoic acid
Thonningiasanguinea, 228–241*t*
Thorotrast accumulation, cancer and, 110
Thymoquinone, 5–9*t*
Thymus capitatus, 228–241*t*
Tinosporacordifolia, 228–241*t*
Tissue inhibitor of metalloproteinases (TIMP-1), 63
Toxic hepatitis, 143
Toxicogenomics, 142
Traditional medicine, 259
Transcription-mediated amplification (TMA), 45
Transfusion-transmitted (TT) viruses, 265
Trianthemaportulacastrum, 228–241*t*
Triglycerides (TGs), 177
Trigonellafoenumgraecum, 228–241*t*
Trimethylamine (TMA), 203
Trimethylamine N-oxide (TMAO), 203
Triterpenes, in *Ganodermalucidum*, 22
Troglitazone, 261
Tumor necrosis factor (TNF-α)
  in alcoholic liver disease, 62
  NAFLD and, 86
Turmeric. *See Curcuma longa*
Two hits hypothesis, 84–85
Tyrosinemia, 109

U

Ultrasonography, hepatic cancer, 111
Ursodeoxycholic acid (UDCA), 210, 210*f*
  primary biliary cirrhosis (PBC), 132
Ursolic acid, 5–9*t*
Urticadioica, 228–241*t*

V

Valerianaofficinalis, 260*t*, 268*f*, 277
Valeric acid, 277
Vascular cell adhesion molecule-1 (VCAM-1), 63
Vetiveriazizanioides, 228–241*t*
Viciacalcarata, 228–241*t*
Viral hepatitis, cancer and, 107
Viruses, hepatotoxicity induced by, 265
Visceral adipose index (VAI), 88–90
Viscum album, 260*t*, 268*f*, 275
Viscum album agglutinin-I (VAA-I), 275
Vitamins, 175
  alcoholic disease treatment, 68
  combinations and liver health, 185–186
Vitamin B$_3$, 177–178
Vitamin C, 175–177, 215, 216*f*
Vitamin C deficiency, 176
Vitamin D, 178–179
  deficiency, 179
  on liver health, 180–182*t*
  receptor, 178
Vitamin E, 182–184, 215, 215*f*
Vitexnegundo, 228–241*t*
Vitextrifolia, 228–241*t*

W

Water dropwort plant. *See Oenanthejavanica*
Wogonin, 5–9*t*, 32
  cancer, 116, 120*t*
Woninone, cancer treatment, 118–119

X

Xanthium strumarium, 260*t*, 268*f*, 275–276

Z

Zanthoxylumarmatum, 228–241*t*
Zatariamultiflora, 228–241*t*
Zingiberofficinale, 228–241*t*
Zizyphus jujube, 228–241*t*